The Phlebotomy Workbook

The Phlebotomy Workbook Second Edition

Susan King Strasinger, DA, MT(ASCP)

Faculty Associate
Medical Technology Program
The University of West Florida
Pensacola, Florida

Marjorie Schaub Di Lorenzo, MT(ASCP)SH

Phlebotomy Program Coordinator
Nebraska Methodist College
Omaha, Nebraska

Adjunct Instructor
Division of Medical Technology
School of Allied Health Professions
University of Nebraska Medical Center
Omaha, Nebraska

Photography by: Scott C. Di Lorenzo, DDS and Frankie Harris-Lyne, MLT(ASCP), CLS(NCA)

Illustrations by: Sherman Bonomelli, MS, and Mary Butters Hukill

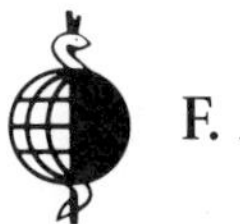

F. A. Davis Company • Philadelphia

F. A. Davis Company
1915 Arch Street
Philadelphia, PA 19103
www.fadavis.com

Printed in the United States of America

Last digit indicates print number: 10 9 8 7 6 5

Acquisitions Editor: Christa Fratantoro
Developmental Editor: Elena Mauceri
Production Editor: Jessica Howie Martin
Cover Designer: Louis J. Forgione

As new scientific information becomes available through basic and clinical research, recommended treatments and drug therapies undergo changes. The authors and publisher have done everything possible to make this book accurate, up to date, and in accord with accepted standards at the time of publication. The authors, editors, and publisher are not responsible for errors or omissions or for consequences from application of the book, and make no warranty, expressed or implied, in regard to the contents of the book. Any practice described in this book should be applied by the reader in accordance with professional standards of care used in regard to the unique circumstances that may apply in each situation. The reader is advised always to check product information (package inserts) for changes and new information regarding dose and contraindications before administering any drug. Caution is especially urged when using new or infrequently ordered drugs.

ISBN 10: 0-8036-1049-1

ISBN 13: 978-0-8036-1049-1

to Harry, my editor-in-chief

SKS

to my husband, Scott, and my children,
Michael, Christopher, and Lauren,
for their encouragement, patience, and support

MSD

Preface

The primary goal of *The Phlebotomy Workbook,* second edition, is to teach the skills required to obtain an optimal blood specimen using state-of-the-art equipment and techniques with minimal trauma to the patient. This edition has been revised to address the latest safety precautions and equipment and the expanded responsibilities of the phlebotomist in today's healthcare system. Additional emphasis has been placed on point-of-care testing, specimen processing, documentation and record keeping, and patient services.

This edition is designed to meet the training needs of structured phlebotomy certification programs, medical laboratory technician and medical technologist programs, medical assisting programs, patient care technician programs, and cross-training of nurses and other allied health personnel. It is an excellent reference for healthcare professionals currently practicing phlebotomy, in-house training programs, and independent study for national certification examinations and employee continuing education.

The book format remains basically the same, with the text divided into three sections covering (one) general phlebotomy, safety, and healthcare information; (two) phlebotomy techniques; and (three) medical terminology, anatomy, and physiology. To provide additional instructional flexibility, medical terminology and anatomy and physiology have been moved to the third section in this edition. The book continues to integrate specific objectives, key terms, the anatomy and physiology of body systems, laboratory tests and their clinical correlations with disorders, safety and special handling, transport and processing procedures, phlebotomy theory and practical techniques, collection and processing of non-blood specimens, interpersonal and communication skills, and quality assurance related to total quality management and continuous quality improvement. Assessment tools, including study questions, clinical situation exercises, and performance evaluation checklists at the end of each chapter, are intended to reinforce key information. These assessment tools are printed on perforated pages, with space for written answers and notes, so that they can be torn out and handed in as homework or tests.

Highlighted features of the second edition include:

- Outlines at the beginning of each chapter.
- Increased numbers of illustrations, photographs, diagrams, charts, and tables.
- Latest safety devices and procedures, including the Standard Precautions and Transmission-Based Precautions and the latest standards of the Needlestick Prevention Act.
- Special collection procedures, including venous access devices.
- An expanded section on age-specific competencies, including special considerations for elderly and pediatric populations.
- The phlebotomist's role in point-of-care testing.
- Color-highlighted Technical Tips to emphasize important points and to help avoid complications such as hematomas and hemolysis.
- Numerous clinical situation exercises to facilitate critical thinking.
- Expanded quality assurance and legal sections on quality management issues, preventing medical errors, confidentiality, malpractice, incident reporting, informed consent, and HIV consent.
- Correlation of laboratory tests, diagnostic procedures, diseases and disorders, and medications for each body system.
- Cross-reference icons that draw attention to related content in other chapters.
- Appendices listing collection requirements for frequently ordered laboratory tests, IV access flush protocols, and abbreviations.
- A complete color tube guide listing the differ-

ent types of collection tubes, the additives, the number of inversions required, and the laboratory uses of the tubes.

- For educators who adopt this text for their course, an Instructor's Resource CD-ROM is available. This valuable CD-ROM contains the following educator ancillaries:
  - Instructor's Guide with Internet resources, lecture outlines, answers to study questions and clinical situation exercises, suggested audiovisual aids and their courses, additional evaluation forms, and sample course schedules.
  - Brownstone ® test generator with 1000 questions.
  - Power Point presentation with lecture points and illustrations.

The Phlebotomy Workbook, second edition, is written to comply with the guidelines established by national certifying organizations and the essentials published by the National Accrediting Agency for Clinical Laboratory Science (NAACLS). All procedures are written in accordance with the standards developed by the National Committee for Clinical Laboratory Sciences (NCCLS) and the Occupational Safety and Health Administration (OSHA), thus enabling this text to be used as a current reference in any healthcare setting.

Susan King Strasinger
Marjorie Schaub Di Lorenzo

Acknowledgments

We wish to thank the many individuals who have spent much time and effort toward the success of this book.

We are truly grateful to our families, not only for their constant encouragement and support, but also for relinquishing their time with us so that we could write this book. We are especially thankful to our husbands: Harry Strasinger, who spent countless hours at the computer typing this manuscript and organizing every detail; and Scott Di Lorenzo, who spent many hours arranging, positioning, and photographing subjects for the numerous illustrations and the book cover.

We are greatly indebted to the many dedicated professionals at Nebraska Methodist Hospital for their enthusiasm and willingness in providing us with technical expertise and photographic opportunities. We would particularly like to thank Diane Wolff, MLT(ASCP), CLS(NCA), Phlebotomy Team Leader, for always being available to share her expertise; to provide charts, forms, and procedures; and to organize the photographic component. We also thank Sharon Terrell, CLPlb(NCA), Phlebotomy Education Coordinator, for her participation in the photographing of technical procedures; Brenda Franks, MT(ASCP), POCT Coordinator, for her invaluable resources; and Patty Janousek, BSN, CRNI, IV Team Leader, for her contribution on venous access devices.

We again thank Mary Butters Hukill and Frankie Harris-Lyne, MLT(ASCP), CLS(NCA), for the illustrations and photography reused from our first edition and Sherman Bonomelli, MS, from the University of West Florida for his current illustrations and power point presentation. Technical information provided by Janet Day, Patient Services/Education and Compliance Supervisor, Baptist Hospital, Pensacola, Florida; and Ruth L. Mills, MD, Orange Beach, Alabama Family Practice, has been a valuable addition to the text.

We also appreciate the encouragement from the supportive team at F. A. Davis. Special thanks go to Christa Fratantoro, Associate Editor, Health Professions; Elena Mauceri, Publishing Consultant; Susan Rhyner, Manager of Creative Development; Michael Bailey, Director of Production; Jack Brandt, Illustration Specialist; Ona Kosmos, Editorial Associate; and Melissa Reed, Developmental Associate.

Reviewers

Frances Cassandra Johnson
BS, MT, M(ASCP), MHS
Meridian Community College
Meridian, Mississippi

Sandra Eisenmenger
BS, MT(ASCP)
Halifax Community College
Halifax, North Carolina

Cheryl Goretti
MT(ASCP), CMA
Quinebaugh Valley Community College
Danielson, Connecticut

Terry Kotrla
MT(ASCP), BB
Austin Community College
Austin, Texas

Jay Wilborn
MEd, MT(ASCP)
Garland Community College
Hot Springs, Arkansas

Diane Wolff, MLT(ASCP), CLS(NCA)
Phlebotomy Team Leader
Nebraska Methodist Hospital
Omaha, Nebraska

Brenda L. M. Franks, MT(ASCP)
Point of Care Coordinator
Nebraska Methodist Hospital
Omaha, Nebraska

Contents

Chapter 6
Routine Venipuncture 113

Chapter 7
Venipuncture Complications 135

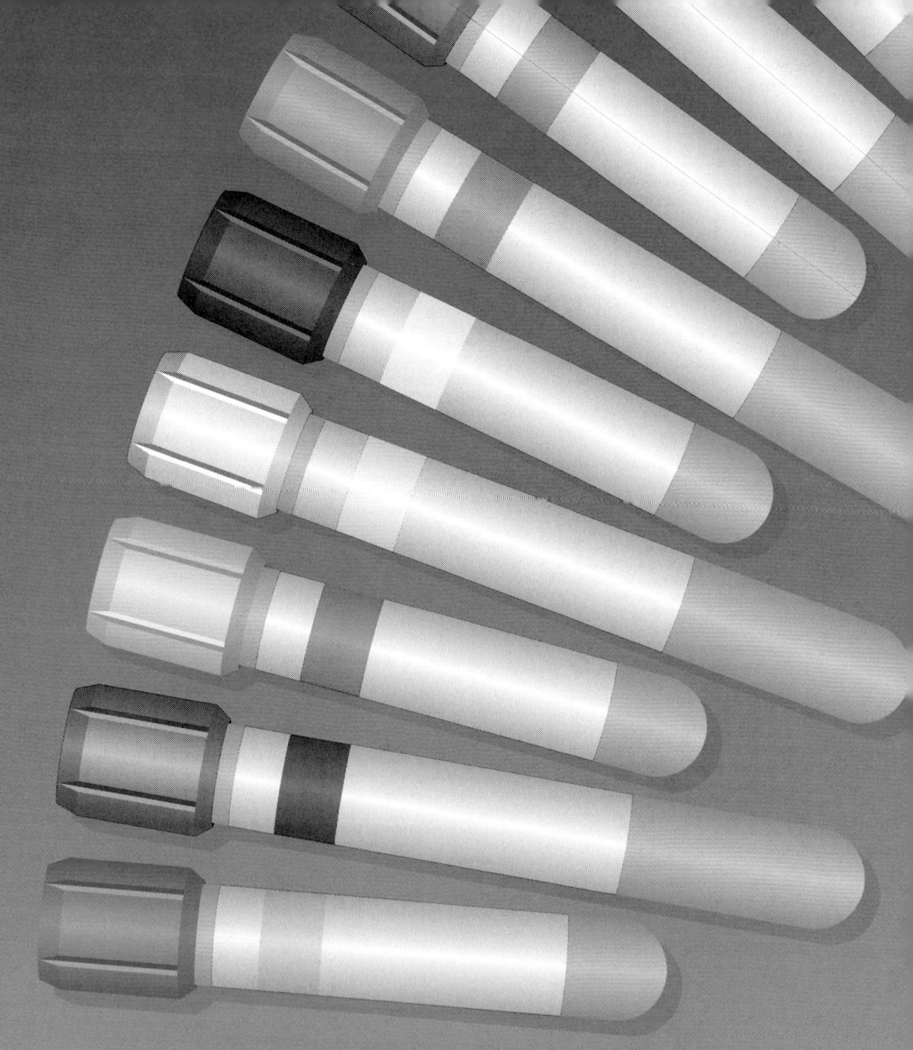

Section One

Phlebotomy and the Healthcare Field

Chapter 1

Phlebotomy and the Healthcare Delivery System

Chapter Outline

Duties of the Phlebotomist

Desirable Personal Characteristics for Phlebotomists
- Communication Skills

Phlebotomy Education and Certification

Healthcare Delivery System
- Hospital Organization

Professional Service Departments
- Radiology and Diagnostic Imaging
- Radiation Therapy
- Nuclear Medicine
- Occupational Therapy
- Pharmacy
- Physical Therapy
- Respiratory Therapy
- Cardiovascular Testing
- Clinical Laboratory

Other Healthcare Settings

Learning Objectives

Upon completion of this chapter, the reader will be able to:

1. Describe the importance of a professional public image for the phlebotomist.
2. Define patient-focused care, decentralization, and cross-training and describe their relationship to phlebotomy.
3. Describe personal characteristics that are important in a phlebotomist.
4. Discuss the importance of communication and interpersonal skills for the phlebotomist within the laboratory, with patients, and with personnel in other departments of the hospital.
5. List four barriers to verbal communication and methods of overcoming them.
6. Describe a phlebotomist using correct listening and body language skills.
7. State six rules of proper telephone etiquette.
8. Discuss the purpose of formal phlebotomy education programs.
9. List the four hospital services.
10. Describe the major functions of the hospital departments.
11. Describe the different types of healthcare settings in which a phlebotomist may be employed.
12. State two valuable characteristics that help a phlebotomist to achieve job security and advancement.

Key Terms

Accreditation	*Cross-training*	*Phlebotomy*
Certification	*Decentralization*	*Professionalism*
Confidentiality	*Patient-focused care*	

Defined as "an incision into a vein," ***phlebotomy*** is one of the oldest medical procedures, dating back to the early Egyptians. The practice of "bloodletting" was used to cure disease and maintain the body in a state of well-being. Hippocrates believed that disease was caused by an excess of body fluids, including blood, bile, and phlegm, and that removal of the excess would cause the body to return to or maintain a healthy state. Techniques for bloodletting included suction cup devices with lancets that pulled blood from the incision; the application of blood-sucking worms, called "leeches," to an incision; and barber surgery, in which blood from an incision produced by the barber's razor was collected in a bleeding bowl. The familiar red and white striped barber pole symbolizes this last technique and represents red blood and white bandages. Bloodletting is now called "therapeutic phlebotomy" and is used as a treatment for only a small number of blood disorders.

At present, the primary role of phlebotomy is the collection of blood specimens for laboratory analysis to diagnose and monitor medical conditions. The use of equipment designed to minimize patient discomfort and of aseptic techniques has replaced the earlier practices.

Because of the increased number and complexity of laboratory tests, phlebotomy has become a specialized area of clinical laboratory practice and has brought about the creation of the job title "phlebotomist." This development supplements, but does not replace, the previous practice, in which laboratory employees both collected and analyzed the specimens. Phlebotomy still remains a part of laboratory training programs for analytical personnel because phlebotomists are not available at all times and in all situations.

The specialization of phlebotomy has expanded rapidly, and with it the role of the phlebotomist, who is no longer just someone who "takes blood" but is recognized as a key player on the healthcare team. In this expanded role, the phlebotomist must be familiar with the healthcare system, the anatomy and physiology related to laboratory testing and phlebotomy, the collection and transport requirements for tests performed in all sections of the laboratory, documentation and patient records, and the interpersonal skills needed to provide quality patient care. These changes have brought about the need to replace on-the-job training with structured phlebotomy training programs leading to certification in phlebotomy. Because the phlebotomist is often the only personal contact a patient has with the laboratory, he or she can leave a lasting impression of the quality of the laboratory and the entire healthcare setting.

Duties of the Phlebotomist

A phlebotomist is a person trained to obtain blood specimens by venipuncture and microtechniques. In addition to technical, clerical, and interpersonal skills, the phlebotomist must develop strong organizational skills to handle a heavy workload efficiently and maintain accuracy, often under stressful conditions.

Major traditional duties and responsibilities of the phlebotomist include:

1. Correct identification of the patient before sample collection
2. Collection of the appropriate amount of blood by venipuncture or dermal puncture for the specified tests
3. Selection of the appropriate specimen containers for the specified tests
4. Correct labeling of all specimens with the required information
5. Appropriate transportation of specimens back to the laboratory in a timely manner
6. Effective interaction with patients and hospital personnel
7. Processing of specimens for delivery to the appropriate laboratory departments
8. Performance of computer operations and record keeping pertaining to phlebotomy
9. Observation of all safety regulations
10. Attendance at continuing education programs

In recent years, changes to increase the efficiency and cost effectiveness of the healthcare delivery system have affected the duties of phlebotomists in many institutions. Terms associated with these changes include ***patient-focused care***, ***decentralization***, and ***cross-training***.

Patient-focused care is designed to increase efficiency by eliminating the need to move patients to centralized testing areas and the necessity for healthcare personnel to travel from a central testing area to the patient's room and then back to the testing area. The scope of patient-focused care can range from the cross-training of persons already located in nursing units to perform basic interdisciplinary bedside procedures to the actual relocation of specialized radiology and clinical laboratory equipment and personnel to the patient-care units.

In many institutions, phlebotomy and the duties and location of phlebotomists have been adapted to meet the needs of patient-focused care. Considering the amount of time spent by phlebotomists traveling to and from the laboratory to patient-care units, decentralization of phlebotomy was one of the first changes associated with patient-focused care. This decentralization has been accomplished by either cross-training personnel working in the patient units to perform phlebotomy or transferring phlebotomists to the patient units and cross-training them to perform basic patient-care tasks. Consequently, additional duties of phlebotomists may include:

1. Training other healthcare personnel to perform phlebotomy
2. Monitoring the quality of specimens collected on the units
3. Evaluation of protocols associated with specimen collection
4. Performing basic bedside laboratory tests (see Chapter 13)
5. Performing electrocardiograms
6. Performing measurement of patient's vital signs
7. Collection of arterial blood specimens

Desirable Personal Characteristics for Phlebotomists

Phlebotomists are part of a service-oriented industry, and specific personal and professional characteristics are necessary for them to be successful in this area.

DEPENDABILITY

Laboratory testing begins with specimen collection and relies on the phlebotomist to report to work whenever scheduled and on time.

COMPASSION

Phlebotomists deal with sick, anxious, and frightened patients every day. They must be sensitive to their needs, understand a patient's concern about a possible diagnosis or just the fear of a needle, and take the time to reassure each patient. A smile and a cheerful tone of voice are simple techniques that can put a patient more at ease.

HONESTY

The phlebotomist should never hesitate to admit a mistake, because a misidentified patient or mislabeled specimen can be critical to patient safety.

INTEGRITY

Patient ***confidentiality*** must be protected, and patient information is never discussed with anyone who does not have a professional need to know it.

FLEXIBILITY

The phlebotomist must be able to adapt to the changes taking place in healthcare delivery. Flexibility and motivation to learn new skills are the key to job security and advancement.

APPEARANCE

Each organization specifies the dress code that it considers most appropriate, but common to all institutions is a neat and clean appearance that portrays a professional attitude to the patient. Uniforms and laboratory coats must be clean and unwrinkled; coats should be completely buttoned. Shoes must be clean and polished. Excessive jewelry, makeup, and perfume should not be worn; long hair must be neatly pulled back; and fingernails must be clean and short. Personal hygiene is extremely important because of close patient contact, and careful attention should be paid to bathing and the use of deodorants and mouthwashes. In general, a sloppy appearance indicates a tendency toward sloppy performance.

Communication Skills

Good communication skills are needed for the phlebotomist to function as the liaison between the laboratory and the patients, their family and visitors, and other healthcare personnel. The three components of communication—verbal skills, listening skills, and nonverbal skills or body language—all contribute to effective communication.

TABLE 1-1
Verbal Communication Barriers

Barrier	Methods to Overcome
Hearing impairment	Speak loudly and clearly Look directly at patient to facilitate lip-reading Communicate in writing
Patient emotions	Speak calmly and slowly Do not appear rushed or disinterested
Age and education levels	Avoid medical jargon Use age-appropriate phrases
Non–English-speaking	Locate a hospital-based volunteer or family member interpreter Use hand signals, show equipment, etc. Remain calm, smiling, and reassuring

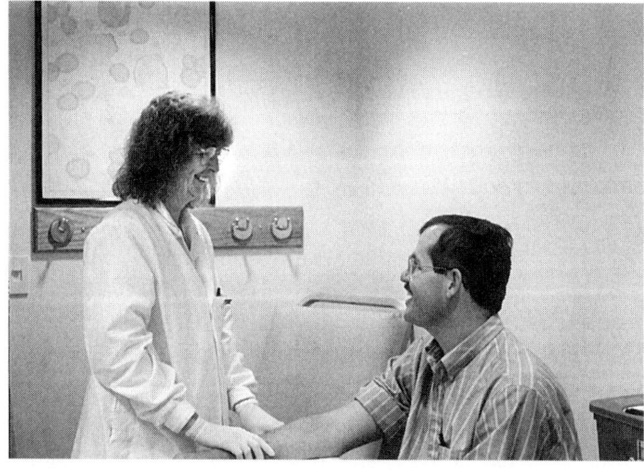

Figure 1–1 Phlebotomist communicating with a patient.

Verbal Skills

Verbal skills enable phlebotomists to introduce themselves, explain the procedure, reassure the patient, and help assure the patient that the procedure is being competently performed. Barriers to verbal communication that must be considered include physical handicaps such as hearing impairment; patient emotions; and the level of patient education, age, and language proficiency. The phlebotomist who recognizes these barriers is better equipped to communicate with the patient. Table 1–1 provides methods to use when verbal communication barriers are encountered.

Listening Skills

Listening skills are a key component of communication. Active listening involves:

- Looking directly and attentively at the patient
- Allowing the patient time to express feelings, anxieties, and concerns
- Providing feedback to the patient through appropriate responses
- Encouraging patient communication by asking questions

Nonverbal Skills

Nonverbal skills or body language include facial expressions, posture, and eye contact. If you walk briskly into the room, smile, and look directly at the patient while talking, you demonstrate positive body language. This makes patients feel that they are important and that you care about them and your work (Fig. 1–1). Conversely, shuffling into the room, avoiding eye contact, and gazing out the window while the patient is talking are examples of negative body language and indicate boredom and disinterest in patients and their tests.

Telephone Skills

Telephone skills are essential for phlebotomists. The phlebotomy department frequently acts as a type of switchboard for the rest of the laboratory because of its location in the central processing area. This is a prime example of the phlebotomist's role as a liaison for the laboratory, and poor telephone skills affect the image of the laboratory. Phlebotomists should have a thorough understanding of the telephone system with regard to transferring calls, placing calls on hold, and paging personnel.

To observe the rules of proper telephone etiquette:

- Answer the phone promptly and politely, stating the name of the department and your name.
- Always check for an emergency before putting someone on hold, and return to calls that are on hold as soon as possible. This may require returning the current call after you have collected the required information.
- Keep writing materials beside the phone to record information such as the location of

emergency blood collections, requests for test results, and numbers for returning calls.

- Make every attempt to help callers, and if you cannot help them, transfer them to another person or department that can. It is also helpful to give callers the number to which you are transferring them.
- Provide accurate and consistent information by keeping current with laboratory policies, looking up information published in department manuals, or asking a supervisor.
- Speak clearly and make sure you understand what the caller is asking and that he or she understands the information you are providing.

Phlebotomy Education and Certification

Structured phlebotomy education programs have been developed by hospitals, community colleges, and technical institutions and are also a part of medical laboratory technician and medical technologist programs. The length and format of these programs vary considerably. However, the goal of providing the healthcare field with phlebotomists who are knowledgeable in all aspects of phlebotomy is universal. The training programs are designed to incorporate a combination of classroom instruction and clinical practice. Most of them follow guidelines developed by national phlebotomy organizations to ensure the quality of the program, to meet national ***accreditation*** requirements, and to prepare graduates for a national certifying examination.

All phlebotomists should obtain ***certification*** from a nationally recognized professional organization because it serves to enhance their position within the healthcare field and documents the quality of their skills and knowledge. Certification examinations can be taken on completion of a structured educational program that meets the standards of the certifying organization or by documentation of experience that meets specified standards. Certification examinations are offered by the organizations listed in Table 1–2. Phlebotomists who attain a satisfactory score can indicate this achievement by placing the initials of the certifying agency behind their names.

TABLE 1–2
Phlebotomist Certifications

Certifying Organization	Phlebotomist Designation
American Medical Technologists (**AMT**)	Registered Phlebotomy Technician, **RPT** (AMT)
American Society of Clinical Pathologists (**ASCP**)	Phlebotomy Technician, **PBT** (ASCP)
American Society of Phlebotomy Technicians (**ASPT**)	Certified Phlebotomy Technician, **CPT** (ASPT)
National Credentialing Agency for Medical Laboratory Personnel (**NCA**)	Clinical Laboratory Phlebotomist, **CLPlb** (NCA)
National Phlebotomy Association (**NPA**)	Certified Phlebotomy Technician, **CPT** (NPA)

Membership in a professional organization enhances the ***professionalism*** of a phlebotomist by providing increased opportunities for continuing education. Professional organizations present seminars and workshops, publish journals containing information on new developments in the field, and represent the profession at state and national levels to influence regulations affecting the profession.

All healthcare professionals are expected to participate in continuing education activities. Attendance at many workshops and seminars is documented by the issuing of certificates containing continuing education units (**CEUs**). Equally important is attending staff meetings, reading pertinent memoranda, and observing notices placed on bulletin boards or in newsletters.

Healthcare Delivery System

As members of the healthcare delivery system, phlebotomists should have a basic knowledge of the various healthcare settings in which they may be employed. Most phlebotomists are employed by hospitals. Other employment settings include physician office laboratories (**POLs**), health maintenance organizations (**HMOs**), reference laboratories, urgent care centers, nursing homes, home healthcare agencies, clinics, and blood donor centers.

Hospital Organization

A typical hospital consists of a Board of Trustees, a Chief of Staff, a hospital administrator, and assistant administrators for service areas. The hospital is governed by the Board of Trustees, who are private citizens. The board is ultimately responsible for the hospital operations and the medical staff. The Chief of Staff is the head of the medical team and acts as the liaison among the physicians, the Board of Trustees, and the hospital administrator. The Board of Trustees hires the hospital administrator to manage the hospital operations. Assistant administrators who head each of the four main services of the hospital may assist this person. These four services are the professional service, nursing service, support service, and fiscal service.

Professional Services

This service consists of the departments of the hospital that assist the physician in the diagnosis and treatment of disease. Radiology, radiation therapy, nuclear medicine, occupational therapy, pharmacy, physical therapy, respiratory therapy, and the clinical laboratory are the main departments in this service. Other branches of professional services include **electrocardiography** and **electroencephalography**. The phlebotomist was traditionally included in this group as part of the clinical laboratory staff.

Nursing Services

This service deals directly with patient care. It consists of the cardiac care unit (**CCU**), central supply, emergency room (**ER**), epidemiology, hospital units, infection control, intensive care unit (**ICU**), nursery, and operating room (**OR**). Healthcare team members associated with this service are registered nurses (**RNs**), licensed practical nurses (**LPNs**), certified nursing assistants (**CNAs**), and the unit secretary or ward clerk. Phlebotomists interact most often with this service and, in decentralized organizations, may be included in it.

Support Services

Support services maintain the hospital and include food service, grounds care, housekeeping, human resources, laundry, maintenance, purchasing, and security.

Fiscal Services

Fiscal services manage the business aspect of a hospital. Included in this service are accounting, admitting, the business office, credit and collection, data processing, and medical health records (health information management).

A hospital organizational chart is shown in Figure 1–2. Organizational charts are designed to define the position of each employee with regard to authority, responsibility, and accountability. Hospital organizational charts are further broken down into department organizational charts. Job descriptions are based on organizational structure.

Hospitals vary in both size and the extent of the services they provide. They may range in size from fewer than 50 beds to more than 300 beds. Smaller hospitals are usually equipped to provide general surgical and medical procedures and emergency procedures. Patients may need to be referred or transferred to a larger hospital if specialized care is needed. Phlebotomists may be required only on the day shift. As the size and specialization of a hospital increases, so does the need for more phlebotomists. Many hospitals also provide clinics to serve patients on an outpatient basis. This service also increases the phlebotomy workload.

The traditional hospital contains many different patient areas and departments to which the phlebotomist must travel to collect specimens. Patient care areas are listed and described in Table 1–3. The location of these patient areas is an important part of the orientation of newly hired phlebotomists.

Professional Service Departments

In addition to patient care areas, phlebotomists may be asked to collect specimens from patients who have been transported to a specialized treatment or testing department. The phlebotomist must be familiar with the location of each department, the nature of the procedures performed there, and the safety precautions pertaining to it. In addition, the phlebotomist interacts with all hospital professionals in each department and projects the professional image of the laboratory to the rest of the hospital staff and the patients.

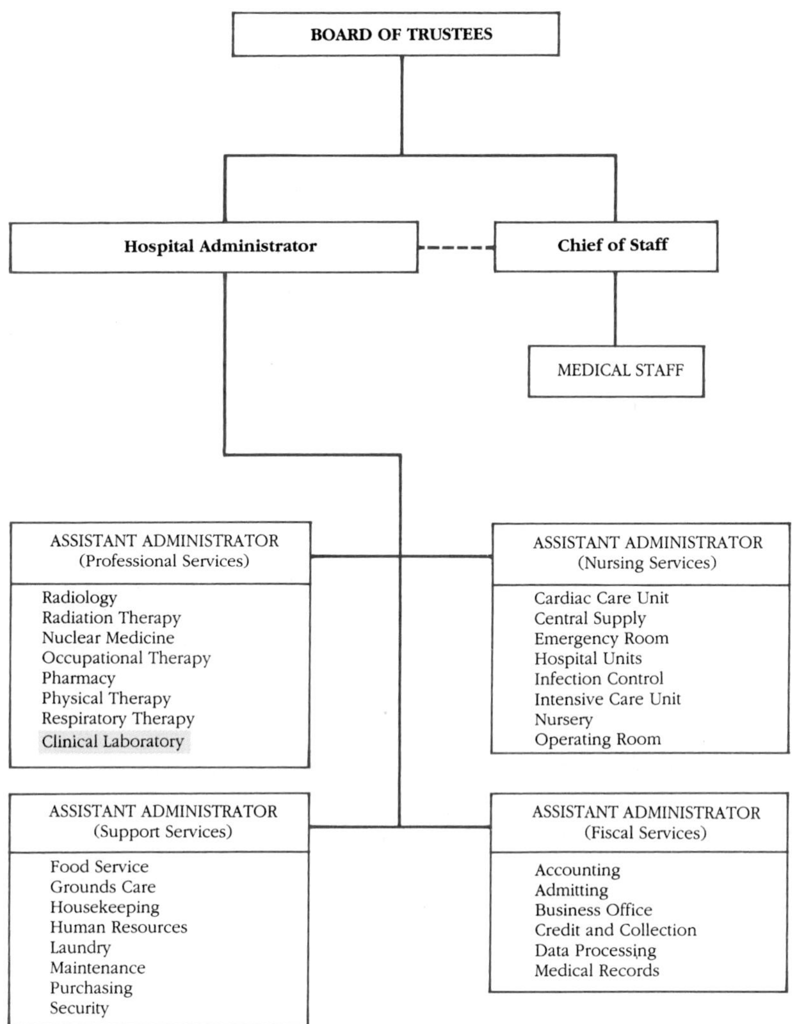

Figure 1–2 Hospital organizational chart.

Radiology and Diagnostic Imaging

The radiology department uses various forms of radiant energy to diagnose and treat disease. Some of the techniques include x-rays of teeth and bones, computerized axial tomography (**CAT or CT scan**), contrast studies using barium sulfate, cardiac catheterization, fluoroscopy, ultrasound, and magnetic resonance imaging (**MRI**). A radiologist, who is a physician, administers diagnostic procedures and interprets radiographs. The allied healthcare professional in this department is a radiographer. Phlebotomists must observe radiation exposure precautions when in this department.

Radiation Therapy

The radiation therapy department uses high-energy x-rays or ionizing radiation to stop the growth of cancer cells. Radiation therapy technologists perform these procedures. Because radiation therapy may affect the bone marrow, blood tests are often performed by the laboratory to monitor the patients. Radiation exposure precautions should be observed.

Nuclear Medicine

The nuclear medicine department uses the characteristics of radioactive substances in the diagnosis and

TABLE 1-3
Hospital Patient Care Areas

Area	Description
Emergency room (ER)	Immediate care
Intensive care unit (ICU)	Critically ill patients
Cardiac care unit (CCU)	Patients with acute cardiac disorders
Pediatrics	Children
Nursery	Infants
Neonatal intensive care nursery	Newborns experiencing difficulty
Labor and delivery (**L & D**)	Childbirth
Operating room (OR)	Surgical procedures
Recovery room	Postoperative patients
Psychiatric unit	Mentally disturbed patients
Dialysis unit	Severe renal disorders
Medical/surgical units	General patient care
Oncology center	Cancer treatment
Short-stay unit	Outpatient surgery

treatment of disease. Radioactive materials, called **radioisotopes**, emit rays as they disintegrate, and the rays are measured on specialized instruments. Two types of tests are used. In vitro tests analyze blood and urine specimens using radioactive materials to detect levels of hormones, drugs, and other substances. In vivo tests involve administering radioactive material to the patient by intravenous (**IV**) injection and measuring the emitted rays to examine organs and evaluate their function. Examples of these procedures are bone, brain, liver, and thyroid scans. Therapeutic doses of radioactive material also can be given to a patient to treat diseases. Nuclear medicine technologists perform these procedures under the supervision of a physician. Radiation exposure precautions should be observed.

Occupational Therapy

The occupational therapy (**OT**) department teaches techniques that enable patients with physical, mental, or emotional disabilities to function within their limitations in daily living. Occupational therapists provide this instruction.

Pharmacy

The pharmacy department dispenses the medications prescribed by physicians. The phlebotomist is often responsible for the collection of specifically timed specimens used to monitor the blood level of certain medications. Persons trained to dispense medications are called pharmacists.

Physical Therapy

The physical therapy (**PT**) department provides treatment to patients who have been disabled as a result of illness or injury by using procedures involving water, heat, massage, ultrasound, and exercise. Physical therapists are the professionals trained to provide this therapy.

Respiratory Therapy

Respiratory therapists provide treatment in breathing disorders and perform testing to evaluate lung function. They may also perform the arterial punctures used to evaluate arterial blood gases that are discussed in Chapter 11.

Cardiovascular Testing

Cardiac technicians under the supervision of a **cardiologist** evaluate cardiac function using electrocardiograms, stress tests, and imaging techniques. Patients must be closely monitored for adverse reactions.

Clinical Laboratory

The clinical laboratory provides data to the healthcare team to aid in determining the diagnosis, treatment, and prognosis of a patient. The organization and functions of the clinical laboratory are discussed in detail in Chapter 2.

Other Healthcare Settings

The healthcare delivery system has experienced many changes in recent years. As a result of technological advances and the increasing cost of health care, a variety of healthcare settings has been created. This development has produced additional places of employment for phlebotomists and, in many settings, also has expanded their duties to include specimen processing, performance of **waived test** procedures (see Chapter 13), and additional record keeping related to processing of insurance claims.

POLs have progressed from single practitioners doing simple screening tests to large group medical practices employing both phlebotomists and medical laboratory personnel authorized to perform tests that are more specialized. This setting also may serve as a designated drawing center for a contracted reference laboratory. The phlebotomist could be responsible for specimen processing.

HMOs are group practice centers that provide a large variety of services. Physicians' offices, a clinical laboratory, radiology, physical therapy, and outpatient surgery are often available at one location. Members are charged a prepaid fee for all services performed during a designated time period. Phlebotomists are employed as part of the clinical laboratory staff.

Large, independent reference laboratories contract with healthcare providers and institutions to perform both routine and highly specialized tests. Phlebotomists are hired to collect samples from patients referred to the reference laboratory. They may be stationed at the laboratory or at off-site designated collection facilities.

Hospital-sponsored specialty clinics, such as cancer, urology, and pediatric clinics, provide more cost-effective delivery of health care to more patients. Increased emphasis on preventive medicine and **alternative medicine** has resulted in the establishment of wellness clinics for health screening. Phlebotomists may be employed in these settings.

Cost effectiveness has reduced the length of time patients stay in a hospital, and more care is being performed on an outpatient basis. The implementation of **diagnostic related groups (DRGs)** by the federal government to control the rising costs of Medicare and Medicaid has limited the length of hospital stays and the number of diagnostic procedures that can be performed. The DRG system classified patients into diagnostic categories related to body systems and the illnesses associated with them. A total of 467 illness categories has been developed and classification of patients is based on primary and secondary diagnoses, age, treatment performed, and status on discharge. This system determines the amount of money the government will pay for a patient's care, regardless of the number of tests performed. Therefore, the length of a hospital stay, laboratory tests, and other procedures must be kept within the specified DRG guidelines or the healthcare institution must absorb the additional cost. Because of the decreased time of hospital stays, home health care has increased to accommodate patients whose conditions are not compatible with frequent outpatient visits to caregivers. Nurses and other healthcare providers, including phlebotomists, make scheduled visits to patients requiring home health care. Phlebotomists also are employed to perform collections at long-term care facilities or nursing homes.

In summary, the current healthcare delivery system offers a variety of employment opportunities for phlebotomists. Phlebotomists must have the motivation to explore these opportunities and the flexibility to adapt to them.

Bibliography

Clerc, JM: An Introduction to Clinical Laboratory Science. CV Mosby, St. Louis, 1992.

Strasinger, SK, and Di Lorenzo, MS: Skills for the Patient Care Technician. FA Davis, Philadelphia, 1999.

Vogel, DP: Patient-Focused Care. Am J Hosp Pharmacol 50:2321–2329, 1993.

Study Questions

1. Number (1 to 5) the following developments in the history of phlebotomy in chronologic order.
   a. _4_ Development of structured phlebotomy training programs
   b. _1_ Hippocrates' theory on the relationship between excess body fluids and disease
   c. ___ Collection of blood for diagnostic testing
   d. _5_ Certification of phlebotomists
   e. _2_ Appearance of the barber pole symbol

2. How does patient-focused care increase the efficiency of phlebotomy?

____

____

3. Why is flexibility an important quality for phlebotomists?

____

____

4. Describe a way in which failure of the phlebotomist to demonstrate the following characteristics could affect the quality of patient care.
   a. Dependability _______________
   b. Compassion _______________
   c. Honesty _______________
   d. Integrity _______________

5. List four barriers to effective verbal communication and state a means to overcome each.
   a. _______________
   b. _______________

c. ______________________________

____

d. ______________________________

____

6. State two behaviors that represent negative body language.

a. ______________________________

b. ______________________________

7. How can a phlebotomist demonstrate good telephone communication skills in the following situations?

a. Placing a call on hold ______________________________

____

b. Providing instructions to a patient ______________________________

____

c. Receiving a request for information about a radiology procedure ______________________________

____

8. On completion of a structured phlebotomy program, does a phlebotomist seek accreditation or certification? ______________________________

9. Name the four services in a hospital and a department of each.

Service	**Department**
a. ______________	______________
b. ______________	______________
c. ______________	______________
d. ______________	______________

10. Match the following professional service departments and their functions.

a. _____ Radiology	1. Teach daily living skills to disabled patients
b. _____ Occupational therapy	2. Provide pulmonary therapy
c. _____ Pharmacy	3. Perform CT scans and MRIs
d. _____ Physical therapy	4. Analyze blood and urine specimens
e. _____ Clinical laboratory	5. Provide massage and exercise therapy
f. _____ Respiratory therapy	6. Dispense medications

11. State two possible duties of a phlebotomist employed in a POL.

a. ______________________________

b. ______________________________

12. How does an HMO bill patients? ______________________________

13. Which nonhospital healthcare setting performs highly specialized laboratory testing?

____

14. How has the implementation of DRGs affected healthcare delivery?

____

____

15. In what type of employment would phlebotomists be required to have a driver's license?

____

Clinical Situation

1. The phlebotomy supervisor at Healthy Hospital holds a meeting to tell the staff that the phlebotomy service is going to be decentralized.
   a. How will this affect the working location of the phlebotomists?

   ____

   ____

   b. How might this affect the duties of the phlebotomists?

   ____

   ____

   c. What is the major benefit for Healthy Hospital of decentralizing phlebotomy?

   ____

   d. The phlebotomy supervisor will be teaching classes on phlebotomy. Who will be attending the classes?

   ____

Chapter 2

The Clinical Laboratory

Chapter Outline

Clinical Laboratory Personnel
- Laboratory Director (Pathologist)
- Laboratory Manager (Administrator)
- Section Supervisor
- Medical Technologist
- Medical Laboratory Technician
- Phlebotomist

Hematology Section
- Specimen Collection and Handling
- Tests Performed in the Hematology Section
- Coagulation Area of the Hematology Section
- Tests Performed in the Coagulation Area of the Hematology Section

Chemistry Section
- Specimen Collection and Handling
- Tests Performed in the Chemistry Section

Blood Bank Section
- Specimen Collection and Handling
- Tests Performed in the Blood Bank Section

Serology (Immunology) Section
- Specimen Collection and Handling
- Tests Performed in the Serology (Immunology) Section

Microbiology Section
- Specimen Collection and Handling
- Tests Performed in the Microbiology Section

Urinalysis Section
- Specimen Collection and Handling
- Tests Performed in the Urinalysis Section

Regulation Of Clinical Laboratories

Learning Objectives

Upon completion of this chapter, the reader will be able to:

1 Describe the qualifications and functions of the personnel employed in a clinical laboratory.

2 Discuss the basic functions of the hematology, chemistry, blood bank (immunohematology), serology (immunology), microbiology, and urinalysis sections.

3 Describe the appropriate collection and handling of specimens analyzed in the individual clinical laboratory sections.

4 Identify the most common tests performed in the individual clinical laboratory sections and state their function.

5 Describe the regulation and accreditation of clinical laboratories.

CLB

The clinical laboratory is divided into two areas, anatomical and clinical. The anatomical area is responsible for the analysis of surgical specimens, frozen sections, **biopsies**, cytologic specimens, and autopsies. Sections of the anatomical area include cytology, histology, and cytogenetics.

In the cytology section, cytologists **(CTs)** process and examine tissue and body fluids for the presence of abnormal cells, such as cancer cells. The Papanicolaou **(Pap)** smear is one of the most common tests performed in cytology. In the histology section, histology technicians **(HTs)** and technologists **(HTLs)** process and stain tissue obtained from biopsies, surgery, autopsies, and frozen sections. A pathologist then examines the tissue. Cytogenetics is the section in which chromosome studies are performed to detect genetic disorders. Blood, **amniotic fluid**, tissue, and bone marrow specimens are analyzed.

The clinical area is divided into specialized sections: hematology and coagulation, chemistry, blood bank (immunohematology), serology (immunology), microbiology, urinalysis, and phlebotomy and central processing. In the clinical sections, blood, bone marrow, microbiology specimens, urine, and other body fluids are analyzed. Figure 2–1 shows a sample organizational chart of a traditional clinical laboratory. In some institutions, certain sections, such as hematology and coagulation, chemistry, and urinalysis may be combined in a core laboratory for more efficient use of personnel.

Clinical Laboratory Personnel

The laboratory employs a large number of personnel, whose qualifications vary with their job descriptions. Most personnel are required to be certified by a national organization. Some states require an additional state licensure, and the number of these states is increasing. See Figure 2–2 for an organizational chart of clinical laboratory personnel.

Laboratory Director (Pathologist)

The director of the laboratory is usually a pathologist, a physician who has completed a 4- to 5-year pathology residency. A pathologist is a specialist in the study of disease and works in both clinical **pathology** and anatomical pathology. Clinical pathology is the interpretation of clinical laboratory test results to diagnose disease. Anatomical pathology is the study of tissue, including surgical and autopsy specimens.

The pathologist is the liaison between the medical staff and the laboratory staff, and acts as a consultant to physicians regarding a patient's diagnosis and treatment. Direct responsibility for the anatomical and clinical areas of the laboratory lies with the pathologist. His or her responsibilities include establishing laboratory policies, interpreting test results, performing bone marrow biopsies and autopsies, and diagnosing disease from tissue specimens or cell

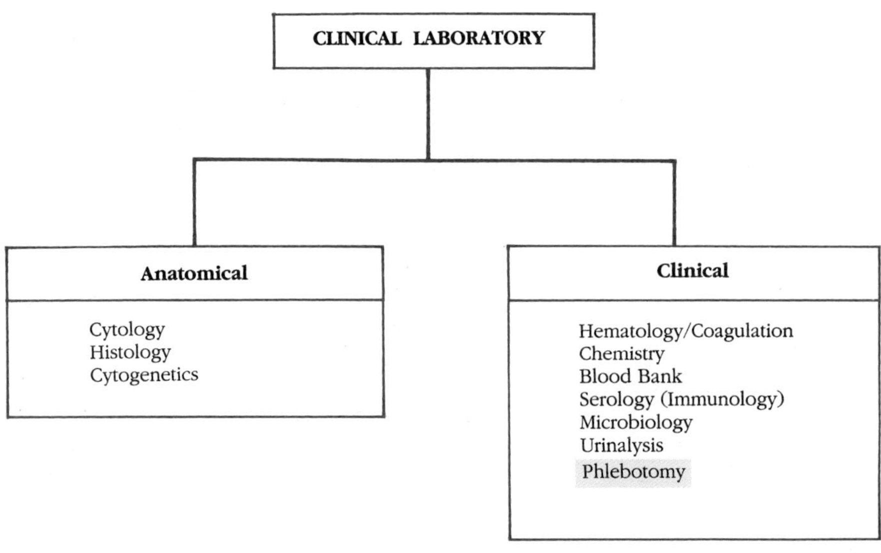

Figure 2–1 Clinical laboratory organizational chart.

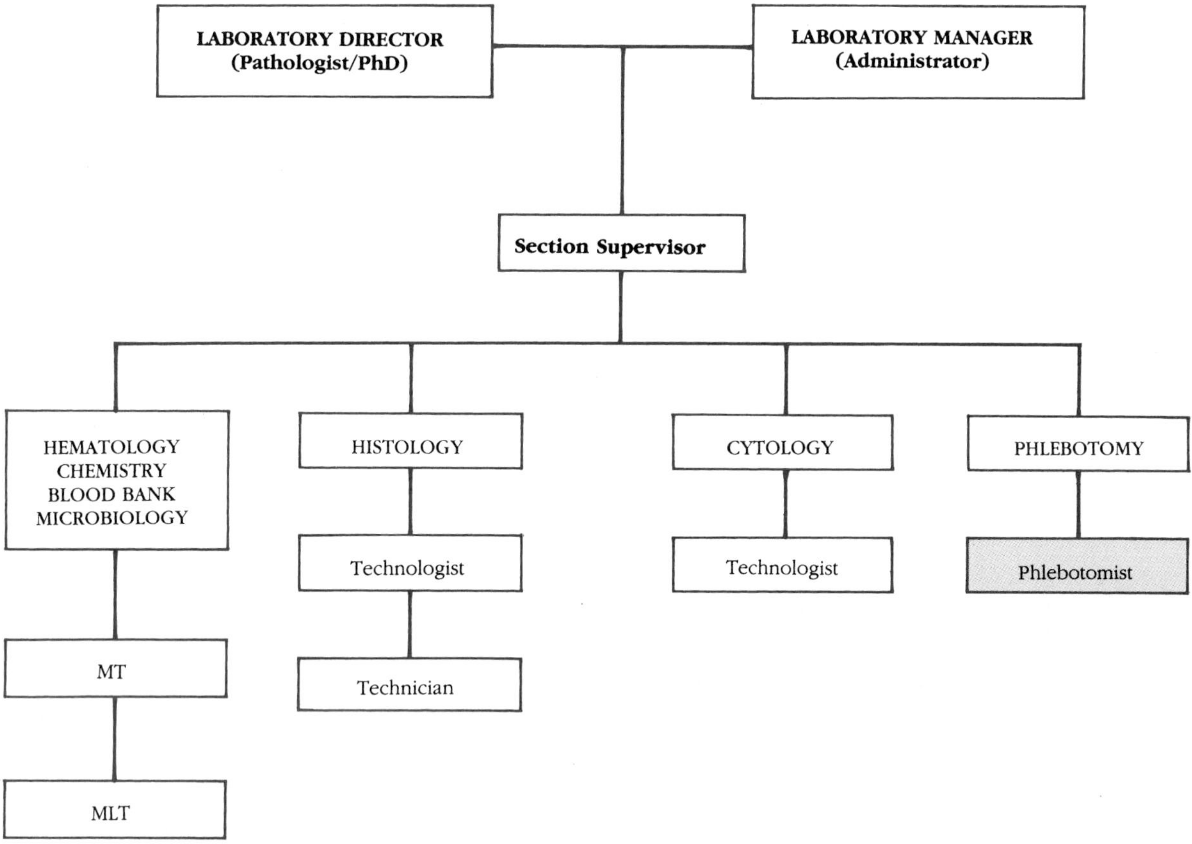

Figure 2–2 Clinical laboratory personnel organizational chart.

preparations. Often the laboratory director has one or more associate pathologists to assist with the laboratory responsibilities. The laboratory director may also be a laboratory specialist who possesses a doctorate degree.

Laboratory Manager (Administrator)

The laboratory manager is responsible for overall technical and administrative management of the laboratory, including personnel and budgets. The laboratory manager is usually a medical technologist with a master's degree and 5 or more years of laboratory experience. The additional education is often in either administration or business. The laboratory manager acts as a liaison between the laboratory staff, the administrator of professional services, and the laboratory director.

Section Supervisor

The section supervisor is a medical technologist **(MT)** with experience and expertise related to the particular laboratory section or sections. Many section supervisors have a specialty certification in hematology, chemistry, blood banking, immunology, or microbiology. The section supervisor is accountable to the laboratory manager. Responsibilities of the section supervisor include reviewing all laboratory test results; consulting with the pathologist on abnormal test results; scheduling personnel; maintaining automated instruments by implementing preventive maintenance procedures and quality control measures; preparing budgets; maintaining reagents and supplies; orienting, evaluating, and teaching personnel; and providing research and development protocols for new test procedures.

Medical Technologist

The MT or clinical laboratory scientist (**CLS**) has a bachelor's degree in medical technology or in a biologic science and 1 year of training in an accredited medical technology program. The technologist performs laboratory procedures that require independent judgment and responsibility with minimal technical supervision; maintains equipment and records; performs quality assurance and preventive maintenance activities related to test performance; and may function as a supervisor, educator, manager, or researcher within a medical laboratory setting. Additional duties of the medical technologist are to evaluate and solve problems related to the collection of specimens, perform complex laboratory procedures, analyze quality control data, report and answer inquiries regarding test results, troubleshoot equipment, participate in the evaluation of new test procedures, and provide education to new employees and students.

Medical Laboratory Technician

A medical laboratory technician (**MLT**) or clinical laboratory technician (**CLT**) usually has a 2-year associate degree from an accredited college medical laboratory program. A medical laboratory technician performs routine laboratory procedures according to established protocol under the supervision of a technologist, supervisor, or laboratory director. The duties of the MLT include collecting and processing biologic specimens for analysis, performing routine analytic tests, recognizing factors that affect test results, recognizing abnormal results and reporting them to a supervisor, recognizing equipment malfunctions and reporting them to a supervisor, performing quality control and preventive maintenance procedures, maintaining accurate records, and demonstrating laboratory technical skills to new employees and students.

Phlebotomist

The phlebotomist collects blood from patients for laboratory analysis. The phlebotomist must have a high school diploma and usually has completed a structured phlebotomy training program. Certified phlebotomy technicians have passed a national certifying examination. The phlebotomist is trained to identify the patient properly; obtain the correct amount of blood by venipuncture or microtechnique, use the correct equipment and collection tubes; properly label and transport specimens to the laboratory; prepare specimens to be delivered to the laboratory sections; and observe all safety and quality control policies. Test collection requirements vary with each department; therefore, the phlebotomist must interact with and have knowledge of all the sections in the laboratory.

Hematology Section

Key Terms

Anemia	*Hemostasis*	*Serum*
Anticoagulant	*Leukemia*	
Hemolysis	*Plasma*	

Hematology is the study of the formed (cellular) elements of the blood. In this section, the cellular elements, red blood cells (**RBCs**), white blood cells (**WBCs**), and platelets (**Plts**) are enumerated and classified in all body fluids and in the bone marrow. These cells, which are formed in the bone marrow, are released into the blood stream as needed to carry oxygen, provide immunity against infection, and aid in blood clotting.

By examining the cells in a blood specimen, the technologist can detect disorders such as ***leukemia***, ***anemia***, other blood diseases, and infection and monitor their treatment (Fig. 2–3).

Specimen Collection and Handling

The most common body fluid analyzed in the hematology section is whole blood (a mixture of cells and plasma). A whole blood specimen is obtained by using a collection tube with an ***anticoagulant*** to prevent clotting of the specimen. Most tests performed in the hematology section require blood that has been collected in tubes with a lavender stopper that contain the anticoagulant ethylenediaminetetraacetic acid (**EDTA**) (see Chapter 5). Immediate inversion of this tube eight times is critical to prevent clotting and ensure accurate blood counts.

Blood is analyzed in the form of either whole blood, ***plasma***, or ***serum***. The liquid portion of blood is called plasma if it is obtained from a specimen that has not been allowed to **clot**. If the specimen is allowed to clot, the liquid portion is called serum. The major difference between plasma and serum is that plasma contains the protein fibrinogen and serum does not. Refer to Figure 4-11 in Chapter 4 to see the role of fibrinogen in the clotting process. Figure 2–4 illustrates the differences between plasma and serum. It is important to differentiate between plasma and serum because many laboratory tests are designed to be performed specifically on either plasma or serum.

Tests Performed in the Hematology Section

A complete blood count (**CBC**) is the primary analysis performed in the hematology section. Very often it is ordered on a **stat** basis. Table 2–1 lists the tests performed in the hematology section, including components of the CBC, which may also be ordered separately. Many of the tests in hematology and coagulation are performed on automated instruments (Fig. 2–5).

Coagulation Area of the Hematology Section

The coagulation laboratory is usually a part of the hematology section, but in larger laboratories it may be a separate section. In this area, the overall process of ***hemostasis*** is evaluated; this includes platelets, blood vessels, coagulation factors, fibrinolysis, inhibitors, and anticoagulant therapy (heparin and Coumadin). Plasma from a specimen drawn in a tube with a light blue stopper that contains the anticoagulant sodium citrate is the specimen most frequently analyzed. The blood specimen must be returned to the laboratory for analysis within 30 minutes, or it can be refrigerated for up to 4 hours.

Tests Performed in the Coagulation Area of the Hematology Section

The tests most frequently performed in the coagulation area of the hematology section and their function are presented in Table 2–2.

Chemistry Section

The clinical chemistry section is the most automated area of the laboratory. Instruments are computerized

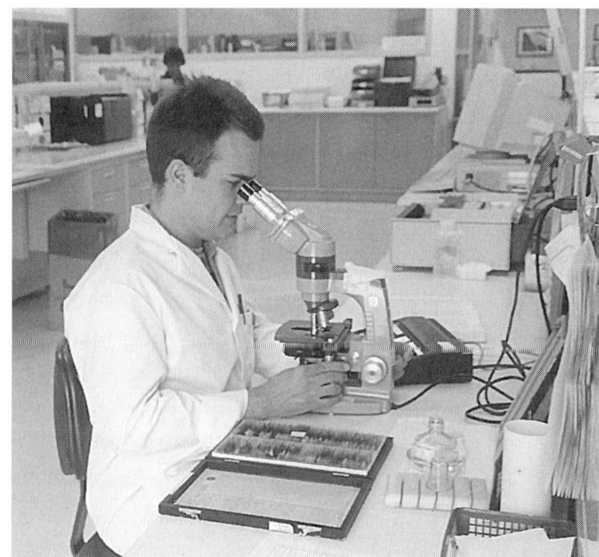

Figure 2–3 A technologist examining blood cells in the hematology section.

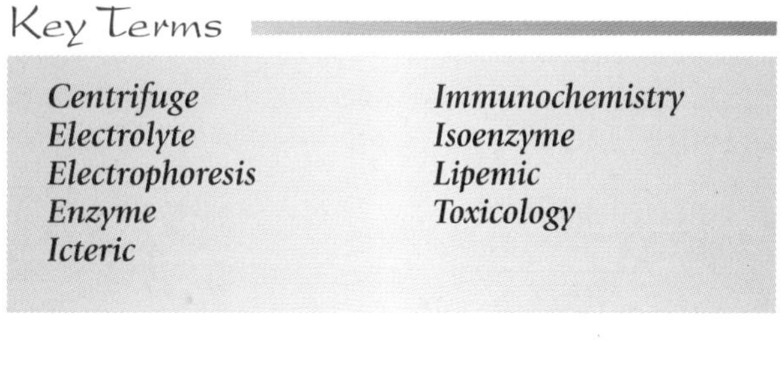

Key Terms

Centrifuge
Electrolyte
Electrophoresis
Enzyme
Icteric
Immunochemistry
Isoenzyme
Lipemic
Toxicology

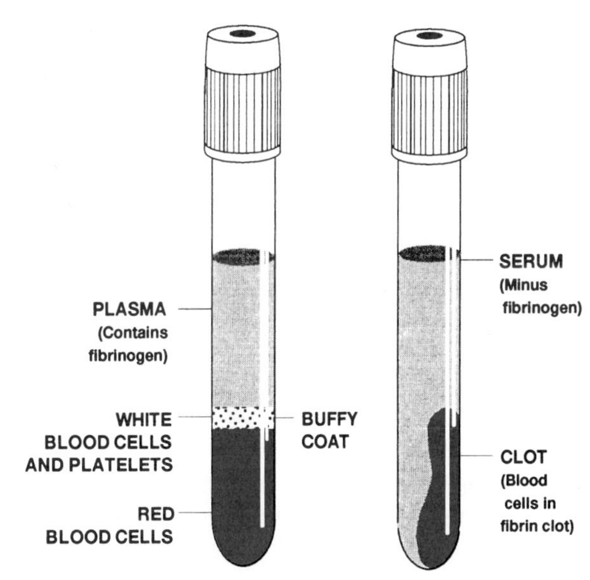

Figure 2–4 Differences between plasma and serum.

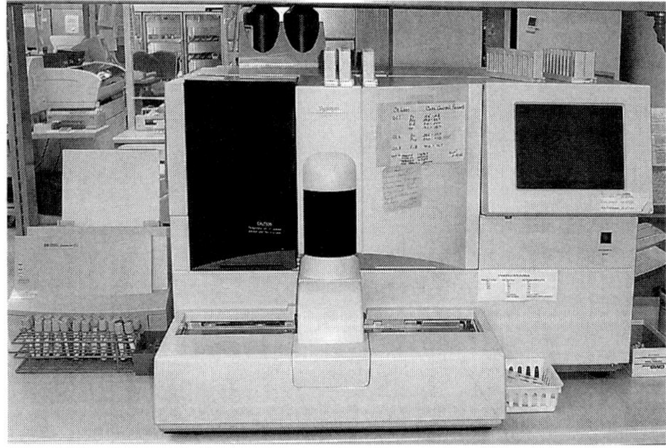

Figure 2–5 An automated coagulation analyzer.

and designed to perform single and multiple tests from small amounts of specimen. Figures 2–6 and 2–7 provide examples of the instrumentation and computerization used in the chemistry section.

The chemistry section may be divided into several areas such as general or automated chemistry, ***electrophoresis***, ***toxicology***, and ***immunochemistry***. The electrophoresis area performs hemoglobin electrophoresis; protein electrophoresis on serum, urine, and cerebrospinal fluid; and ***isoenzyme*** detection. In toxicology, therapeutic drug monitoring (**TDM**) and the identification of drugs of abuse are performed. Examples of substances analyzed include alcohol, lead, salicylate, phenobarbital, Dilantin, and cocaine. Immunochemistry uses the techniques of radio-

TABLE 2–1
Tests Performed in the Hematology Section

Test	Function
Complete Blood Count	
Differential (**Diff**)	Determines the percentage of the different types of white blood cells and evaluates red blood cell and platelet morphology (may be examined microscopically on a peripheral blood smear stained with Wright's stain)
Hematocrit (**Hct**)	Determines the volume of red blood cells packed by centrifugation (expressed as a percent)
Hemoglobin (**Hgb**)	Determines the oxygen-carrying capacity of red blood cells
Indices	Calculations to determine the size of red blood cells and amount of hemoglobin
Mean corpuscular hemoglobin (**MCH**)	Determines the amount of hemoglobin in a red blood cell
Mean corpuscular hemoglobin concentration (**MCHC**)	Determines the weight of hemoglobin in a red blood cell and compares it with the size of the cell (expressed as a percent)
Mean corpuscular volume (**MCV**)	Determines the size of red blood cells
Platelet (PLT) count	Determines the number of platelets in circulating blood
Red blood cell (RBC) count	Determines the number of red blood cells in circulating blood
Red cell distribution width (**RDW**)	Calculation to determine the differences in the size of red blood cells (expressed as a percent)
White blood cell (WBC) count	Determines the number of white blood cells in circulating blood
Body fluid analysis	Determines the number and type of cells in various body fluids
Bone marrow	Determines the number and type of cells in the bone marrow
Eosinophil count	Determines the number of eosinophils in blood or nasal secretions (elevated in allergies or parasitic infection)
Erythrocyte sedimentation rate (**ESR**)	Determines the rate of red blood cell sedimentation (nonspecific test for inflammatory disorders)
Kleihauer-Betke	Measures fetal maternal bleeding for Rh immune globulin administration
Osmotic fragility	Determines the ability of red blood cells to absorb liquid without lysing
Plasma hemoglobin	Detects intravascular ***hemolysis***
Reticulocyte (**Retic**) count	Evaluates bone marrow production of red blood cells
Sickledex	Screening test for Hgb S (sickle cell anemia)
Special stains	Determine the type of leukemia or other cellular disorders

TABLE 2-2
Tests Performed in the Coagulation Area of the Hematology Section

Test	Function
Activated partial thromboplastin time [**APTT** (**PTT**)]	Evaluates the intrinsic system of the coagulation cascade and monitors heparin therapy
Antithrombin III	Screening test for increased clotting tendencies
Bleeding time (**BT**)	Evaluates the function of platelets
D-dimer	Measures abnormal blood clotting and fibrinolysis
Factor assays	Detect factor deficiencies that prolong coagulation
Fibrin degradation products (**FDP**)	Test for increased fibrinolysis (usually a stat test drawn in a special tube)
Fibrinogen	Determines the amount of fibrinogen in plasma
Platelet aggregation	Evaluates the function of platelets
Prothrombin time (**PT**)	Evaluates the extrinsic system of the coagulation cascade and monitors Coumadin therapy
Thrombin time (**TT**)	Determines if adequate fibrinogen is present for normal coagulation

immunoassay (**RIA**) and ***enzyme*** immunoassay (**EIA**) to measure substances such as digoxin, thyroid hor-mones, cortisol, vitamin B_{12}, folate, carcinoembryonic antigen, and creatine kinase (**CK**) isoenzymes.

Specimen Collection and Handling

Clinical chemistry tests are performed primarily on serum collected in serum separator tubes, but the serum may also be collected in tubes with red, green, gray, or royal blue stoppers. Tests are also performed on plasma, urine, and other body fluids. Serum and plasma are obtained by ***centrifugation***, which should be performed within 1 to 2 hours of collection.

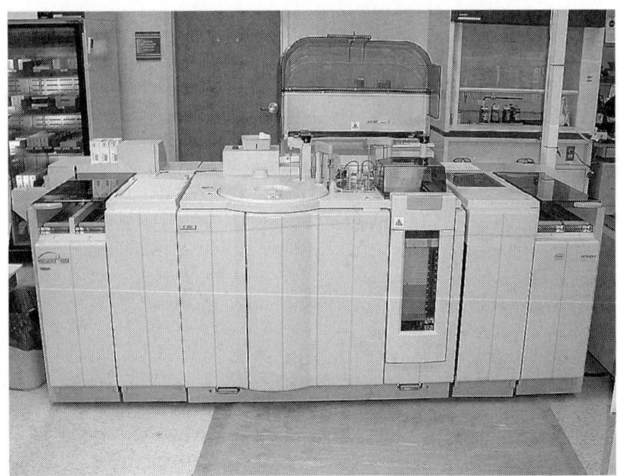

Figure 2–6 Example of a clinical chemistry analyzer.

Because many tests are performed on instruments that take photometric readings, differences in the appearance or color of a specimen may adversely affect the test results. Specimens of concern include hemolyzed specimens that appear red because of the release of hemoglobin from RBCs, ***icteric*** specimens that are yellow because of the presence of excess bilirubin, and ***lipemic*** specimens that are cloudy because of increased lipids. Fasting specimens drawn from patients who have not eaten for 8 to 12 hours are preferred.

Serum separator tubes contain an inert gel that prevents contamination of the specimen by RBCs or

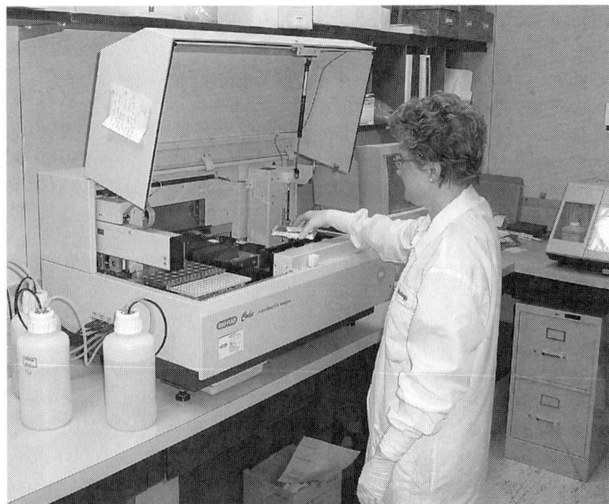

Figure 2–7 Technologist operating an automated instrument.

their metabolites. Specimens must be allowed to clot fully before centrifugation to ensure complete separation of the cells and serum. Many chemistry tests require special collection and handling procedures, such as chilling and protection from light, and these tests are discussed in Chapter 8.

Tests Performed in the Chemistry Section

The tests most frequently performed in the chemistry section and their functions are presented in Table 2–3.

Chemistry profiles or panels are groups of tests used to evaluate a particular organ, body system, or the general health of a patient. The specific tests included in a profile vary among institutions.

Blood Bank Section

Key Terms

Antibody	*Cryoprecipitate*
Antigen	*Fresh frozen plasma*
Blood group	*Immunohematology*
Compatibility (crossmatch)	*Packed cells*
	Unit of blood

TABLE 2–3
Tests Performed in the Chemistry Section

Test	Function
Acid phosphatase	Elevated levels indicate prostatic cancer
Alanine aminotransferase [**ALT** (**SGPT**)]	Elevated levels indicate liver disorders
Albumin	Decreased levels indicate liver or kidney disorders or malnutrition
Alcohol	Elevated levels indicate intoxication
Alkaline phosphatase (**ALP**)	Elevated levels indicate bone or liver disorders
Ammonia	Elevated levels indicate severe liver disorders
Amylase	Elevated levels indicate pancreatitis
Apo-A lipoprotein	Elevated levels indicate cardiac risk
Apo-B lipoprotein	Elevated levels indicate cardiac risk
Arterial blood gases (**ABGs**)	Determine the acidity or alkalinity and oxygen and carbon dioxide levels of blood
Aspartate aminotransferase [**AST(SGOT)**]	Elevated levels indicate myocardial infarction or liver disorders
Bilirubin	Elevated levels indicate liver or hemolytic disorders
Blood urea nitrogen (**BUN**)	Elevated levels indicate kidney disorders
Brain natriuretic peptide (**BNP**)	Elevated levels indicate congestive heart failure
Calcium (**Ca**)	Mineral associated with bone, musculoskeletal, or endocrine disorders
Cholesterol	Elevated levels indicate coronary risk
Creatine kinase [**CK(CPK)**]	Elevated levels indicate myocardial infarction or other muscle damage
Creatine kinase [**CK(CPK)**] isoenzymes	Determine the extent of muscle or brain damage (elevated in myocardial infarction)
Creatinine	Elevated levels indicate kidney disorders
Creatinine clearance	Urine and serum test to measure glomerular filtration rate
Drug screening	Detects drug abuse and monitors therapeutic drugs
Electrolytes (**Lytes**)	Evaluate body fluid balance
Ferritin	Low levels indicate iron deficiency anemia
Gamma-glutamyltransferase (**GGT**)	Elevated levels indicate early liver disorders
Glucose	Elevated levels indicate diabetes mellitus
Glucose tolerance test (**GTT**)	Detects diabetes mellitus or hypoglycemia
Haptoglobin	Used to evaluate hemolytic anemia and certain chronic diseases
Hemoglobin A_1C	Monitors diabetes mellitus
Hemoglobin (Hgb) electrophoresis	Detects abnormal hemoglobins

TABLE 2-3
Tests Performed in the Chemistry Section (Continued)

Test	Function
High-density lipoprotein **(HDL)**	Assesses coronary risk
Iron	Decreased levels indicate iron deficiency anemia
Lactic dehydrogenase **[LD(LDH)]**	Elevated levels indicate myocardial infarction or lung or liver disorders
Lead	Elevated levels indicate poisoning
Lipase	Elevated levels indicate pancreatitis
Lithium **(Li)**	Monitors antidepressant drug
Low-density lipoprotein **(LDL)**	Assesses coronary risk
Magnesium	Cation involved in neuromuscular excitability of muscle tissue
Myoglobin	Early indicator of myocardial infarction
Phosphorus **(P)**	Mineral associated with skeletal or endocrine disorders
Prostate-specific antigen **(PSA)**	Screening for prostatic cancer
Protein	Decreased levels associated with liver or kidney disorders
Total protein **(TP)**	Decreased levels indicate liver or kidney disorders
Transferrin	Used in the differential diagnosis of anemia
Triglycerides	Used to assess coronary risk
Troponin I and T	Early indicators of myocardial infarction
Uric acid	Elevated levels indicate kidney disorders or gout

The blood bank (**BB**) is the section of the laboratory where blood is collected, stored, and prepared for transfusion. It is also called the ***immunohematology*** section because the testing procedures involve RBC ***antigens*** (**Ag**) and ***antibodies*** (**Ab**).

Common Chemistry Profiles

PROFILE	**TESTS**
Comprehensive	Glucose, BUN, creatinine, sodium (**Na**), potassium (**K**), AST, LD, cholesterol, triglycerides, uric acid, total protein/albumin, bilirubin, Ca, and ALP
Hepatic	ALP, ALT, AST, bilirubin, and GGT
Myocardial infarction (**MI**)	AST, CK, CK isoenzymes, LD, troponin I and T, and myoglobin
Coronary risk	Cholesterol, triglycerides, HDL, LDL, and cholesterol/HDL ratio
Basic metabolic	Glucose, BUN, creatinine, Na, chloride (**Cl**), K, and carbon dioxide (**CO_2**)

ALP = alkaline phosphatase; ALT = alanine aminotransferase; AST = aspartate aminotransferase; BUN = blood urea nitrogen; CK = creatine kinase; GGT = gamma glutamyltransferase; HDL = high-density lipoproteins; LD = lactic dehydrogenase; LDL = low-density lipoproteins.

In the blood bank, blood from patients and donors is tested for its ***blood group*** (**ABO**) and **Rh** type (See Table 4-1 in Chapter 4), the presence and identity of abnormal antibodies, and its ***compatibility*** (**crossmatch**) for use in a transfusion (Fig. 2-8). ***Units*** (pints) ***of blood*** are collected from donors, tested for the presence of bloodborne pathogens such as hepatitis viruses and human immunodeficiency virus (HIV), and stored for transfusions (Fig. 2-9). Donor blood may also be separated into components including ***packed cells***, platelets, ***fresh frozen plasma***, and ***cryoprecipitate***. These components are stored separately and used for patients with specific needs. Patients may come to the blood bank to donate their own blood so that they can receive an **autologous transfusion** if blood is needed during surgery.

Specimen Collection and Handling

Blood bank specimens are collected in plain red glass (serum) or pink (plasma) stopper tubes. Serum separator tubes containing gel are not acceptable because the gel will coat the RBCs and interfere with testing. Hemolysis also interferes with the interpretation of test results.

Patient identification is critical in the blood bank, and phlebotomists must carefully follow all patient

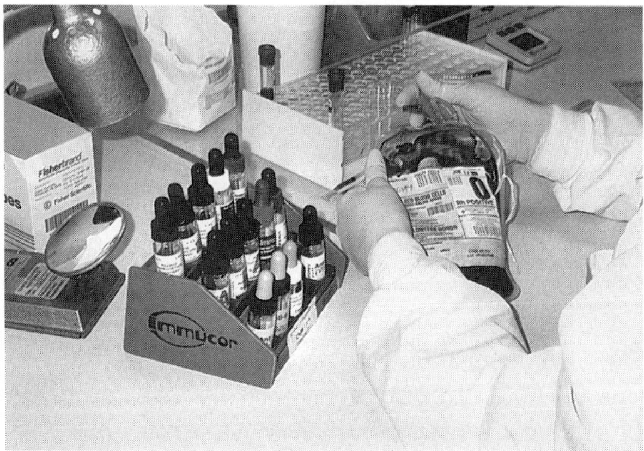

Figure 2–8 A technologist tests a unit of blood before it is transfused.

identification and specimen labeling procedures to ensure that a patient does not receive a transfusion with an incompatible blood type.

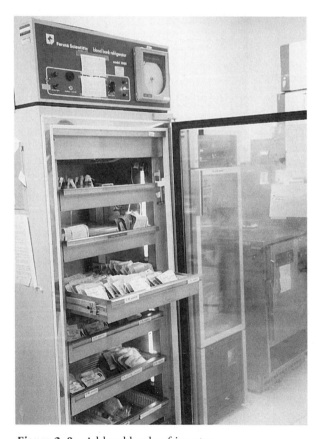

Figure 2–9 A blood bank refrigerator.

Tests Performed in the Blood Bank Section

The tests most frequently performed in the blood bank section and their function are presented in Table 2–4.

Serology (Immunology) Section

Key Terms

Autoimmunity	*Immunology*
Immunoglobulin	*Serology*

The ***serology*** (***immunology***) section performs tests to evaluate the body's immune response; that is, the production of antibodies (***immunoglobulins***) and cellular activation. Because the majority of tests performed in this section analyze for the presence of antibodies in serum, the section is frequently called serology rather than by the broader term immunology.

Tests in the serology section detect the presence of antibodies to bacteria, fungi, parasites, viruses, and antibodies produced against body substances (***autoimmunity***).

Specimen Collection and Handling

Blood for serologic testing is collected in tubes with red stoppers. Serum separator tubes are not used

TABLE 2–4
Tests Performed in the Blood Bank Section

Test	Function
Antibody (Ab) screen (indirect antiglobulin test)	Detects abnormal antibodies in serum
Direct antihuman globulin test (DAT) or direct Coombs	Detects abnormal antibodies on red blood cells
Group and type	ABO and Rh typing
Panel	Identifies abnormal antibodies in serum
Type and crossmatch (T & C)	ABO, Rh typing, and compatibility test
Type and screen	ABO, Rh typing, and antibody screen

because the gel can interfere with the antigen-antibody reactions.

Tests Performed in the Serology (Immunology) Section

The tests most frequently performed in the serology (immunology) section and their functions are presented in Table 2–5.

Microbiology Section

Key Terms

Bacteria	*Microorganism*
Bacteriology	*Mycology*
Culture and sensitivity	*Parasitology*
Gram stain	*Virology*
Microbiology	

The ***microbiology*** section is responsible for the identification of pathogenic microorganisms and for hospital infection control. In large laboratories the section may be divided into ***bacteriology***, ***mycology***, ***parasitology***, and ***virology***.

A ***culture and sensitivity*** (C & S) test is the primary procedure performed in microbiology. It is used to detect and identify ***microorganisms*** and to determine the most effective antibiotic therapy. Results are available within 2 days for most bacteria; however, cultures for tuberculosis and fungi may require several weeks for completion.

Identification of ***bacteria*** is based on morphology, ***Gram stain*** reactions, oxygen and nutritional requirements, and biochemical reactions. Fungi are identified by culture growth and microscopic morphology. Stool specimens are concentrated and examined microscopically for the presence of parasites, ova, or larvae. Viruses must be cultured in living cells, and most laboratories send viral specimens to specialized reference laboratories or perform serological testing.

Specimen Collection and Handling

Most microbiology specimens are obtained from the blood, urine, throat, sputum, genitourinary tract, wounds, cerebrospinal fluid, and feces. Correct

TABLE 2–5
Tests Performed in the Serology (Immunology) Section

Test	Function
Anti-**HIV**	Screening test for human immunodeficiency virus
Antinuclear antibody (**ANA**)	Detects nuclear autoantibodies
Antistreptolysin O (**ASO**) titer	Detects a previous streptococcus infection
C-reactive protein (**CRP**)	Elevated levels indicate inflammatory disorders
Cold agglutinins	Elevated levels indicate atypical (Mycoplasma) pneumonia
Complement levels	Evaluate the function of the immune system
Cytomegalovirus antibody (**CMV**)	Detects cytomegalovirus infection
Febrile agglutinins	Detect antibodies to microorganisms causing fever
Fluorescent antinuclear antibody (**FANA**)	Detects and identifies nuclear autoantibodies
Fluorescent treponemal antibody-absorbed (**FTA-ABS**)	Confirmatory test for syphilis
Hepatitis A antibody	Detects hepatitis A current or past infection
Hepatitis B surface antigen (**HBsAg**)	Detects hepatitis B infection
Hepatitis C antibody	Detects hepatitis C infection
Human chorionic gonadotropin (**HCG**)	Hormone found in the urine and serum during pregnancy
Immunoglobulin (IgG, IgA, IgM) levels	Evaluate the function of the immune system
Monospot	Screening test for infectious mononucleosis
Rapid plasma reagin (**RPR**)	Screening test for syphilis
Rheumatoid arthritis (**RA**)	Detects autoantibodies present in rheumatoid arthritis
Rubella titer	Evaluates immunity to German measles
Venereal Disease Research Laboratory (**VDRL**)	Screening test for syphilis
Western blot	Confirmatory test for human immunodeficiency virus

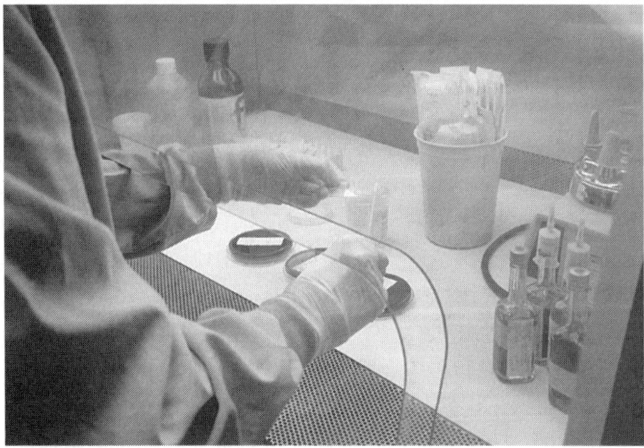

Figure 2–10 Technologist plating a culture and preparing a Gram stain.

identification of pathogens depends on proper collection and prompt transport to the laboratory for processing. Figures 2–10 and 2–11 provide examples of specimen processing in the microbiology section. Phlebotomists may be asked to transport specimens to the laboratory.

Phlebotomists are responsible for collecting blood cultures and may be required to obtain throat cultures (TCs) and instruct patients in the procedure for collecting urine specimens for culture. Specific **sterile** techniques must be observed in the collection of culture specimens to prevent bacterial contamination. These procedures are covered in Chapters 8 and 12.

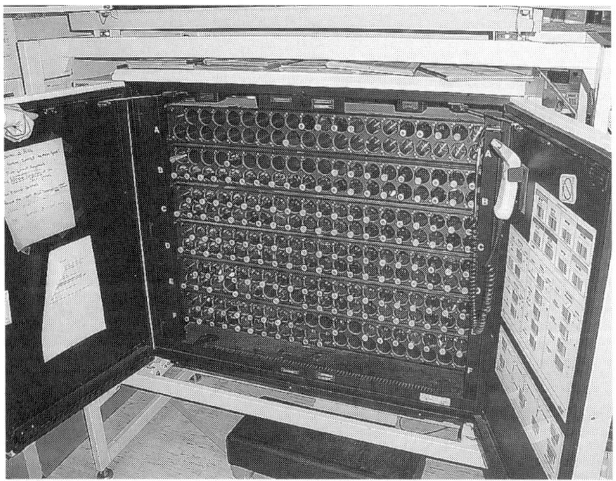

Figure 2–11 Automated blood culture incubator.

Tests Performed in the Microbiology Section

The tests most frequently performed in the microbiology section and their functions are presented in Table 2–6.

Urinalysis Section

Key Terms

Cast	*Ketonuria*
First morning specimen	*Proteinuria*
Glycosuria	*Reagent strip (dipstick)*
Hematuria/hemoglobinuria	*Urinalysis*

Urinalysis (UA) may be a separate laboratory section or a part of the hematology or chemistry sections. UA is a routine screening procedure to detect disorders and infections of the kidney and to detect metabolic disorders such as diabetes mellitus and liver disease.

A routine UA consists of physical, chemical, and microscopic examination of the urine. The physical

TABLE 2–6
Tests Performed in the Microbiology Section

Test	Function
AFB culture	Detects acid-fast bacteria, including mycobacteria tuberculosis
Blood culture	Detects bacteria and fungi in the blood
Culture and sensitivity (C & S)	Detects microbial infection and determines antibiotic treatment
Fungal culture	Detects the presence of and determines the type of fungi
Gram stain	Detects the presence of and aids in the identification of bacteria
Occult blood	Detects nonvisible blood (performed on stool specimens)
Ova and parasites (O & P)	Detects parasitic infection (performed on stool specimens)

examination evaluates the color, clarity, and specific gravity of the urine. The chemical examination is performed using chemical ***reagent strips*** (***dipsticks***) to determine pH, glucose, ketones, protein, blood, bilirubin, urobilinogen, nitrite, and leukocytes (Fig. 2-12). The microscopic examination identifies the presence of cells, ***casts***, bacteria, crystals, yeast, and parasites.

Specimen Collection and Handling

Phlebotomists may be requested to deliver urine specimens to the laboratory. This should be done promptly because many changes can take place in a urine specimen that sits at room temperature for longer than 2 hours. Different types of specimens are required for testing. Random specimens are most frequently collected for routine screening; however, a ***first morning specimen*** is more concentrated and may be required for certain tests. Other types of urine specimens include timed or 24-hour collections for quantitative chemistry tests, and midstream clean-catch and catheterized specimens for cultures (see Chapter 12).

Tests Performed in the Urinalysis Section

The primary test performed in the urinalysis section is the routine urinalysis. As shown in Table 2–7, the test has multiple parts.

Regulation of Clinical Laboratories

All healthcare organizations are governed by guidelines and rules designed to ensure a high standard of patient care. To receive reimbursement for Medicare and Medicaid, facilities must be accredited by an accrediting agency.

The preferred overall accrediting agency for hospitals and organizations is the Joint Commission on Accreditation of Healthcare Organizations (**JCAHO**). Accreditation must be renewed every 3 years. Compliance with regulations is ensured by an on-site visit to the facility by an inspection team. If deficiencies are present, they must be corrected within a specified time frame and the facility may be reinspected.

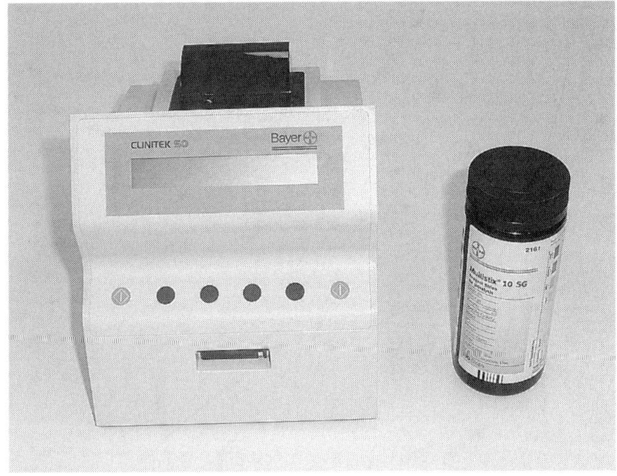

Figure 2–12 Automated urinalysis reagent strip reader.

A primary accrediting agency for clinical laboratories is the College of American Pathologists (**CAP**), which provides on-site inspection and proficiency testing. Samples for proficiency testing are periodically sent to each laboratory section and specified tests are performed. The test results are compared with the range of results from all participating laboratories throughout the country. Incorrect results indicate a problem with the procedures, which must be corrected and the corrective action documented. Inspection teams, made up of pathologists and medical technologists, visit the laboratory every 2 years to review procedures, personnel qualifications, and required documentation. Usually, a laboratory that is accredited by CAP is recognized by JCAHO and does not undergo two inspections.

The National Committee for Clinical Laboratory Standards (**NCCLS**) is a nonprofit organization that publishes recommendations by nationally recognized experts for the performance of laboratory testing.

In 1988, a bill called the Clinical Laboratory Improvement Amendments of 1988 (**CLIA '88**) was introduced in Congress. The regulations in the bill went into effect in 1992 and require that all laboratories performing testing on human specimens for the purposes of diagnosis, treatment, monitoring, or screening must be licensed. The regulations apply to all independent and hospital laboratories, physicians' office laboratories, clinics, nursing homes, outpatient laboratories, mobile health screening, and government laboratories.

TABLE 2–7
Routine Urinalysis

Test	Function
Color	Detects blood, bilirubin, and other pigments
Appearance	Detects cellular and crystalline elements
Specific gravity (**SG**)	Measures the concentration of urine
pH	Determines the acidity of urine
Protein	Elevated levels indicate kidney disorders **(proteinuria)**
Glucose	Elevated levels indicate diabetes mellitus **(glycosuria)**
Ketones	Elevated levels indicate diabetes mellitus or starvation **(ketonuria)**
Blood	Detects red blood cells or hemoglobin **(hematuria/hemoglobinuria)**
Bilirubin	Elevated levels indicate liver disorders
Urobilinogen	Elevated levels indicate liver or hemolytic disorders
Nitrite	Detects bacterial infection
Leukocyte esterase	Detects white blood cells
Microscopic	Determines the number and type of cellular elements

CLIA '88 classifies laboratory tests into categories and specifies the educational requirements and training required for the personnel performing the testing. The categories are waived, provider-performed microscopy, moderate complexity, and high complexity.

Waived tests are considered easy to perform and interpret, require no special training or educational background, and require only a minimum of standardization and **quality control**. Phlebotomists are qualified to perform waived tests, and many of these procedures are covered in Chapter 13. Tests are continually being modified to meet the requirements for waived testing. Table 2–8 lists the most common tests in this category.

TABLE 2–8
Common CLIA-Waived Tests

Test	Function
Activated clotting time (ACT)	
Activated partial thromboplastin time (APTT)	
Arterial blood gases (**ABGs**)	
Cholesterol	
Fecal occult blood	
Glucose	
Group A Streptococcus	
Helicobacter pylori	
HemoCue hemoglobin	
i-STAT instrumentation (chemistry panels, electrolytes)	
Microhematocrit	
Monotest	
Pregnancy	
Prothrombin time (PT)	
Transcutaneous bilirubins	
Troponin T and I	
Urinalysis—physical and chemical	

Tests categorized as provider-performed microscopy, moderate complexity, and high complexity require additional education and training. Laboratories in which this testing is performed must participate in proficiency testing and undergo on-site inspections. Documentation of phlebotomy procedures is included in these inspections.

CLIA '88 is administered by the Centers for Medicare and Medicaid Services (**CMS**), which conducts the on-site inspections and proficiency testing. Accrediting agencies, including JCAHO, CAP, and the Commission on Laboratory Assessment (**COLA**), have been approved by CMS, and laboratories accredited by one of these agencies do not receive an additional inspection.

Bibliography

Clerc, JM: An Introduction to Clinical Laboratory Science. CV Mosby, St Louis, 1992.

Study Questions

1. Differentiate between the two areas of the hospital laboratory. Indicate the sections in each.

Area	Section
a. ______________	______________
	______________
b. ______________	______________
	______________
	______________

2. Which person associated with the clinical laboratory has an MD degree?

   ____

3. Who in the clinical laboratory is responsible for personnel and budgeting?

   ____

4. What are the educational requirements for an MT? ______________

5. Using the laboratory organizational chart, answer the following questions.
   a. To whom would the phlebotomist report the failure to obtain a blood specimen?

      ____

   b. Would a medical technologist report to a medical laboratory technician or a section supervisor?

      ____

6. To which laboratory department would the following tests be taken?
   a. Type and screen ______________
   b. C & S ______________
   c. Electrolytes ______________
   d. Fasting blood sugar ______________
   e. Sedimentation rate ______________
   f. Rapid plasma reagin and Venereal Disease Research Laboratory tests ______________
   g. Gram stain ______________
   h. Bilirubin ______________
   i. CBC ______________
   j. Direct antihuman globulin test (DAT) ______________
   k. Human immunodeficiency virus ______________
   l. Crossmatch ______________

7. What is the major difference between serum and plasma?

____

8. The three cellular elements found in whole blood are ______________________.

9. Name the components of a CBC. Place a checkmark beside the components primarily associated with RBCs.

Components **Checkmark**

a. ____

b. ____

c. ____

d. ____

e. ____

f. ____

g. ____

h. ____

10. Name two tests performed in the coagulation area to monitor anticoagulant therapy.

a. ____

b. ____

11. Name three areas of the chemistry section and give an example of a test performed in each.

Area	Test
a. ____________	____________
b. ____________	____________
c. ____________	____________

12. Name six tests used to diagnose a myocardial infarction.

a. ____

b. ____

c. ____

d. ____

e. ____

f. ____

13. List the tests that measure coronary risk.

a. ____

b. ______________________________

c. ______________________________

d. ______________________________

e. ______________________________

14. Compare a type and screen request with a type and crossmatch request.

____

15. Describe a situation in which an autologous transfusion is performed.

____

16. What volume of blood is routinely collected from a blood donor?

____

17. Define autoimmune disease and give two examples of related tests.

____

____

18. Name two screening tests and one confirmatory test for syphilis.

a. ______________________________

b. ______________________________

c. ______________________________

19. Name a microbiology test in which the phlebotomist would collect blood.

____

20. Name four subsections of microbiology and give an example of a test performed in each.

	Subsection	**Test Performed**
a.	______________	______________
b.	______________	______________
c.	______________	______________
d.	______________	______________

21. What is the most common procedure performed in the microbiology section?

____

22. Name the three parts of a routine urinalysis.

    a. ____________________

    b. ____________________

    c. ____________________

23. In what part of the routine urinalysis must the reagent strip be used?

    ____

24. Match the accrediting agencies with their primary inspection site.

    a. ______ JCAHO 1. Hospital laboratories

    b. ______ CAP 2. POLs

    c. ______ COLA 3. Hospitals

25. What organization publishes recommendations for performance of laboratory tests?

    ____

26. List the four CLIA '88 classifications of laboratory tests.

    a. ____________________

    b. ____________________

    c. ____________________

    d. ____________________

27. Which CLIA category might a phlebotomist perform? ____________________

Clinical Situations

1. A phlebotomist with a high school diploma has completed a structured phlebotomy program and obtained national certification. After working in a hospital for a year, the phlebotomist asks the phlebotomy supervisor how he or she can continue on with a clinical laboratory career.

   a. What would be the quickest education and training route the supervisor could recommend?

   ____

   b. What would be the next step in education and training for this person's advancement?

   ____

   c. How might specialist certification help this person's career?

   ____

d. Name two categories of educational courses that could help this person's advancement to a laboratory manager.

____

2. State whether the following situations are acceptable or not acceptable procedure and explain your answer.

   a. A phlebotomist delivering a specimen to the coagulation section is instructed to place the tube in the refrigerator.

   ____

   b. A histology technician is examining Pap smears to detect cancerous cells.

   ____

   c. A phlebotomist delivers a gel serum separator tube to the blood bank for a type and cross-match.

   ____

   d. A phlebotomist is asked to deliver a urine specimen to microbiology for a C & S.

   ____

   e. A phlebotomist working in a POL is performing dipstick urinalysis.

   ____

   f. A phlebotomist delivers a CBC to the chemistry section.

   ____

   g. A hospital laboratory receives yearly inspections by JCAHO and CAP.

   ____

Chapter 3

Safety

Chapter Outline

Biologic Hazards
- Transmission Prevention Procedures
- Patient Isolation
- Biologic Waste Disposal

Sharp Hazards
- Government Regulations
- Occupational Exposure to Bloodborne Pathogens

Chemical Hazards

Radioactive Hazards

Electrical Hazards

Fire/Explosive Hazards

Physical Hazards

Learning Objectives

Upon completion of this chapter, the reader will be able to:

1. List the components of the chain of infection and the safety precautions that will break the chain.
2. Correctly perform routine handwashing.
3. List and state the purpose of the personal protective equipment used by phlebotomists.
4. Describe the symptoms of latex allergy.
5. Correctly put on and remove personal protective equipment.
6. Describe the three isolation categories used in transmission-based precautions.
7. Differentiate between transmission-based isolation and protective isolation.
8. Differentiate among universal precautions, body substance isolation, and standard precautions.
9. Describe the procedures followed by phlebotomists in isolation areas.
10. Name a common blood and body fluid disinfectant.
11. Safely dispose of sharp objects.
12. Describe the components of the Occupational Exposure to Bloodborne Pathogens Standard and state three additions mandated by the Needlestick Safety and Prevention Act.
13. List in order the actions to be taken if an exposure to bloodborne pathogens occurs.
14. Describe safety precautions used when handling chemicals.
15. Identify the symbol for radiation.
16. Discuss electrical safety and the procedure to follow in cases of electrical shock.
17. List the basic steps to follow when a fire is discovered (RACE).
18. Correlate the classifications of fires to types of fire extinguishers.
19. Interpret the warnings of the National Fire Protection Association symbol.
20. List six precautions observed by phlebotomists to avoid physical hazards.

CLB

Key Terms

Airborne precautions	*Nosocomial infection*	*Standard precautions*
Biohazardous	*Personal protective equipment*	*Transmission-based precautions*
Contact precautions	*Postexposure prophylaxis*	*Universal precautions*
Droplet precautions	*Radioactivity*	

The healthcare setting contains a wide variety of safety hazards, many capable of producing serious injury or life-threatening disease. To work safely in this environment, the phlebotomist must learn what hazards exist, the basic safety precautions associated with them, and finally to apply the basic rules of common sense required for everyday safety. Some hazards are unique to the healthcare environment and others are encountered routinely throughout life. One must also keep in mind that these hazards affect not only the phlebotomist but also the patient. Therefore, phlebotomists must be prepared to protect both themselves and the patients (Table 3-1).

Biologic Hazards

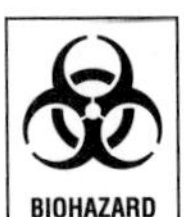

The healthcare setting provides an abundant source of potentially harmful microorganisms including bacteria, fungi, parasites, and viruses. An understanding of the transmission (chain of infection) of microorganisms is necessary to prevent infection. The chain of infection requires a continuous link between three elements—a source, a method of transmission, and a susceptible host. The source refers to the location of the potentially harmful microorganisms and may be a person or a contaminated object. Microorganisms from the source must then be transferred to the host. This may occur through direct contact (e.g., host touches or is touched by the contaminated source), inhaling infected material (e.g., **aerosol** droplets released by an infected patient or an uncapped tube in a centrifuge), ingesting contaminated food or water (e.g., food poisoning), or by means of a **vector** (e.g., malaria transmitted by mosquitoes). Although patients are considered the most logical susceptible host, anyone can serve as the host. Therefore, safety precautions are designed for both healthcare workers and patients. Keep in mind that once the chain of infection is completed, the susceptible host becomes the new source. The ultimate goal of biologic safety is to prevent completion of the chain. Figure 3–1 uses the universal symbol for ***biohazardous*** material to illustrate the chain of infection and demonstrates how it can be broken by following safety practices.

Previously uninfected patients who become infected during hospitalization represent approximately 5% of the patient population. The term ***nosocomial infection*** designates an infection contracted by a patient during a hospital stay. Although some of these **infections** may be caused by visitors, the majority are the result of personnel not following infection control practices.

In addition to observing infection control procedures, phlebotomists must report all cases of personal illness to a supervisor and keep immuniza-

TABLE 3–1
Types of Safety Hazards

Type	Source	Possible Injury
Biologic	Infectious agents	Bacterial, fungal, viral, or parasitic infections
Sharp	Needles, lancets, and broken glass	Cuts, punctures, or bloodborne pathogen exposure
Chemical	Preservatives and reagents	Exposure to poisonous, caustic, or carcinogenic agents
Radioactive	Equipment and radioisotopes	Damage to a fetus or generalized exposure to radiation
Electrical	Ungrounded or wet equipment and frayed cords	Burns or shock
Fire/explosive	Bunsen burners and organic chemicals	Burns or dismemberment
Physical	Wet floors, heavy boxes and patients	Falls, sprains, or strains

tions current. A phlebotomist with a contagious disease can easily transmit it to a patient, and institutions have regulations limiting patient contact in certain conditions.

Transmission Prevention Procedures

Preventing the transmission of microorganisms from infected sources to susceptible hosts is critical in controlling the spread of infection. Procedures used to prevent microorganism transmission include handwashing, the wearing of ***personal protective equipment*** (**PPE**), isolation of highly infective or highly susceptible patients, and proper disposal of contaminated materials. Strict adherence to guidelines published by the Centers for Disease Control and Prevention (**CDC**) and the Occupational Safety and Health Administration (**OSHA**) is essential. These procedures are designed to protect the phlebotomist when encountering infectious patients, prevent the phlebotomist from transferring microorganisms among patients, and protect highly susceptible patients.

Handwashing

Notice the emphasis on handwashing in Figure 3–1. Hand contact represents the number one method of infection transmission. Phlebotomists circulate from one patient to another throughout their working hours, and without the observance of proper precautions, such contact can provide an unlimited vehicle for the transmission of infection. It is essential to *change gloves and wash hands between patients*.

The importance of handwashing extends away from the patient setting to include the protection of coworkers, family and friends, and the phlebotomist. Hands should always be washed before patient contact, when gloves are removed, before leaving the work area, at any time when they have been knowingly contaminated, and before going to designated break areas, as well as before and after using bathroom facilities.

Correct routine handwashing technique (see Fig. 3–2) includes:

1 Wetting hands with warm water
2 Applying soap, preferably antimicrobial
3 Rubbing to form a lather, create friction, and loosen debris

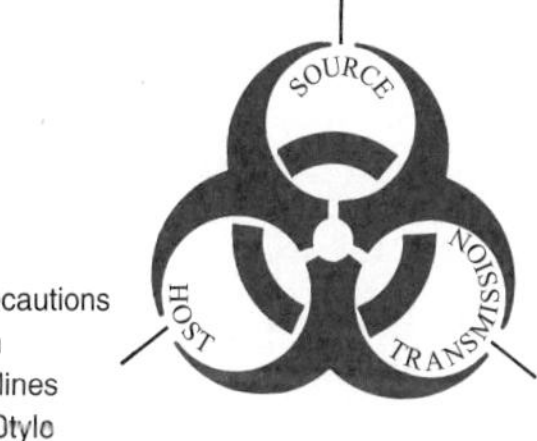

Figure 3–1 Chain of infection and safety practices related to the biohazard symbol. (From Strasinger, SK, and Di Lorenzo, MS: Urinalysis and Body Fluids, ed 4. FA Davis, Philadelphia, 2001, p. 3, with permission.)

4 Thoroughly cleaning between fingers and under fingernails and rings for at least 15 seconds and up to the wrist.
5 Rinsing hands in a downward position
6 Drying hands with a paper towel
7 Turning off faucets with the paper towel to prevent recontamination

More stringent procedures are used in surgery and in areas with highly susceptible patients, such as burn patients, immunocompromised patients, and newborns.

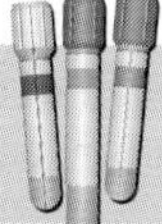

Transmission Prevention Guidelines for Phlebotomists

- Wear appropriate PPE.
- Change gloves between patients.
- Wash hands after removing gloves.
- Dispose of biohazardous material in designated containers.
- Properly dispose of sharps in puncture-resistant containers.
- Do not recap needles.
- Do not activate needle safety device using both hands.
- Follow institutional protocol governing working during personal illness.
- Maintain personal immunizations.
- Decontaminate work areas and equipment.
- Do not centrifuge uncapped tubes.
- Do not eat, drink, smoke, or apply cosmetics in the work area.

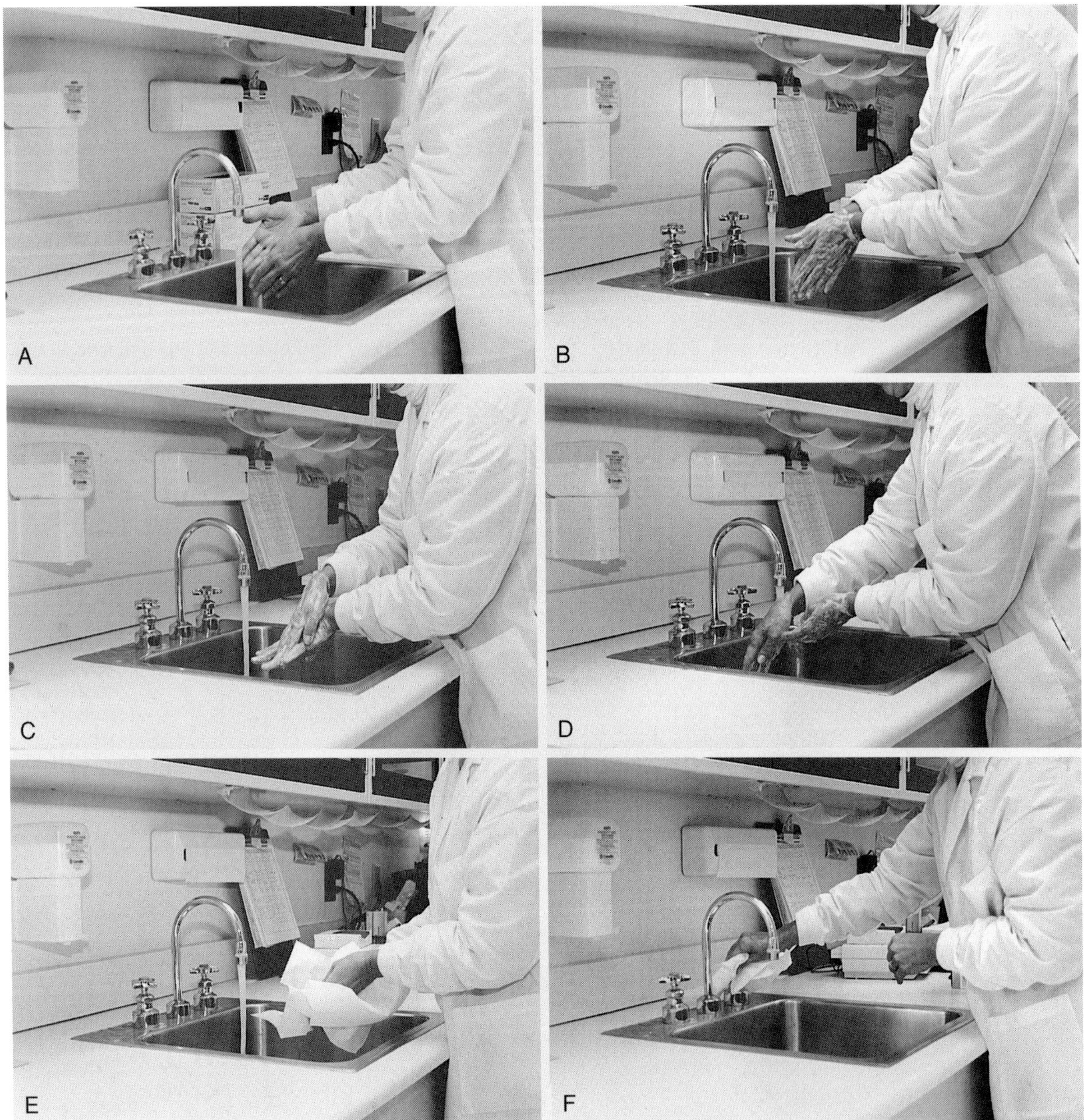

Figure 3–2 Handwashing technique. (*A*) Wetting hands. (*B*) Lathering hands and creating friction. (*C*) Cleaning between fingers. (*D*) Rinsing hands. (*E*) Drying hands. (*F*) Turning off water. (From Strasinger, SK, and Di Lorenzo, MS: Skills for the Patient Care Technician. FA Davis, Philadelphia, 1999, p. 24, with permission.)

Personal Protective Equipment

Personal protective equipment encountered by the phlebotomist includes gloves, gowns, masks, goggles, face shields, and respirators.

Gloves are worn to protect the healthcare worker's hands from contamination by patient body substances and to protect the patient from possible microorganisms on the healthcare worker's hands. Wearing gloves is not a substitute for handwashing. Hands must always be washed when gloves are removed. A variety of gloves are available including sterile and nonsterile, powdered and unpowdered, and latex and nonlatex.

Allergy to latex is increasing among healthcare workers, and phlebotomists should be alert for symptoms of reactions associated with latex contact. Reactions to latex include irritant contact dermatitis that produces patches of dry, itchy irritation on the hands, delayed hypersensitivity reactions resembling poison ivy that appear 24 to 48 hours following exposure, and true immediate hypersensitivity reactions often characterized by respiratory difficulty. Handwashing immediately after removal of gloves and avoiding powdered gloves may aid in preventing the development of latex allergy. Replacing latex gloves with nitrile or vinyl gloves provides an acceptable alternative. Phlebotomists should report any signs of a latex reaction to a supervisor because true latex allergy can be life-threatening.

technical tip Be alert for warnings of latex allergy in patients and take appropriate precautions.

Gowns are worn to protect the clothing and skin of healthcare workers from contamination by patient body substances and to prevent the transfer of microorganisms between patient rooms. Fluid-resistant gowns should be worn when the possibility of encountering splashes or large amounts of body fluids is anticipated. Gowns usually tie in the back at the neck and the waist and have tight-fitting cuffs. They should be large enough to provide full body coverage, including closing completely at the back.

technical tip Laboratory coats worn while processing specimens in the laboratory must not be worn when leaving the area.

Masks are worn to protect against inhalation of droplets containing microorganisms from infective patients. Masks and goggles are worn to protect the mucous membranes of the mouth, nose, and eyes from splashing of body substances (Fig. 3–3). Face shields also protect the mucous membranes from splashes. They are most commonly worn when processing blood and body fluids in the laboratory. Respirators may be required when collecting blood from patients who have airborne diseases, such as tuberculosis.

DONNING AND REMOVING PERSONAL PROTECTIVE EQUIPMENT

Specific procedures must be followed when putting on and removing protective apparel. To prevent contact with or the spread of infectious microorganisms, apparel is put on before entering a room and removed and disposed of before leaving the room. An exception to these procedures is observed for patients requiring sterile conditions and is discussed later in this chapter. Care must be taken to avoid touching the outside of contaminated areas of apparel when it is being removed.

Gowns are put on first and tied in the back. Masks are tied first above the ears, securely molded to the face, and then tied at the neck. To provide maximum effectiveness be sure the side labeled "outside" is facing outward. Gloves are put on last and stretched over the cuffs of the gown (Fig. 3–4).

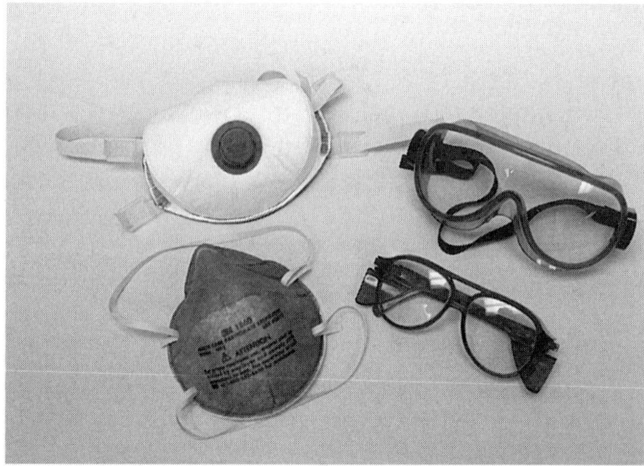

Figure 3–3 Face protective equipment. (From Strasinger, SK, and Di Lorenzo, MS: Skills for the Patient Care Technician. FA Davis, Philadelphia, 1999, p. 29, with permission.)

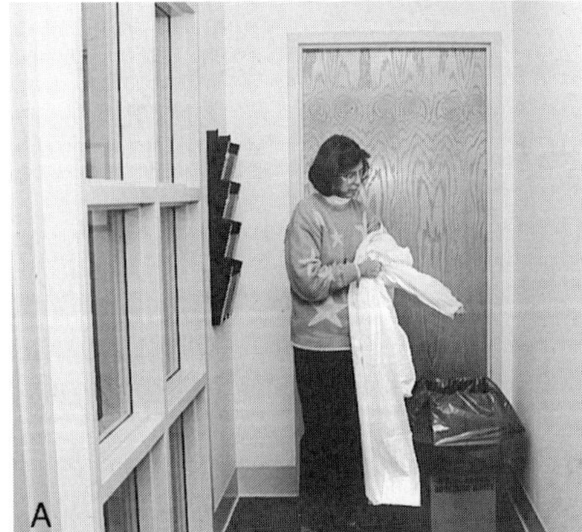

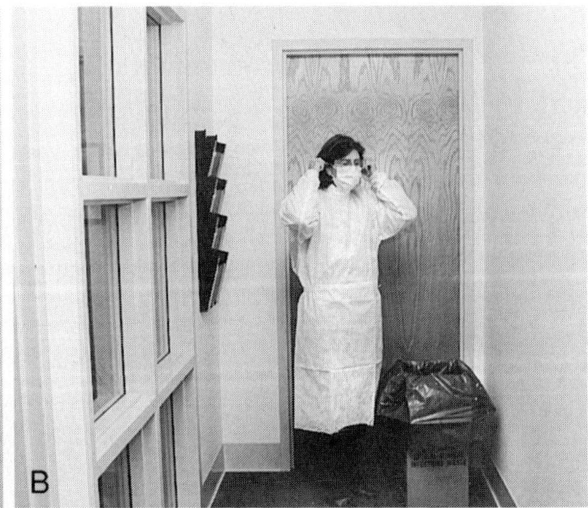

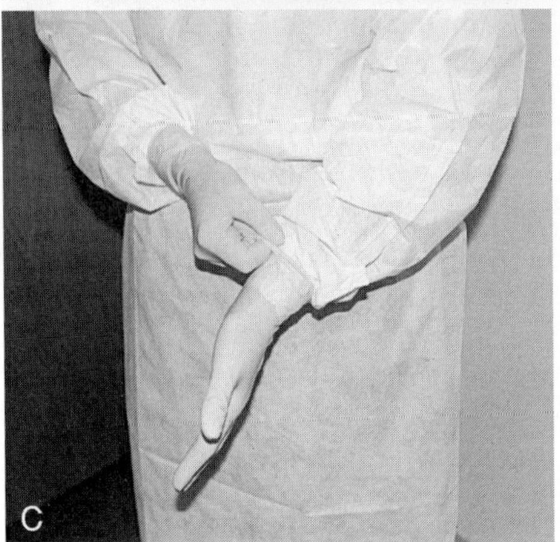

Figure 3–4 Donning PPE. (*A*) Putting on gown. (*B*) Putting on mask. (*C*) Stretching glove over cuff of gown. (From Strasinger, SK, and Di Lorenzo, MS: Skills for the Patient Care Technician. FA Davis, Philadelphia, 1999, p. 30, with permission.)

PPE is removed in reverse order: gloves, mask, and gown. To avoid touching the outside of gloves with an ungloved hand, the first glove is pulled off using the gloved hand so that it will end up inside out. While holding the removed glove in the palm of the gloved hand, one ungloved finger is slipped inside the second glove and is pulled off the hand and over the removed glove without touching the outside (Fig. 3–5). Gloves are discarded in a designated container. Masks are untied by holding only the ends of the ties and dropped into designated disposal bags. Gowns are untied at the waist before the gloves are removed. For removal, the gown is untied at the neck and removed by turning it inside out. Hands are washed immediately after removing PPE.

Patient Isolation

In addition to the protective barriers provided by PPE, the spread of infection can be controlled by placing highly infectious or highly susceptible patients in private rooms. Guidelines for isolation practices are published by the CDC and have been periodically revised to meet the ever-changing healthcare environment.

technical tip Pay strict attention to all warning signs posted outside or inside patient rooms.

Classification of isolation has evolved from category-specific isolation to disease-specific isolation to the current practice of ***transmission-based precautions*** instituted in 1995. The type of PPE worn by phlebotomists when entering an isolation room is determined by the isolation classification. Warning signs containing specific instructions for the type of PPE required are posted on the doors of isolation rooms (Fig. 3–6).

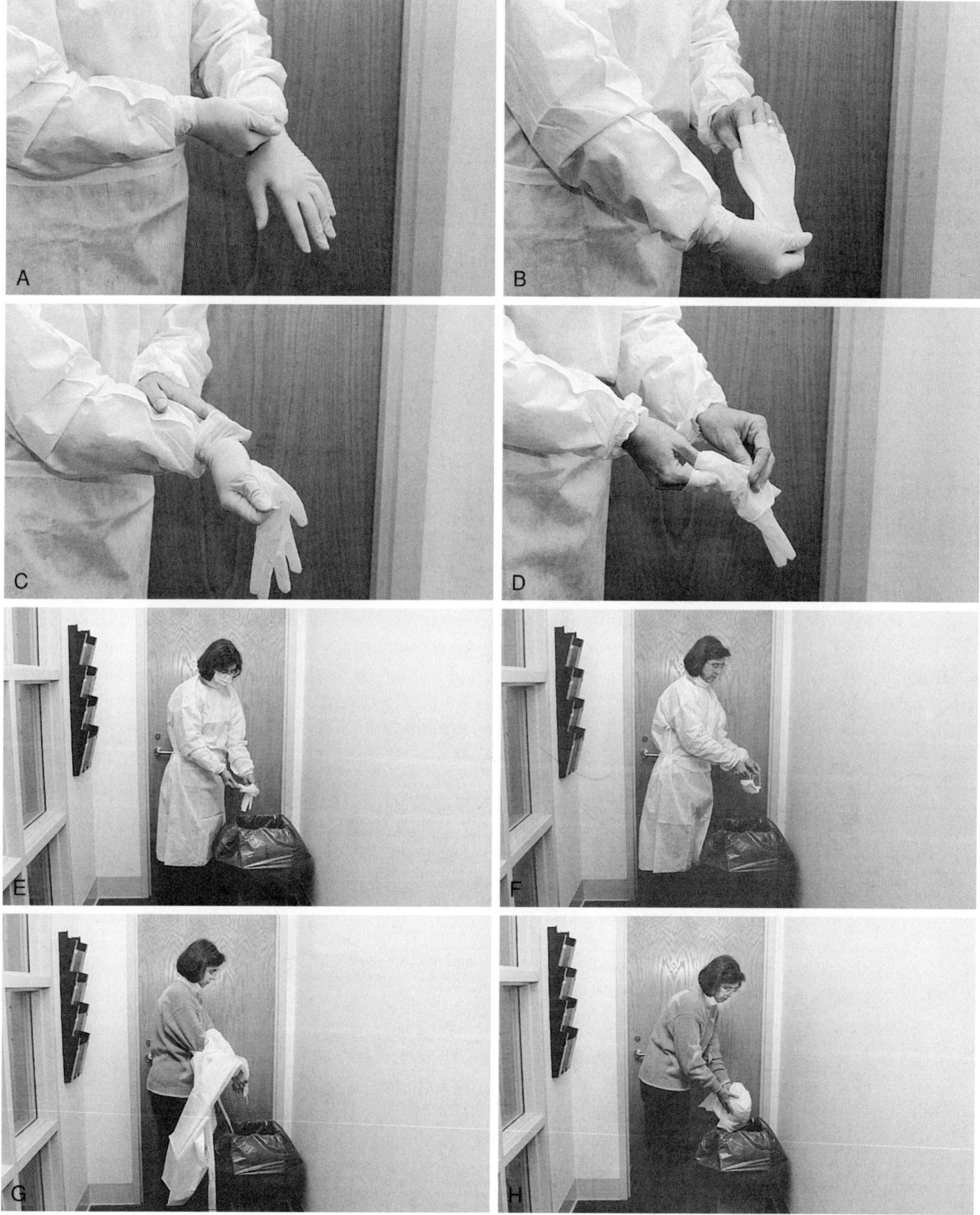

Figure 3–5 Removing PPE. (*A*) Beginning glove removal. (*B*) Removing first glove. (*C*) Beginning removal of second glove. (*D*) Removing second glove. (*E*) Disposing of gloves. (*F*) Disposing of mask. (*G*) Removing gown. (*H*) Disposing of gown. (From Strasinger, SK, and Di Lorenzo, MS: Skills for the Patient Care Technician. FA Davis, Philadelphia, 1999, p. 31, with permission.)

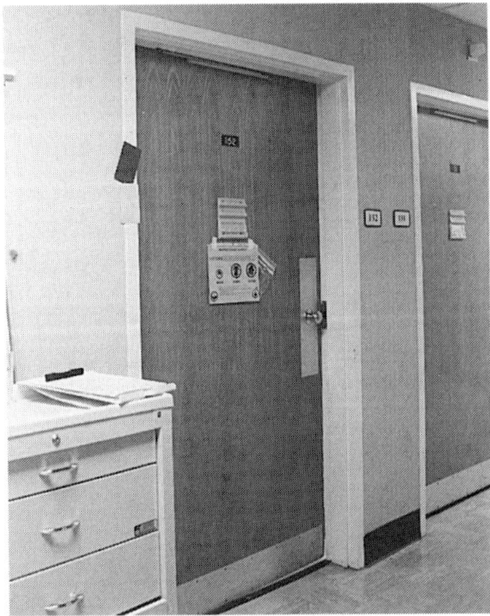

Figure 3–6 Isolation room with posted procedures and equipment stand. (From Strasinger, SK, and Di Lorenzo, MS: Skills for the Patient Care Technician. FA Davis, Philadelphia, 1999, p. 28, with permission.)

Category-specific isolation groups diseases together based on their mode of transmission. Disease-specific isolation considers the mode of transmission of individual diseases. Examples of these earlier classifications are shown in Table 3–2. Modifications were made to adapt to changing disease conditions, such as the emergence of antibiotic-resistant strains of microorganisms. These modifications, in conjunction with development of standard precautions to be used with all patients, produced the current transmission-based precautions guideline.

The three remaining isolation categories used in transmission-based precautions are airborne, droplet, and contact. They are implemented in addition to standard precautions for patients known or suspected to be infected by certain microorganisms that are transmitted by these routes (Table 3–3).

Airborne precautions are necessary when microorganisms can remain infective while being carried through the air on the dried residue of a droplet or on a dust particle. Personal protective equipment should include a mask or respirator. Filtration systems may be required in the patients' room.

Droplet precautions are required for persons infected with microorganisms transmitted on moist particles such as those produced during coughing and sneezing. Droplets are capable of traveling only short distances through the air, less than 3 feet; therefore, masks are worn when procedures requiring close patient contact are performed.

Contact precautions are used when patients have an infection that can be transmitted by direct skin-to-skin contact or by indirect contact by touching objects in the patient's room. Gloves should be worn even if no contact with moist body substances is anticipated. Gowns are worn when entering the room and removed before leaving the room. After removing the gown and washing the hands, care must be taken to avoid touching objects in the room.

TABLE 3–2
Category-Specific Isolation Classifications

Type of Isolation	Possible Conditions	PPE
Strict	Infectious diseases: chickenpox, measles, diphtheria, rabies, and staphylococcal and streptococcal pneumonia	Gown, mask, and gloves
Respiratory	Airborne infections: tuberculosis, mumps, whooping cough, diphtheria, and meningococcal meningitis	Mask and gloves for body substance contact
Enteric	Organisms that cause disease through ingestion: *Salmonella, Shigella, Yersinia,* and intestinal parasites	Gown and gloves
Drainage/secretion	Skin, wound, and surgical infections	Gown and gloves
Blood/body fluid	Bloodborne pathogens: hepatitis, AIDS, and syphilis	Gloves
Protective (reverse)	Immunocompromised patients: burns, nursery, and chemotherapy	Sterile gown, mask, gloves, and equipment

PPE = personal protective equipment.

TABLE 3-3
Transmission-Based Precautions Classifications

Type	Possible Conditions	PPE
Airborne	Tuberculosis, measles, and chickenpox	Standard precautions Mask or respirator
Droplet	Infection with *Neisseria meningitides*, pertussis, and diphtheria	Standard precautions Mask
Contact	*Clostridium difficile*, enteric pathogens, draining wounds, antibiotic-resistant infections, scabies, impetigo, herpes simplex, and herpes zoster	Standard precautions Gown and gloves

PPE = personal protective equipment.

Protective/Reverse Isolation

In addition to preventing transmission of microorganisms from infected patients to other persons, patients with compromised immunity must be protected from microorganisms routinely encountered by persons with intact immune systems. Protective isolation procedures may be required for severely burned patients, patients receiving chemotherapy, organ and bone marrow transplant patients, and in the nursery.

PPE worn by phlebotomists entering protective isolation includes gowns, gloves, and masks. All PPE must be sterile instead of the routinely used chemically clean PPE that is acceptable in other situations.

Procedure Precautions

Universal precautions were instituted by CDC in 1985 to protect healthcare workers from exposure to bloodborne **pathogens**, primarily hepatitis B virus (**HBV**) and human immunodeficiency virus (HIV). Under universal precautions, all patients are assumed to be possible carriers of bloodborne pathogens. Transmission may occur by skin puncture from a contaminated sharp object or by passive contact through open skin lesions or mucous membranes. The guideline recommends wearing gloves when collecting or handling blood and body fluids contaminated with blood, wearing face shields when there is danger of blood splashing on mucous membranes, and disposing of all needles and sharp objects in puncture-resistant containers without recapping.

A modification of universal precautions, **body substance isolation (BSI)** is not limited to bloodborne pathogens, and considers all body fluids and moist body substances to be potentially infectious. Personnel should wear gloves at all times when encountering moist body substances. A disadvantage of the BSI guideline is that it does not recommend handwashing following removal of gloves unless visual contamination is present.

The major features of universal precautions and BSI have now been combined and are called ***standard precautions***. Standard precautions should be used for the care of all patients and include the following:

1 Handwashing
Wash hands after touching blood, body fluids, secretions, excretions, and contaminated items, whether or not gloves are worn. Wash hands immediately after gloves are removed, between patient contacts, and when otherwise indicated to avoid transfer of microorganisms to other patients or environments. It may be necessary to wash hands between tasks and procedures on the same patient to prevent cross-contamination of different body sites.

2 Gloves
Wear gloves (clean, nonsterile gloves are adequate) when touching blood, body fluids, secretions, excretions, and contaminated items. Put on gloves just before touching mucous membranes and open wounds. Change gloves between tasks and procedures on the same patient after contact with material that may contain a high concentration of microorganisms. Remove gloves promptly after use, before touching noncontaminated items and environmental surfaces, and before going to another patient, and wash hands immediately to avoid transfer of microorganisms to other patients or environments.

3 Mask, Eye Protection, and Face Shield
Wear a mask and eye protection or a face shield to protect mucous membranes of the eyes, nose, and mouth during procedures and patient-care activities that are likely to generate splashes or sprays of blood, body fluids, secretions, and excretions.

4 Gown
Wear a gown (a clean, nonsterile gown is adequate) to protect skin and to prevent soiling of clothing during procedures and patient-care activities that are likely to generate splashes of blood, body fluids, secretions, or excretions. Select a gown that is appropriate for the activity and amount of fluid likely to be encountered. Remove a soiled gown as promptly as possible, and wash hands to avoid transfer of microorganisms to other patients or environments.

5 Patient-Care Equipment
Handle used patient-care equipment soiled with blood, body fluids, secretions, and excretions in a manner that prevents skin and mucous membrane exposures, contamination of clothing, and transfer of microorganisms to other patients and environments. Ensure that reusable equipment is not used for the care of another patient until it has been cleaned and reprocessed appropriately. Ensure that single-use items are discarded properly.

6 Environmental Control
Ensure that the hospital has adequate procedures for the routine care, cleaning, and disinfection of environmental surfaces, beds, bed rails, bedside equipment, and other frequently touched surfaces and ensure that these procedures are being followed.

7 Linen
Handle, transport, and process used linen soiled with blood, body fluids, secretions, and excretions in a manner that prevents skin and mucous membrane exposures and contamination of clothing, and that avoids transfer of microorganisms to other patients and environments.

8 Occupational Health and Bloodborne Pathogens
Take care to prevent injuries when using needles, scalpels, and other sharp instruments; when handling sharp instruments after procedures; when cleaning used instruments; and when disposing of used needles. Never recap used needles, or otherwise manipulate them using both hands, or use any other technique that involves directing the point of a needle toward any part of the body. Do not remove used needles from disposable syringes by hand, and do not bend, break, or otherwise manipulate used needles by hand. Place used disposable syringes and needles, scalpel blades, and other sharp items in appropriate puncture-resistant containers, which are located as close as practical to the area in which the items were used, and place reusable syringes and needles in a puncture-resistant container for transport to the reprocessing area.
Use mouthpieces, resuscitation bags, or other ventilation devices as an alternate to mouth-to-mouth resuscitation methods in areas where the need for resuscitation is predictable.

9 Patient Placement
Place a patient who contaminates the environment or who does not (or cannot be expected to) assist in maintaining appropriate hygiene or environmental control in a private room. If a private room is not available, consult with infection control professionals regarding patient placement or other alternatives.

Phlebotomy Procedures in Isolation

Special precautions must be taken with phlebotomy equipment and specimens collected in isolation areas. Bring only necessary equipment (not the phlebotomy tray) into isolation rooms. Be sure, however, to include duplicate collection tubes and enough supplies to perform a second venipuncture if necessary. All equipment, including PPE, taken into the room must be left in the room and, when appropriate, deposited in labeled waste containers. Tourniquets, gauze, alcohol pads, and pens may already be present in the room.

Specimens taken from the room should be cleaned of any blood contamination and placed in plastic bags located near or just outside the door (Fig. 3–7). Bags should be folded open to allow tubes to be added to the bag without touching the outside of the bag with contaminated gloves or tubes. If double bagging is required, a clean open bag must be available immediately outside the room.

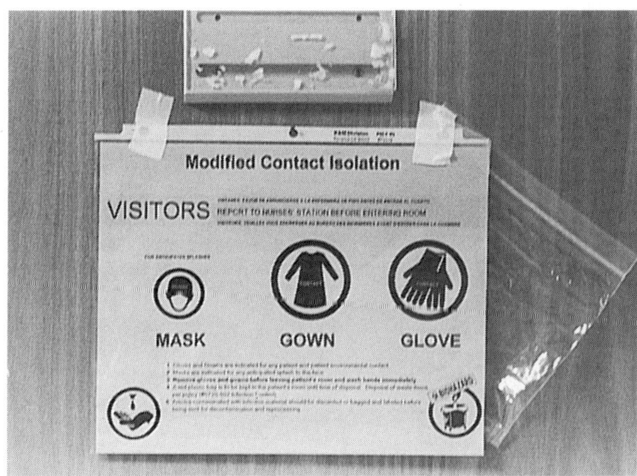

Figure 3–7 Contact isolation sign with specimen bags. (From Strasinger, SK, and Di Lorenzo, MS: Skills for the Patient Care Technician. FA Davis, Philadelphia, 1999, p. 28, with permission.)

technical tip Double-bagging may require a second person to stand outside the room to hold the second bag open.

When performing phlebotomy under conditions of protective isolation, necessary equipment brought in the room is taken out of the room and PPE is removed after leaving the room.

Biologic Waste Disposal

Phlebotomy equipment and supplies contaminated with blood and body fluids must be disposed of in containers clearly marked with the biohazard symbol or red or yellow color coding. These items include alcohol pads, gauze, bandages, disposable tourniquets, gloves, masks, and gowns. Disposal of needles and other sharp objects is discussed in the next section.

Contaminated nondisposable equipment, blood spills, and blood and body fluid processing areas must be disinfected. The most commonly used **disinfectant** is a 1:10 dilution of sodium hypochlorite (household bleach) prepared weekly and stored in a plastic, not a glass, bottle. The bleach should be allowed to air dry on the contaminated area before removal.

Sharp Hazards

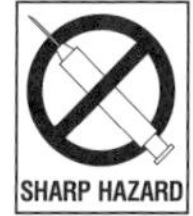

A primary concern for phlebotomists is possible exposure to bloodborne pathogens caused by accidental puncture with a contaminated needle or lancet. Although bloodborne pathogens also are transmitted through contact with mucous membranes and nonintact skin, a needle or lancet used to collect blood has the capability to produce a very significant exposure to bloodborne pathogens. It is essential that safety precautions be followed at all times when sharp hazards are present.

The number one personal safety rule when using needles is to *never* recap a needle manually. Many safety devices are available for needle disposal, and they provide a variety of safeguards, including needle holders that become a sheath, needles that automatically resheath or become blunt, and needles with attached sheaths (see Chapter 5). Needle safety devices must be activated before disposing of the entire blood collection assembly. All sharps must be disposed of in puncture-resistant, leak-proof containers labeled with the biohazard symbol. Containers should be located in close proximity to the phlebotomist's work area. Portable containers can be carried on phlebotomy trays or placed at specified blood collection areas. Containers may be attached to the walls in patient rooms. Do not reach into these containers when discarding material, because accidental puncture may occur from a previously discarded sharp device. Containers must always be replaced when the safe capacity mark is reached.

technical tip The availability of safety needles and devices should make the one-handed "scoop" technique past history.

Government Regulations

The federal government has enacted regulations to protect healthcare workers from exposure to bloodborne pathogens. These regulations are monitored and enforced by the OSHA. The Occupational Exposure to Bloodborne Pathogens Standard became law in 1991. It requires all employers to have a written Bloodborne Pathogen Exposure Control Plan and to provide necessary protection, free of charge for employees. Specifics of the OSHA standard include the following:

1 Requiring all employees to practice universal (standard) precautions.
2 Providing laboratory coats, gowns, face shields, and gloves to employees and laundry facilities for nondisposable protective clothing.
3 Providing sharps disposal containers and prohibiting recapping of needles.
4 Prohibiting eating, drinking, smoking, and applying cosmetics in the work area.
5 Labeling all biohazardous materials and containers.
6 Providing immunization for the hepatitis B virus free of charge.
7 Establishing a daily work surface disinfection protocol. The disinfectant of choice for bloodborne pathogens is sodium hypochlorite (household bleach diluted 1:10).
8 Providing medical follow-up to employees who have been accidentally exposed to bloodborne pathogens.
9 Documenting regular training of employees in safety standards. The exposure control plan must be available to employees. It must be updated annually and identify procedures and individuals at risk of exposure to bloodborne pathogens. The plan must identify the engineering controls, that is, sharps containers, and the procedures in place to prevent exposure incidents.

In 1999, OSHA issued a new compliance directive, called the Enforcement Procedures for the Occupational Exposure to Bloodborne Pathogens Standard. The new directive placed more emphasis on the use of engineering controls to prevent accidental exposure to bloodborne pathogens. Additional changes to the directive were mandated by passage of the Needlestick Safety and Prevention Act, signed into law in 2001. Under the new law employers must do the following:

1 Document their evaluations and implementation of safer needle devices.
2 Involve employees in the selection and evaluation of new devices.
3 Maintain a log of all injuries from contaminated sharps.

Phlebotomists should be prepared to assist in the evaluation of new needlestick prevention devices.

In June 2002, OSHA issued a revision to the Bloodborne Pathogens Standard compliance directive. In the revised directive, the agency requires that all blood holders (adapters) with needles attached be immediately discarded into a sharps container after the device's safety feature is activated. The rationale for the new directive is based on the exposure of workers to the unprotected stopper-puncturing end of evacuated tube needles, the increased needle manipulation required to remove it from the holder, and the possible worker or patient exposure from the use of contaminated holders.

technical tip Always become thoroughly proficient with the operation of new devices before using them when drawing blood from patients.

Accidental breakage of glass capillary tubes used by phlebotomists when collecting samples from a dermal puncture can present a major risk of bloodborne pathogens exposure. A 1999 government safety advisory recommends using the following items:

1 Capillary tubes wrapped in puncture-resistant film (Mylar)
2 Plastic capillary tubes
3 Sealing methods that do not require pushing the tubes into a sealant to form a plug

Occupational Exposure to Bloodborne Pathogens

Any accidental exposure to blood through needlestick, mucous membranes, or nonintact skin must be reported to a supervisor and a confidential medical examination immediately be started. Evaluation of the incident must begin right away to ensure appropriate ***postexposure prophylaxis*** **(PEP)**. Needlesticks are the most frequently encountered exposure in phlebotomy and place the phlebotomist in danger of contracting HIV, hepatitis B virus (HBV), and hepatitis C virus (**HCV**).

technical tip Never, never hesitate to report a possible bloodborne pathogen exposure.

The CDC has recommended procedures to follow for the initial examination and for any necessary PEP.

Initial procedures include the following:

1 Draw a baseline blood sample from the employee and test it for HBV, HCV, and HIV.
2 If possible, identify the source patient, collect a blood sample, and test it for HBV, HCV, and HIV. Patients must usually give informed consent for these tests, and they do not become part of the patient's record. In some states a physician's order can replace patient consent.
3 Testing must be completed within 24 hours for maximum benefit from PEP.

Source patient tests positive for HIV:

1 Employee is counseled about receiving PEP using zidovudine (**ZDV**) and one or two additional anti-HIV medications.
2 Medications are started within 24 hours.
3 Employee is retested at intervals of 6 weeks, 12 weeks, 3 months, and 6 months.
4 Additional evaluation and counseling is needed if the source patient is unidentified or untested.

Source patient tests positive for HBV:

1 Unvaccinated employees can be given hepatitis B immune globulin (**HBIG**) and HBV vaccine.
2 Vaccinated employees are tested for immunity and receive PEP, if necessary.

Source patient tests positive for HCV:

1 No PEP is available.
2 Employee is monitored for early detection of HCV infection and treated appropriately.

Any exposed employee should be counseled to report any symptoms related to viral infection that occur within 12 weeks of the exposure.

Chemical Hazards

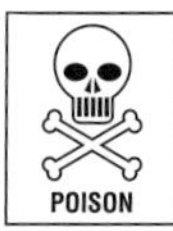

Phlebotomists may come in contact with chemicals while accessioning or processing specimens in the laboratory and preparing containers for urine specimens that require preservatives. Many of these preservatives can be hazardous when they are not properly handled. General rules for safe handling of chemicals include taking precautions to avoid getting chemicals on your body, clothes, and work area; wearing PPE, such as safety goggles when pouring chemicals, observing strict labeling practices, and carefully following instructions.

Chemicals should never be mixed together unless specific instructions are followed, and they must be added in the order specified. This is particularly important when combining acid and water, because acid should always be added to water to avoid the possibility of sudden splashing.

When skin or eye contact occurs, the best first aid is to flush the area immediately with water for at least 15 minutes and then seek medical attention. Phlebotomists must know the location of the emergency shower and eyewash station in the laboratory. Do not try to neutralize chemicals spilled on the skin.

technical tip Learn how to use the emergency shower and eyewash station.

All chemicals and reagents containing hazardous ingredients in a concentration greater than 1% are required to have a Material Safety Data Sheet (**MSDS**) on file in the work area. By law, vendors must provide these sheets to purchasers; however, it is the responsibility of the facility to obtain and

Healthcare Worker Immunizations/Tests

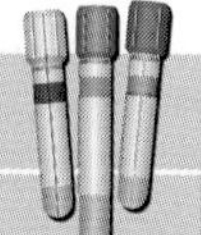

- Hepatitis B Vaccination
  Completion of three-shot immunization protocol
  Positive antibody titer
- Measles, Mumps, and Rubella (MMR)
  Immunization
  Current positive antibody titer
- Varicella (Chickenpox)
  Immunization
  Current positive antibody titer
- Tetanus
  Immunization within the past 10 years
- Annual Tuberculosis Skin Test (PPD)
  Positive tests followed by chest radiograph

keep them available to employees. An MSDS contains information on physical and chemical characteristics, fire, explosion reactivity, health hazards, primary routes of entry, exposure limits and **carcinogenic** potential, precautions for safe handling, spill clean-up, and emergency first-aid information. Containers of chemicals that pose a high risk must be labeled with a chemical hazard symbol representing the possible hazard, such as flammable, poison, or corrosive. Examples of chemical safety equipment and information are shown in Figure 3–8.

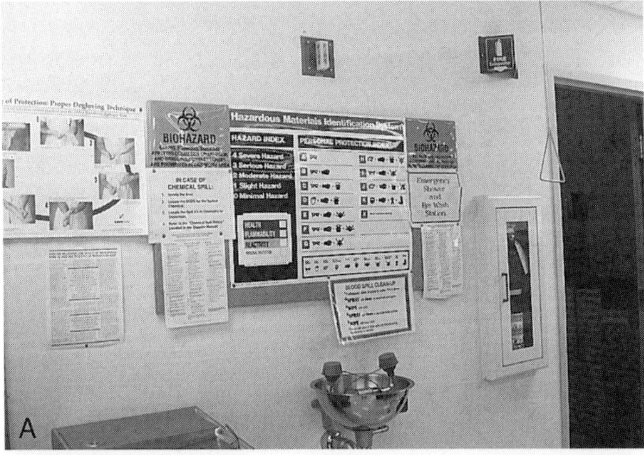

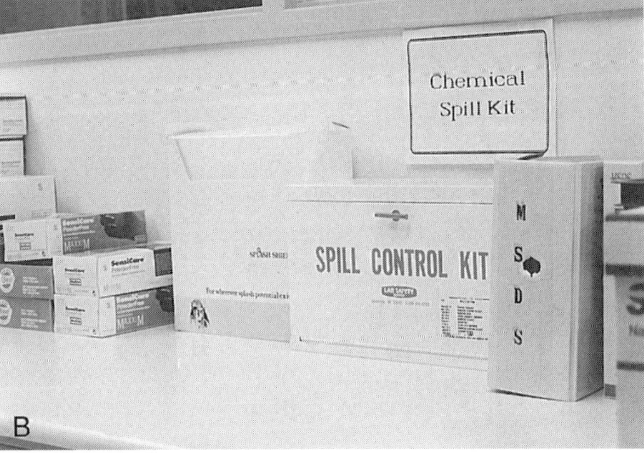

Figure 3–8 Chemical safety aids. (*A*) Equipment. (*B*) Information and supplies. (From Strasinger, SK, and Di Lorenzo, MS: Skills for the Patient Care Technician. FA Davis, Philadelphia, 1999, p. 34, with permission.)

Radioactive Hazards

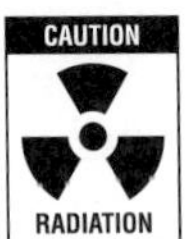

Phlebotomists may come in contact with ***radioactivity*** while drawing blood from patients in the radiology department or from patients receiving radioactive treatments, and in the laboratory when procedures using radioisotopes are performed.

The amount of radioactivity present in most medical situations is very small and represents little danger; however, the effects of radiation are related to the length of exposure and are cumulative. Exposure to radiation is dependent on the combination of time, distance, and shielding. Persons working in a radioactive environment are required to wear measuring devices to determine the amount of radiation they are accumulating.

Phlebotomists should be familiar with the radioactive symbol shown in the margin. This symbol must be displayed on the doors of all areas where radioactive material is present. Exposure to radiation during pregnancy presents a danger to the fetus, and phlebotomists who are pregnant or think they may be should avoid areas with this symbol.

Electrical Hazards

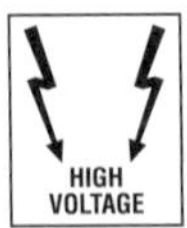

The healthcare setting contains a large amount of electrical equipment with which phlebotomists are in contact, both in patients' rooms and in the laboratory. The same general rules of electrical safety observed outside the work place apply. Keep in mind that the danger of water or fluid coming in contact with equipment is greater in the hospital setting.

technical tip Do not operate electrical equipment with wet hands or while in contact with water.

Electrical equipment is closely monitored by designated hospital personnel. However, phlebotomists should be observant for any dangerous conditions such as frayed cords and overloaded circuits, and they should report these items to the appropriate persons. Equipment that has become wet should be unplugged and allowed to dry completely before reusing. Equipment should also be unplugged before cleaning. It is required that all electrical equipment be grounded with a three-pronged plug.

As an additional precaution when drawing blood or performing other procedures, phlebotomists should avoid contact with electrical equipment in the patient's room because current from improperly grounded equipment can pass through the phlebotomist and metal needle to the patient.

When a situation involving electrical **shock** occurs, it is important to remove the electrical source immediately. This must be done without touching the person or the equipment because the current will pass on to you. Turning off the circuit breaker and moving the equipment using a nonconductive glass or wood object are safe procedures to follow. The victim should receive immediate medical assistance following discontinuation of the electricity. Cardiopulmonary resuscitation (**CPR**) may be necessary.

technical tip Phlebotomists should maintain current CPR certification.

Fire/Explosive Hazards

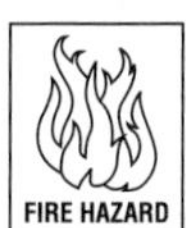

The Joint Commission on Accreditation of Healthcare Organizations (JCAHO) requires that all healthcare institutions have posted evacuation routes and detailed plans to follow when a fire occurs. Phlebotomists should be familiar with these procedures and with the basic steps to follow when a fire is discovered. Initial steps to follow when a fire is discovered are identified by the code word RACE.

1 *R*escue—anyone in immediate danger
2 *A*larm—activate the institutional fire alarm system
3 *C*ontain—close all doors to potentially affected areas
4 *E*xtinguish/*E*vacuate—extinguish the fire, if possible, or evacuate, closing the door

The laboratory uses many chemicals that may be volatile or explosive, and special procedures for handling and storage are required. Designated chemicals are stored in safety cabinets or explosion-proof refrigerators and are used under vented hoods. Fire blankets should be present in the laboratory. Persons with burning clothes should be wrapped in the blanket to smother the flames.

technical tip Always return chemicals to their designated storage area.

The National Fire Protection Association (**NFPA**) classifies fires with regard to the type of burning material and also classifies the type of fire extinguisher that is used to control them. This information is summarized in Table 3–4. The multipurpose ABC fire extinguishers are the most common, but the label should always be checked before using. Phlebotomists should be thoroughly familiar with the operation of the fire extinguishers. The code word PASS can be used to remember the steps in the operation.

1 *P*ull pin
2 *A*im at base of fire
3 *S*queeze handles
4 *S*weep nozzle, side to side

Standard System for the Identification of the Fire Hazards of Materials, NFPA 704, is a symbol system used to inform firefighters of the hazard they may encounter when fighting a fire in a particular area. The color-coded areas contain information relating to health, flammability, reactivity, use of water, and personal protection. These symbols are placed on doors, cabinets, and reagent bottles. An example of hazardous material symbols is shown in Figure 3–9.

TABLE 3–4
Types of Fires and Fire Extinguishers

Fire Type	Composition of Fire	Type of Fire Extinguisher	Extinguishing Material
Class A	Wood, paper, or clothing	Class A	Water
Class B	Flammable organic chemicals	Class B	Dry chemicals, carbon dioxide, foam, or halon
Class C	Electrical	Class C	Dry chemicals, carbon dioxide, or halon
Class D	Combustible metals	None	Sand or dry powder
		Class ABC	Dry chemicals

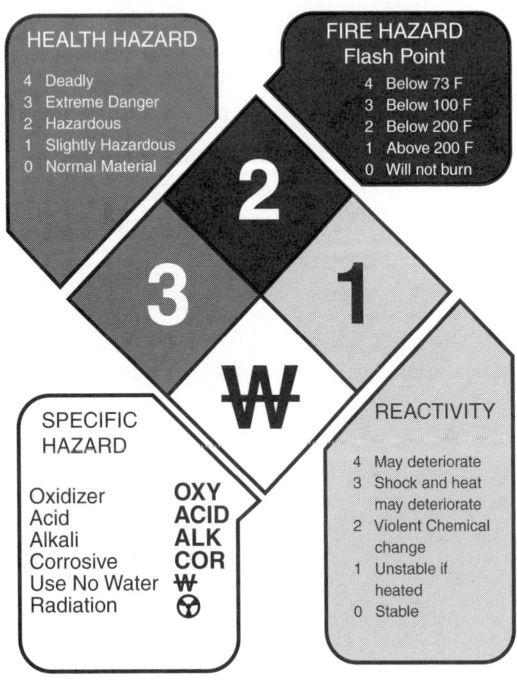

Figure 3–9 NFPA hazardous material symbols. (Adapted from Strasinger, SK, and Di Lorenzo, MS: Urinalysis and Body Fluids, ed. 4. FA Davis, Philadelphia, 2001, p. 6.)

Physical Hazards

Physical hazards are not unique to the healthcare setting, and routine safety precautions observed outside the workplace can usually be applied. General precautions that phlebotomists should observe include:

1 Avoid running in rooms and hallways.
2 Be alert for wet floors.
3 Bend the knees when lifting heavy objects or patients.
4 Keep long hair tied back and remove dangling jewelry to avoid contact with equipment and patients.
5 Wear comfortable, closed-toe shoes with nonskid soles that provide maximum support.
6 Maintain a clean, organized work area.

Bibliography

CDC, Updated U.S. Public Health Service Guidelines for the Management of Occupational Exposures to HBV, HCV, and HIV and Recommendations for Post-exposure Prophylaxis. MMWR 2001:50(RR11); 1-42. Website: *http:// www.cdc.gov*

FDA, NIOSH, OSHA. Glass Capillary Tubes: Joint Safety Advisory About Potential Risks. FDA, Rockville, MD, 1999. Website: *http://www.fda.gov/cdrh/safety/capssa9.html*

Guidelines for Isolation Precautions in Hospitals. Parts I and II. Atlanta, 1996. Website: *http://www.cdc.gov*

National Committee for Clinical Laboratory Standards. Protection of Laboratory Workers from Instrument Biohazards and Infectious Disease Transmitted by Blood, Body Fluids, and Tissue: Approved Guideline M29-A, NCCLS, Wayne, PA, 1997.

National Fire Protection Association. Hazardous Chemical Data, No. 49. NFPA, Boston, 1991.

NIOSH Alert. Preventing Allergic Reactions to Natural Rubber Latex in the Workplace. DHHS (NIOSH) Publication 97-135. National Institute for Occupational Safety and Health, Cincinnati, OH, 1997.

Occupational Exposure to Bloodborne Pathogens, Final Rule. Federal Register, 29 (Dec 6), 1991.

OSHA: Enforcement Procedures for the Occupational Exposure to Bloodborne Pathogens Standard. Directive 2-2.44D. Washington, DC, 1999. Website: *http://www.asha.slc.gov/oshdoc/Directive data/cpl_2-2_69.html*

OSHA: Needlestick Requirements Take Effect April 18. OSHA, Washington, DC, 2001. Website: *http://www.oshasle.gov/medic/oshnews/apr01/national-20010412.html*

OSHA. OSHA Clarifies Position on the Removal of Contaminated Needles. OSHA, Washington, DC, 2002. Website: *http://www.osha.gov/media/oshnews/june02/trade-20020612A.html*

Study Questions

1. List the three components of the chain of infection.
   a. ______________________________
   b. ______________________________
   c. ______________________________

2. List four methods by which infection can be transferred from the source to the host.
   a. ______________________________
   b. ______________________________
   c. ______________________________
   d. ______________________________

3. What is the significance of a rash appearing on the hands after wearing gloves?
   ____

4. Indicate the correct order for putting on and removing protective apparel by placing a 1, 2, or 3 opposite the listed apparel.

Putting On	Removing
a. Gown ____________	____________
b. Gloves ____________	____________
c. Mask ____________	____________

5. List the three categories of transmission-based isolation requirements.
   a. ______________________________
   b. ______________________________
   c. ______________________________

6. State the isolation category associated with each of the following:
   a. ____________ phlebotomists may need a respirator
   b. ____________ gowns and gloves are always worn
   c. ____________ close contact requires a mask

7. Define the following:
   a. Body substance isolation ______________________________
   b. Universal precautions ______________________________
   c. Standard precautions ______________________________

8. The recommended disinfectant for blood and body fluid spills is

____.

9. To avoid an accidental needlestick, a phlebotomist should never _______________.

10. True or False. Employers are required to provide hepatitis B vaccine to phlebotomists free of charge.

11. List three viruses transmitted by needlestick.

a. ____

b. ____

c. ____

12. When a caustic solution such as hydrochloric acid is spilled on the skin, what is the recommended first aid treatment? ____

13. True or False. Water should always be added to acid.

14. Give an example of when a phlebotomist should avoid areas with a radiation symbol.

____

15. State two ways to remove the source of an electrical shock.

a. ____

b. ____

16. Define the code words RACE and PASS.

a. R _______________ e. P _______________

b. A _______________ f. A _______________

c. C _______________ g. S _______________

d. E _______________ h. S _______________

17. What is the most common type of fire extinguisher used in the laboratory? What does it contain?

____

18. What NFPA type of fire can be prevented by using an explosion-proof refrigerator?

____

19. When a fire occurs in the laboratory, does the MSDS or the NFPA symbol provide the most important information? ____

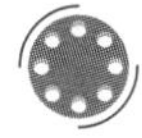

Clinical Situations

1. A phlebotomist with an exceptionally heavy workload decides to save time by not changing gloves and washing his/her hands between patients.
   a. What type of infection could be spread to previously uninfected patients?
   ____
   b. Who would be considered the source of these infections? ______________
   c. Who would be considered the host of these infections? ______________
   d. How were these infections transmitted? ______________

2. For each of the following actions taken by a phlebotomist, place a "T" for transmission-based precautions, a "P" for protective isolation, or a "PT" for both situations in the blank.
   a. ______________ Only necessary equipment is brought into the room
   b. ______________ Sterile gloves are worn
   c. ______________ PPE is removed and disposed of inside the room
   d. ______________ Duplicate tubes are taken into the room
   e. ______________ Specimens may require double bagging
   f. ______________ Equipment taken into the room is taken out of the room

3. A phlebotomist using a new safety device for the first time receives an accidental needlestick while activating the safety feature on the used needle.
   a. How could this accident possibly have been avoided?
   ____
   b. What should the phlebotomist do first? ______________
   c. What tests are performed on the phlebotomist?
   ____
   d. If necessary, when should the phlebotomist receive PEP?
   ____

4. As a phlebotomy supervisor you are evaluating a new needlestick prevention device. State three requirements of the Needlestick Safety and Prevention Act with which you must comply:
   a. ______________________________
   b. ______________________________
   c. ______________________________

Laboratory Safety Exercise

Instructions

Explore the student laboratory or the area designated by the instructor, and provide the following information.

1. Location of the fire extinguishers

   ____

2. State the instructions for operation of the fire extinguisher.

   ____

   ____

   ____

3. Location of the fire blanket

   ____

4. Location of the eyewash station

   ____

5. Location of the emergency shower

   ____

6. Location of the first aid kit

   ____

7. Location of the master electrical panel

   ____

8. Location of the fire alarm

   ____

9. The emergency exit route

   ____

10. Location of the MSDS pertaining to phlebotomy

    ____

11. Location of the emergency spill kit

    ____

12. Location of the Bloodborne Pathogen Exposure Control Plan

___

13. Locate an NFPA sign and list the following:

Location ___

Health Rating ___

Fire Rating ___

Reactivity Rating

___

14. What disinfectants are available for cleaning work areas?

___

___

NAME ____________________

Evaluation of Handwashing Technique

RATING SYSTEM 2 = SATISFACTORILY PERFORMED 1 = NEEDS IMPROVEMENT 0 = INCORRECT/DID NOT PERFORM

__________ 1. Turns on warm water

__________ 2. Dispenses an adequate amount of soap on to palm

__________ 3. Creates a lather

__________ 4. Creates friction, rubbing both sides of hands

__________ 5. Rubs between fingers and under nails

__________ 6. Rinses hands in a downward position

__________ 7. Obtains paper towel, touching only the towel

__________ 8. Dries hands with paper towel

__________ 9. Turns off water using paper towel

__________ 10. Does not recontaminate hands

TOTAL POINTS __________

MAXIMUM POINTS = 20

Comments:

NAME ______________________

Evaluation of Personal Protective Equipment (Gowning, Masking, and Gloving)

RATING SYSTEM 2 = SATISFACTORILY PERFORMED 1 = NEEDS IMPROVEMENT
0 = INCORRECT/DID NOT PERFORM

________ 1. Correctly washes hands

________ 2. Puts on gown with opening at the back

________ 3. Assures that gown is large enough to close in the back

________ 4. Ties neck strings

________ 5. Ties waistband

________ 6. Positions mask with proper side facing outward and ties top string above the ears

________ 7. Securely positions mask over nose

________ 8. Ties bottom string at back of neck

________ 9. Puts on gloves

________ 10. Pulls gloves over cuffs of gown

________ 11. Unties gown at the waist

________ 12. Removes gloves touching only the inside

________ 13. Deposits gloves in biohazard container

________ 14. Unties mask at neck and then head

________ 15. Touches only strings of mask

________ 16. Deposits mask in biohazard container

________ 17. Unties gown at neck

________ 18. Removes gown touching only the inside

________ 19. Deposits gown in biohazard container

________ 20. Correctly washes hands

TOTAL POINTS ________

MAXIMUM POINTS = 40

Comments:

Chapter 4

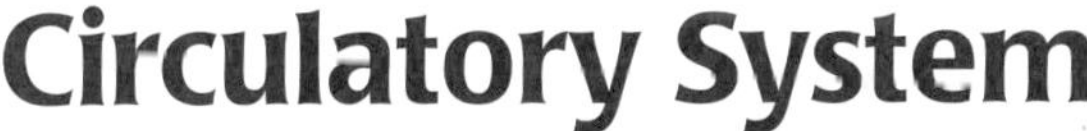

Circulatory System

Chapter Outline

Blood Vessels

Heart
- Pathway of Blood Through the Heart

Blood
- Erythrocytes
- Leukocytes
- Thrombocytes

Coagulation

Disorders
- Blood Vessels
- Heart
- Blood
- Coagulation

Diagnostic Tests

Medications

Learning Objectives

Upon completion of this chapter, the reader will be able to:

1. Briefly describe the functions of the blood vessels, heart, and blood.
2. Differentiate between arteries, veins, and capillaries by structure and function.
3. Locate the femoral, radial, brachial, and ulnar arteries.
4. Locate the basilic, cephalic, median cubital, radial, and saphenous veins.
5. Trace the pathway of blood through the heart and define the function of each chamber.
6. Identify the components of blood.
7. State the major function of red blood cells, white blood cells, and platelets.
8. Briefly explain the coagulation process.
9. Describe the major disorders associated with the circulatory system.
10. State the clinical correlations of laboratory tests associated with the circulatory system.
11. Recognize the primary medications associated with the circulatory system.

Key Terms

Arteriole	*Capillary*	*Leukocyte*	*Vein*
Artery	*Cardiovascular*	*Thrombocyte*	*Ventricle*
Atrium	*Erythrocyte*	*Vascular*	*Venule*

The circulatory (*cardiovascular*) system consists of the heart, blood vessels, and the blood. Blood is circulated through the blood vessels by the heart to deliver oxygen and nutrients to the cells and transport waste products to the organs that remove them from the body.

Blood Vessels

The three types of blood vessels that transport blood throughout the body are ***arteries, veins***, and ***capillaries***. Arteries and veins are composed of three layers. The outer layer is a connective tissue called **tunica adventitia**. The middle layer is a smooth muscle tissue called **tunica media**. The inner layer is called the **tunica intima** and is composed of endothelial cells. The space within a blood vessel through which the blood flows is called a **lumen**. Figure 4–1 shows the differences between arteries, veins, and capillaries.

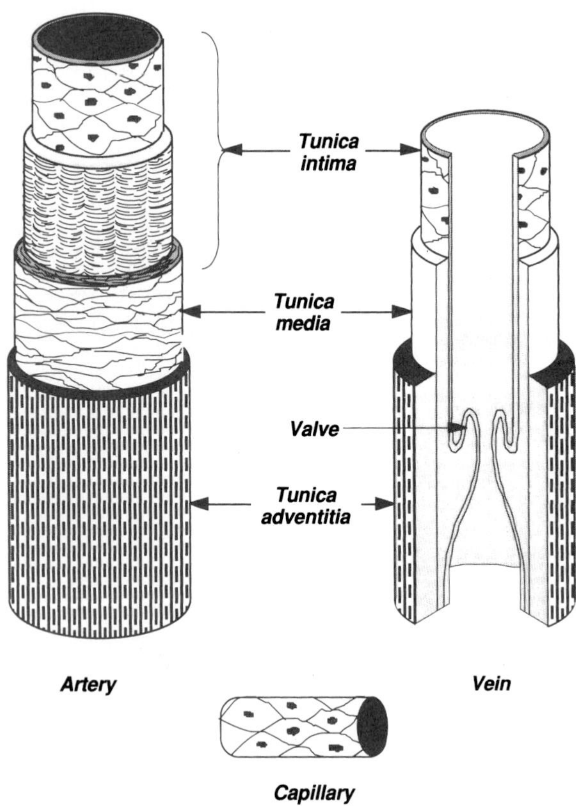

Figure 4–1 Comparison of arteries, veins, and capillaries.

Arteries are large thick-walled blood vessels that propel oxygen-rich blood away from the heart to the capillaries. Arteries branch into smaller thinner vessels called ***arterioles*** that connect to capillaries. The walls of arteries consist of tough connective tissue, elastic fibers, and an inner layer of endothelial cells. The thicker walls aid in the pumping of blood, maintain normal blood pressure (**BP**), and give arteries the strength to resist the high pressure caused by the contraction of the heart ventricles. The elastic walls expand as the heart pushes blood through the arteries. A **pulse** is the wave of increased pressure felt along arteries each time the heart ***ventricle*** contracts.

The radial artery located near the thumb side of the wrist is the most common site for obtaining a pulse rate. The brachial artery located in the **antecubital** space of the elbow is the most common site to obtain a BP. The carotid artery located near the side of the neck is the most accessible site in an emergency, such as cardiac arrest, to check for a pulse rate. The femoral artery located near the groin and the temporal artery located at the temple are other major arteries. The aorta is the largest artery and branches into the smaller arteries to distribute oxygen-rich blood throughout the body. The pulmonary artery is the only artery that does not carry oxygenated blood. Figure 4–2 shows the major arteries in the body.

Capillaries are the smallest vessels, one epithelial cell thick, that connect arterioles and ***venules***. The blood in capillaries consists of a mixture of arterial and venous blood. The thin walls of capillaries allow the exchange of oxygen, carbon dioxide, and nutrients between the blood and tissue cells.

Venules are small veins that connect capillaries to larger veins. Veins have thinner walls than arteries and carry oxygen-poor blood, carbon dioxide, and other waste products back to the heart. No gaseous exchange takes place in the veins, only in the capillaries. The thinner walls of veins have less elastic tissue and less connective tissue than arteries because the BP in the veins is very low. Veins have one-way **valves** to keep blood flowing in one direction as the blood flows through the veins by skeletal muscle contraction. The leg veins have numerous valves to return the blood to the heart against the force of gravity.

The main veins in the arm are the basilic, cephalic, and median cubital veins. The great saphe-

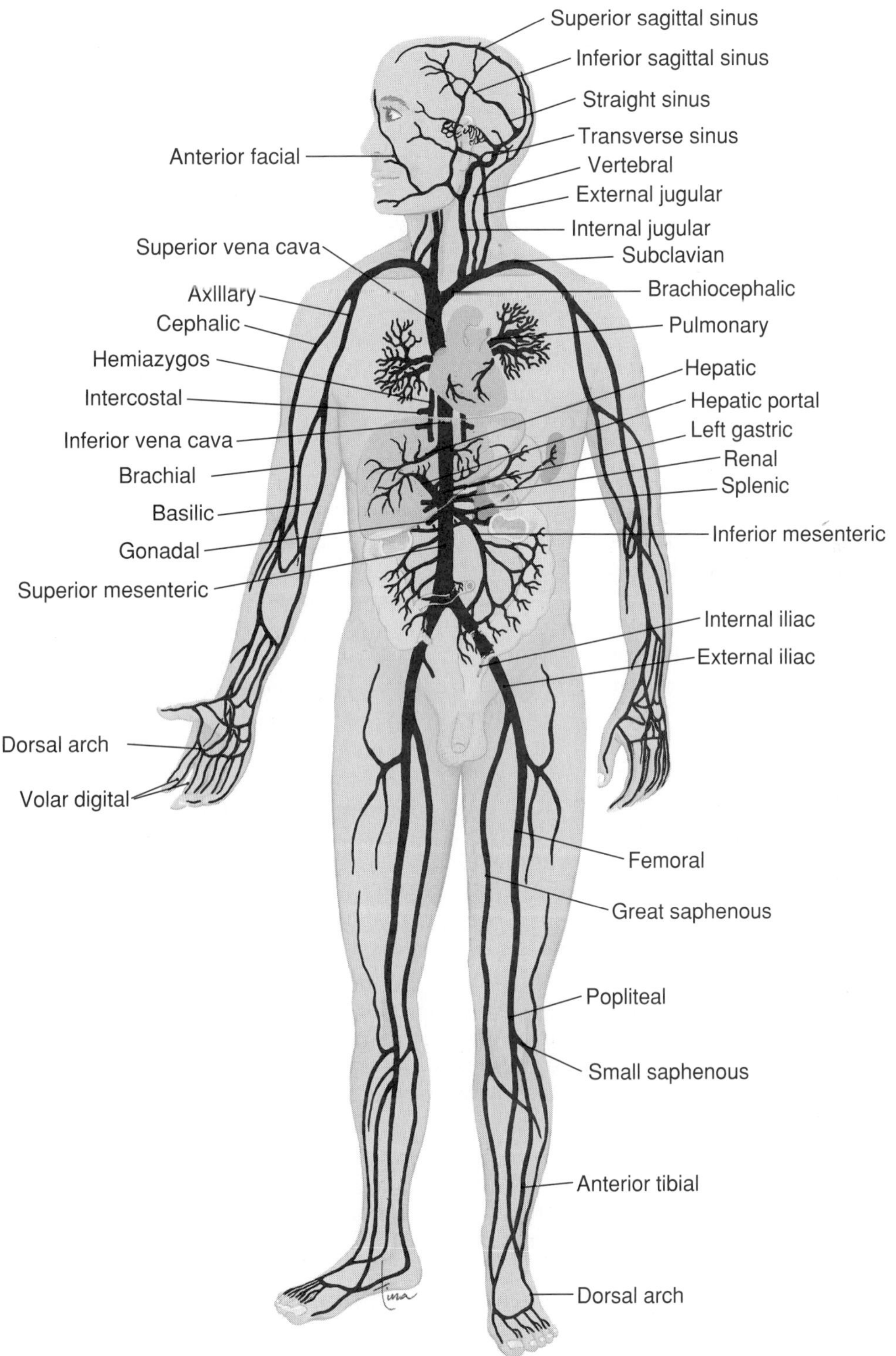

Figure 4–2 The major veins. (From Scanlon, VC, and Sanders, T: Essentials of Anatomy and Physiology, ed. 3. FA Davis, Philadelphia, 1999, p. 281, with permission.)

nous vein is the principal vein in the leg and the longest in the body. The largest veins, the superior and inferior venae cavae, carry the oxygen-poor blood back to the heart. The pulmonary vein is the only vein that carries oxygenated blood. Figure 4–3 shows the principal veins of the body.

Most blood tests are performed on venous blood. Venipuncture is the procedure for removing blood from a vein for analysis. The veins of choice for venipuncture are the basilic, cephalic, and median cubital veins located in the antecubital area of the elbow, as shown in Figure 4–4.

Heart

The heart is a hollow muscular organ located in the thoracic cavity between the lungs and slightly to the left of the body midline that consists of two pumps to circulate blood throughout the circulatory system. The heart has three layers of tissue. The thin outer layer of the heart is the **epicardium**. Lining the walls of each heart chamber is a thick muscle tissue called the **myocardium,** and lining the cavities of the heart is a smooth tissue called the **endocardium**. The **pericardium** is a fibrous membrane sac that surrounds the heart to hold it in position.

The heart has four chambers and is divided into right and left halves by a partition called the **septum**. Each side has an upper chamber called the ***atrium*** to collect blood and a lower chamber called the ventricle to pump blood from the heart. The right side is the "pump" for the **pulmonary circulation,** and the left side is the "pump" for the **systemic circulation**. The heart contracts and relaxes to pump deoxygenated blood through the heart to the lungs and return oxygenated blood to the heart for distribution throughout the body. Refer to Figure 4–5 to follow the circulation of blood through the heart.

Valves located at the entrance and exit of each ventricle prevent a backflow of blood and keep it flowing in one direction. The right **atrioventricular (AV) valve** or **tricuspid valve**, located at the entrance to the right ventricle, lets blood flow into the right ventricle and prevents backflow into the right atrium. The **pulmonary semilunar valve**, located at the exit of the right ventricle, allows blood to flow from the right ventricle through the pulmonary artery to the lungs. The left AV valve or **bicuspid valve**, also called the **mitral valve**, located at the entrance of the left ventricle, prevents the backflow of blood to the left atrium, forcing blood into the left ventricle. The **aortic semilunar valve**, located at the exit of the left ventricle, permits blood to leave the left ventricle and flow into the aorta. Heart sounds created by the cardiac cycle are the "lub-dup" sounds heard with a **stethoscope**. The first sound, the "lub," is the closure of the AV valves as the ventricles contract. The second sound, the "dup," is the closure of the semilunar valves. A heart murmur is an abnormal heart sound that occurs when the valves close incorrectly.

The heart has its own ***vascular*** system to nourish the heart muscle. The heart receives its oxygenated blood through the right and left coronary arteries. Both coronary arteries obtain their blood from the aorta just above the aortic semilunar valve. The coronary arteries are the first branching of blood vessels off the aorta, but they receive their blood supply during the relaxation phase of the cardiac cycle, rather than during the contraction phase. The coronary arteries are angled downward in a self-preservation manner. Even if the heart is capable only of a minimal ventricular contraction, the heart muscle itself will benefit as blood flows downward into the coronary arteries during relaxation. When the coronary arteries become obstructed, heart muscle dies because of lack of oxygen, and a heart attack can occur.

The left coronary artery divides into two major branches, the circumflex artery and the left anterior descending artery. The circumflex branch curves to the posterior portion of the heart and supplies blood through various branches to the posterior wall of the left atrium and ventricle. The left anterior descending branch travels down the anterior portion of the left ventricle and supplies, through branching, the right and left walls with blood. The right coronary artery travels across the heart to the right side and branches to supply blood to the posterior and anterior walls of the right ventricle and atrium (Fig. 4–6).

Pathway of Blood Through the Heart

Two large veins, the superior vena cava and the inferior vena cava, transport blood to the right atrium of the heart. The superior vena cava collects blood from the upper portion of the body, and the inferior vena cava collects blood from the lower portion of the body. The blood passes through the tricuspid valve

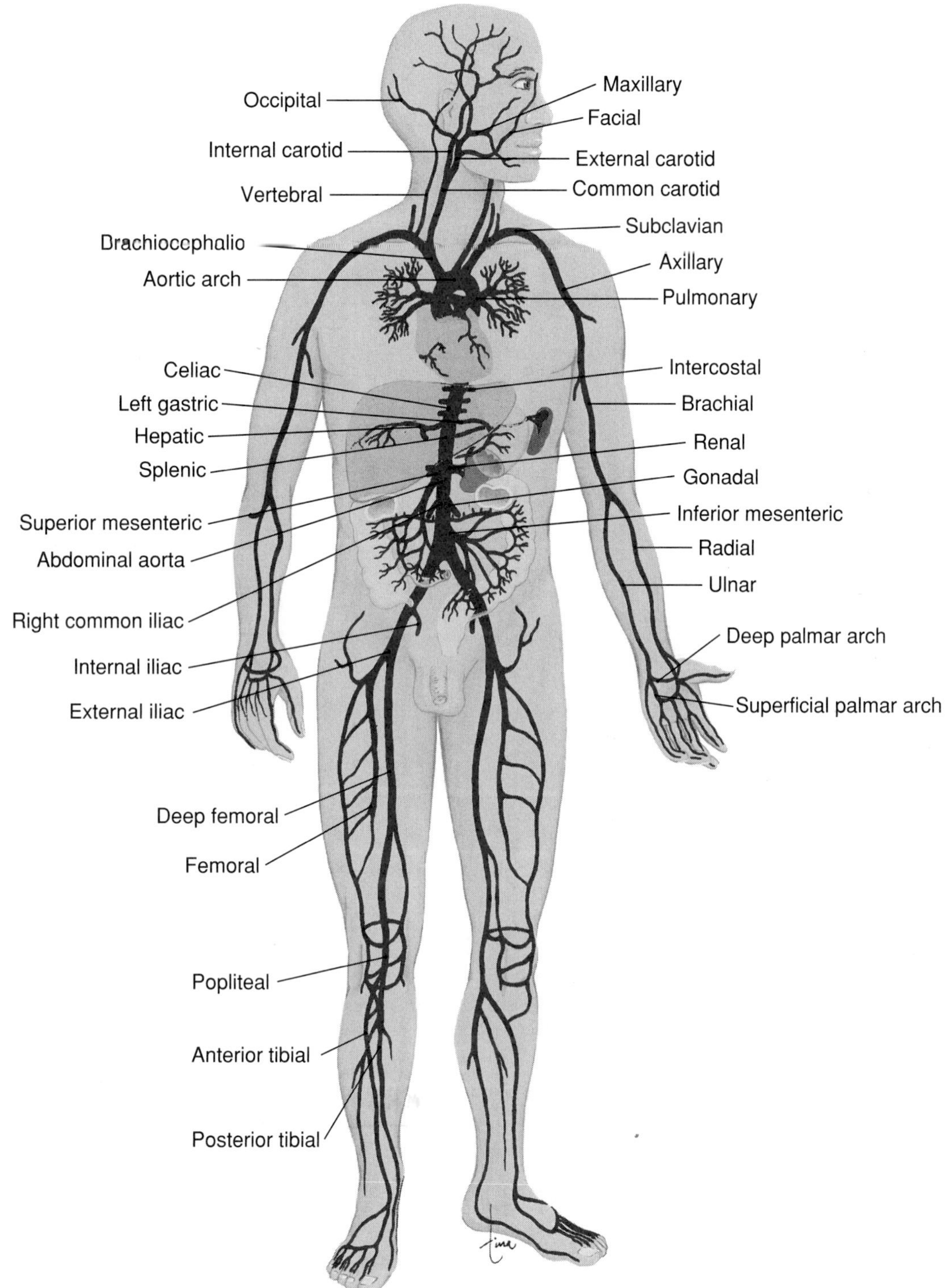

Figure 4–3 The major arteries. (From Scanlon, VC, and Sanders, T: Essentials of Anatomy and Physiology, ed. 3. FA Davis, Philadelphia, 1999, p. 282, with permission.)

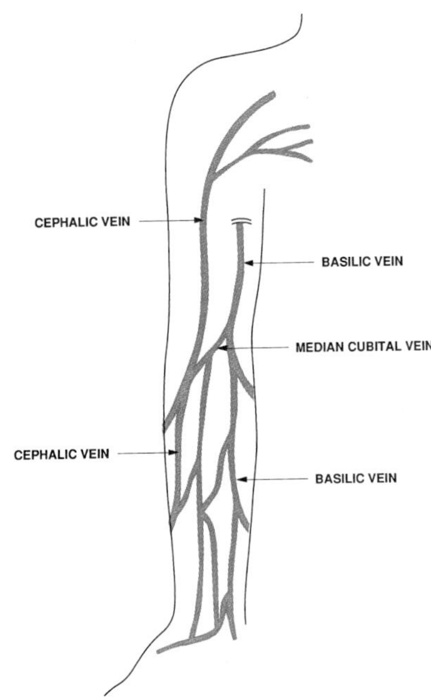

Figure 4–4 Veins in the arm used for venipuncture.

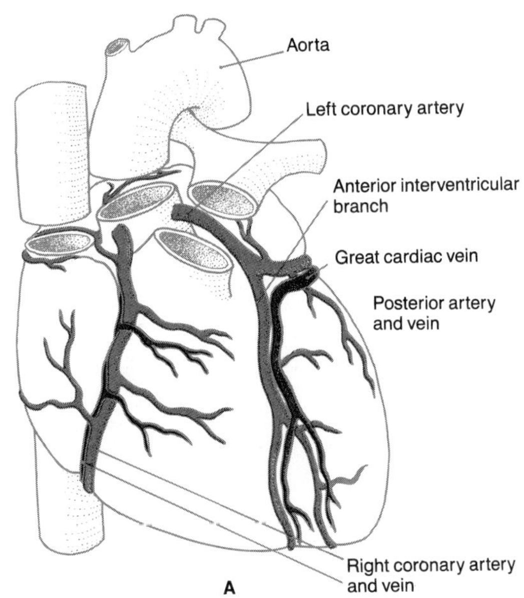

Figure 4–6 Coronary blood vessels. (Adapted from Scanlon, VC, and Sanders, T: Essentials of Anatomy and Physiology, ed. 3. FA Davis, Philadelphia, 1999, p. 262.)

to the right ventricle. The right ventricle contracts to pump the blood through the pulmonary semilunar valve into the right and left pulmonary arteries that carry it to each lung. In the lung capillaries, blood releases carbon dioxide and acquires oxygen. The right and left pulmonary veins carry the oxygenated blood from the lungs to the left atrium of the heart. The blood flows through the mitral valve into the left ventricle that contracts to pump blood through the aortic semilunar valve into the aorta. Blood travels throughout the body to the capillaries by arteries that branch off the aorta.

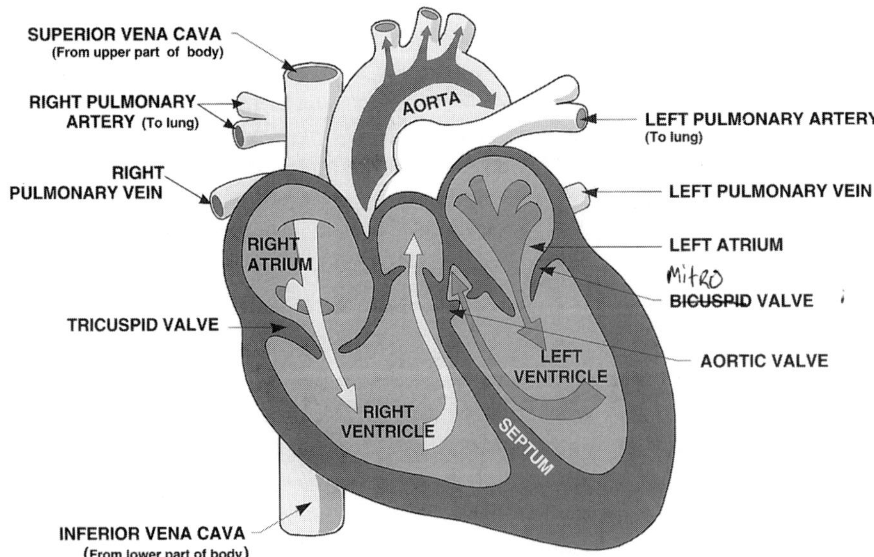

Figure 4–5 Pathway of blood through the heart.

Summary of Blood Circulation

- Oxygen-poor blood from the venae cavae enters the right atrium of the heart.
- The right atrium contracts to force the blood through the tricuspid valve to the right ventricle.
- The right ventricle contracts to force the blood through the pulmonary semilunar valve into the pulmonary artery, which divides to each lung.
- The red blood cells release carbon dioxide and absorb oxygen in the lungs.
- The oxygen-rich blood returns to the heart through the pulmonary veins and enters the left atrium.
- The left atrium contracts to force the blood through the mitral valve into the left ventricle.
- The left ventricle contracts to force the blood through the aortic semilunar valve into the aorta.
- The aorta divides into arteries, which branch into arterioles, to deliver blood throughout the body.
- The arterioles connect to capillaries, where oxygen and nutrients leave the blood and carbon dioxide and waste products enter the blood.
- The blood from the capillaries returns to the heart through venules, which fuse into larger veins.
- The blood enters the heart through the largest veins, the superior vena cava and the inferior vena cava.

The cardiac cycle is the contraction phase (**systole**) and the relaxation phase (**diastole**) of the cardiac muscle that occurs in one heartbeat. Specialized cardiac conductive tissue initiates electrical impulses that cause the heart muscle to rhythmically contract. The **sinoatrial (SA) node**, located in the upper right atrium, is the pacemaker of the heart and initiates the heartbeat. An electrical impulse travels from the SA node to the AV node located in the lower right atrium. This causes the right and left atria to contract, forcing the blood through the AV valves into the ventricles. The impulse travels to the AV bundle (**Bundle of His**), located in the upper interventricular septum, where it divides into right and left branches. The impulse continues to travel to the Purkinje fibers in the ventricles, causing them to contract. This forces blood through the semilunar valves into the pulmonary artery and the aorta. After a brief relaxation, the cycle starts again (Fig. 4–7). An electrocardiogram (**ECG**) detects and records the electrical activity of the atria and ventricles by leads placed on the patient's skin. An ECG detects cardiac abnormalities and heart muscle damage.

The heart contracts approximately
per minute, which represents the hear
rate. The cardiac output is the quantity of bl
pumped by the heart ventricle in 1 minute and averages about 5 liters of blood per minute. Cardiac output increases to meet the body's need for more oxygen.

The arterial pulse is a rhythmic recurring wave that occurs through the arteries during normal pumping action of the heart. The pulse is most easily detected by palpation where an artery crosses over a bone or firm tissue. Common pulse sites are the temporal, carotid, brachial, and radial arteries. In adults and children older than 3 years of age, the radial artery is usually the easiest to locate. Two fingers are pressed against the radius just above the wrist on the thumb side (Fig. 4–8).

The pulse reveals heart function and, therefore, is considered a vital sign and is taken routinely. When taking the pulse, the rate (number of beats per minute), the rhythm (pattern of beats or regularity), and volume are determined. If the patient's pulse is irregular, it should always be counted for a full 60 seconds.

BP is the pressure exerted by the blood on the walls of blood vessels during contraction and relaxation of the ventricles. Systolic and diastolic readings are taken and reported in millimeters of mercury (**mm Hg**). The systolic pressure is the higher of the two numbers and indicates the BP during contraction of the ventricles. The diastolic pressure is the lower number and is the BP when the ventricles are relaxed.

To measure the BP, a BP cuff called a **sphygmomanometer** is placed over the upper arm and a stethoscope is placed over the brachial artery to listen for heart sounds (Fig. 4–9). The BP cuff is inflated to restrict the blood flow in the brachial artery and then slowly deflated until loud heart sounds are heard with the stethoscope. The first heart sounds represent the systolic pressure during contraction of the ventricles and is the top number of a BP reading. The cuff continues to be deflated until the sound is no longer heard, which represents the diastolic pressure during the relaxation of the ventricles and is the bottom number of a BP reading. An average BP for an adult is 120/80, representing a systolic pressure of 120 mm Hg and a diastolic pressure of 80 mm Hg.

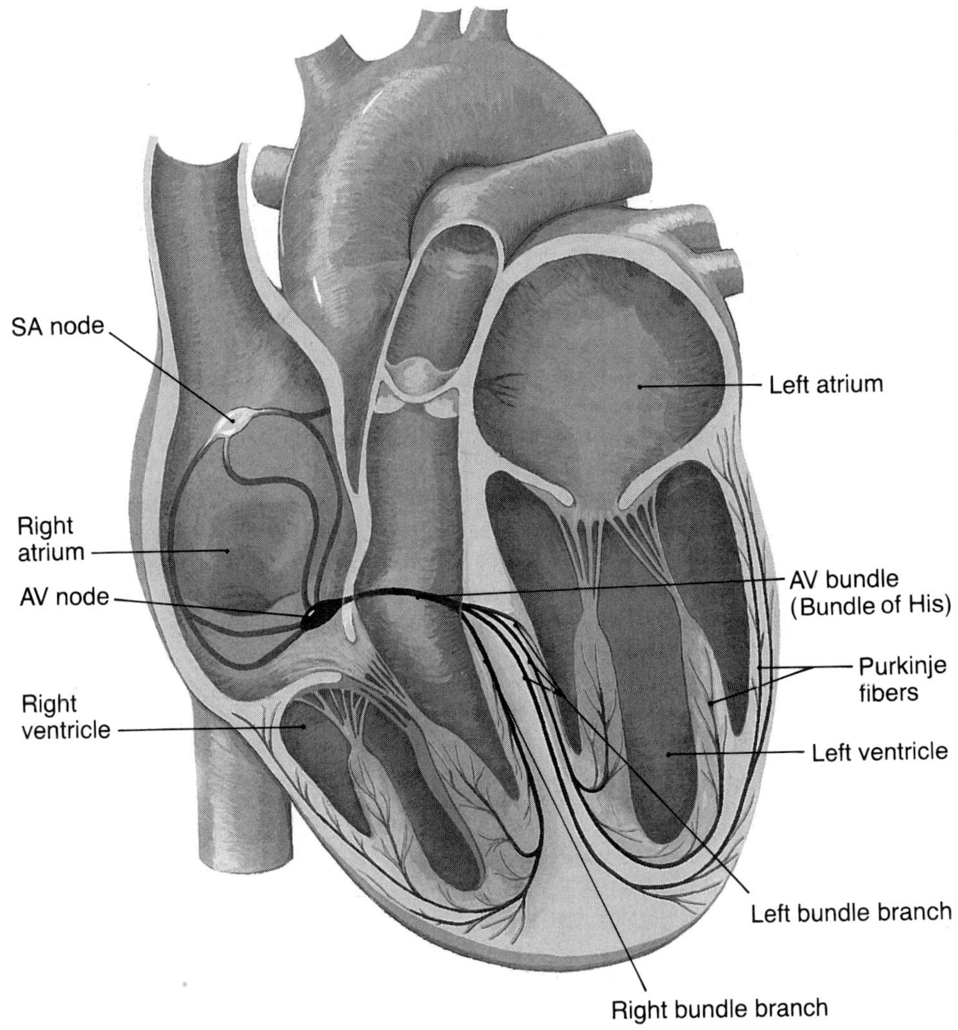

Figure 4–7 Conduction pathway of the heart. (Adapted from: Scanlon, VC, and Sanders, T: Essentials of Anatomy and Physiology, ed. 3. FA Davis, Philadelphia, 1999, p. 266.)

Blood

Blood is the body's main fluid for transporting nutrients, waste products, gases, and hormones through the circulatory system. Blood assists in the regulation of body temperature and protection against pathogens, acid-base, fluid and electrolyte balance, and blood clotting. An average adult has a blood volume of 5 to 6 L. Blood consists of two parts: a liquid portion called plasma, and a cellular portion called the formed elements.

Plasma comprises approximately 55% of the total blood volume. It is a clear, straw-colored fluid that is about 91% water and 9% dissolved substances. It is the transporting medium for the plasma proteins (albumin, globulin, fibrinogen, and prothrombin); the nutrients (glucose and lipids); the minerals (sodium, potassium, calcium, and magnesium); the gases (oxygen, carbon dioxide, and nitrogen); vitamins, hormones, and blood cells, as well as waste products of metabolism (blood urea nitrogen, creatinine, and uric acid).

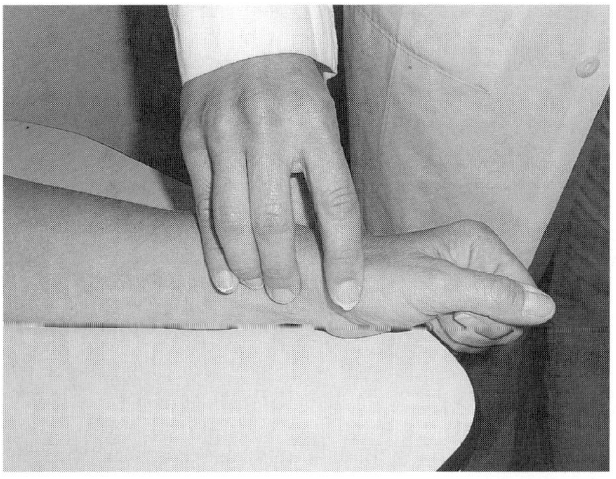

Figure 4–8 Proper placement of fingers along the radial artery.

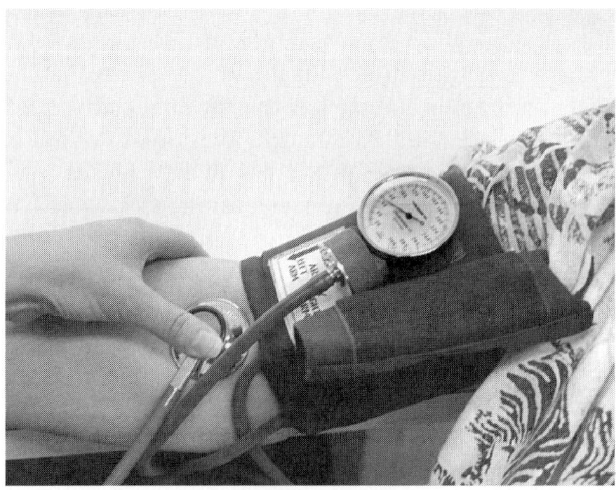

Figure 4–9 Sphygmomanometer. (From Strasinger, SK, and Di Lorenzo, MS: Skills for the Patient Care Technician. FA Davis, Philadelphia, 1999, p. 336, with permission.)

The formed elements constitute 45% of the total blood volume and include the ***erythrocytes*** (red blood cells [RBCs]), ***leukocytes*** (white blood cells [WBCs]), and ***thrombocytes*** (**platelets**). Blood cells are produced in the bone marrow, which is the spongy material that fills the inside of the major bones of the body. Cells originate from stem cells in the bone marrow, differentiate, and mature through several stages in the bone marrow and lymphatic tissue until they are released to the circulating blood.

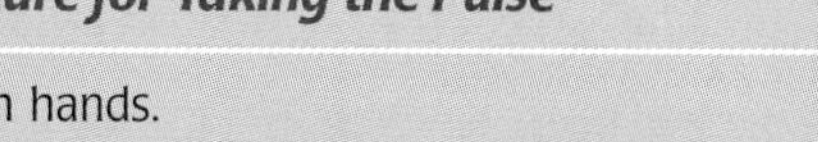

Procedure for Taking the Pulse

1. Wash hands.
2. Obtain a watch with a second hand.
3. Have the patient sitting or lying down with the arm at the side or across the chest.
4. Gently press the fingers on the radial artery inside the patient's wrist on the thumb side.
5. When the pulse is located, count the beats for a full 60 seconds.
6. Record the pulse rate, rhythm, and volume and the time the pulse was taken.

Examination of the bone marrow is used to diagnose many blood disorders.

Erythrocytes

Erythrocytes (RBCs) are anuclear biconcave disks that are approximately 7.2 microns in diameter. Erythrocytes contain the protein hemoglobin to transport oxygen and carbon dioxide. Hemoglobin consists of two parts, heme and globin. The heme portion requires iron for its synthesis.

Erythrocytes mature through several stages in the bone marrow and enter the circulating blood as reticulocytes that contain fragments of nuclear material. There are approximately 4.5 to 6.0 million erythrocytes per microliter (μL) of blood, with men having slightly higher values than women. The normal life span for an erythrocyte is 120 days. **Macrophages** in the liver and spleen remove the old erythrocytes from the blood stream and destroy them. The iron is reused in new cells.

The surface of erythrocytes contains antigens that determine the blood group and type of an individual, frequently referred to as the person's ABO group and Rh type. As shown in Table 4–1, four blood types exist based on the antigens present on the erythrocyte membrane. Type A blood has the "A" antigen (Ag), and type B blood has the "B" antigen. Type AB blood has both the "A" and "B" antigens, and type O blood has neither the "A" nor "B" antigens. Types O and A are the most common, and type AB is the least common.

The plasma of an individual contains natural-occurring antibodies (Abs) for those antigens not present on the erythrocytes. Type A blood has anti-B

Procedure for Measuring Blood Pressure

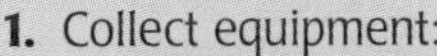

1. Collect equipment:
   Sphygmomanometer (blood pressure cuff)
   Stethoscope
   Alcohol wipes
2. Wash hands.
3. Identify the patient.
4. Explain the procedure to the patient.
5. Clean stethoscope diaphragm and ear pieces with alcohol wipes.
6. The patient may lie supine or sit erect with the arm extended and supported at the level of the heart.
7. The mercury measuring device should be at eye level and the gauge should be directly in front of you.
8. Expose the upper arm and place the arrow of the cuff over the brachial artery, wrapping the cuff around the arm at least an inch above the elbow.
9. With thumb and index finger close the valve on the rubber inflation bulb.
10. Put the stethoscope in your ears, and place the diaphragm over the brachial artery.
11. With the tips of your fingers, locate the radial artery and inflate the cuff until you no longer feel the pulse. Inflate to between 160 and 170 mm Hg.
12. Using thumb and index finger, carefully open the bulb valve and slowly deflate the cuff—no faster than 5 mm Hg/second.
13. When you hear the first beat, note the pressure on the gauge. This is the systolic pressure reading.
14. Continue to deflate slowly, listening carefully for the sound. Note the point where the sound disappears. This is the diastolic pressure reading.
15. Completely deflate the cuff. Remove it from the patient's arm.
16. Record the patient's blood pressure.
17. Return the equipment to its proper place.

TABLE 4–1
ABO Blood Group System

Blood Type	RBC Antigen	Plasma Antibodies
A	A	Anti-B
B	B	Anti-A
AB	A and B	Neither anti-A nor anti-B
O	Neither	Anti-A and anti-B

antibodies in the plasma, and type B blood has anti-A antibodies. Type O blood has both the anti-A and anti-B antibodies, and type AB blood has neither anti-A nor anti-B antibodies. The naturally occurring antibodies react with erythrocytes carrying antigens that are not present on the individual's own erythrocytes.

A transfusion reaction may occur when a person receives a different type of blood because a person's natural antibodies will destroy the donor RBCs that contain the antigen specific for the antibodies. For example, if a type A person received type B blood, the anti-B antibodies of the type A person would bind to the B antigens of the type B donor blood and destroy the donor cells. Patients receive type-specific blood to avoid this type of transfusion reaction. Misidentification of patients during phlebotomy is a major cause of transfusion reactions.

The presence or absence of the RBC antigen called the Rh factor or D antigen determines whether a person is Rh-positive or Rh-negative. Approximately 85% of the population has the Rh factor. Rh-negative people do not have natural antibodies to the Rh factor but will form antibodies if they receive Rh-positive blood. A second transfusion of Rh-positive blood will cause a transfusion reaction. **Hemolytic disease of the newborn (HDN)** occurs when an incompatibility is present between maternal and fetal blood Rh antigens.

Leukocytes

Leukocytes, or WBCs, provide immunity to certain diseases by producing antibodies and destroying harmful pathogens by **phagocytosis**. Leukocytes are produced in the bone marrow from a stem cell and develop in the thymus and bone marrow. They differentiate and mature through several stages before being released into the blood stream. Leukocytes circulate in the peripheral blood for several hours and then migrate to the tissues through the capillary walls. The normal number of leukocytes for an adult is 4500 to 11,000 per μL of blood.

Five types of leukocytes are present in the blood, each with a specific function. They are distinguished by their morphology, as shown in Figure 4–10. When stained with Wright's stain, the cells are examined microscopically for granules in the cytoplasm, the shape of the nucleus, and the size of the cell. A differential cell count determines the percentage of each type of leukocyte. The five normal types of leukocytes are neutrophils, lymphocytes, monocytes, eosinophils, and basophils.

Neutrophils (40%–60%)

Neutrophils, the most numerous leukocytes, provide protection against infection through phagocytosis. Neutrophils are called segmented or polymorphonuclear cells because the nucleus has several lobes. The nucleus stains dark purple, and the cytoplasm stains pink with fine granules. The number of neutrophils increases in bacterial infections.

Lymphocytes (20%–40%)

Lymphocytes, the second most numerous leukocytes, provide the body with immune capability. The lymphocyte has a large round purple nucleus with a rim of sky blue cytoplasm. There are two main types of lymphocytes: B cells and T cells. The B lymphocyte develops in the bone marrow, becomes a **plasma cell**, and produces antibodies for defense against bacterial infections. T lymphocytes mature in the thymus, act in delayed hypersensitivity reactions and graft rejections, and assist B lymphocytes in the production of antibodies. The number of lymphocytes increases in viral infections.

Monocytes (3%–8%)

Monocytes are the largest circulating leukocytes and act as powerful phagocytes to digest foreign material. The cytoplasm has a fine blue-gray appearance with vacuoles and a large, irregular nucleus. A tissue monocyte is known as a macrophage. The number of monocytes increases in intracellular infections and tuberculosis.

Eosinophils (1%–3%)

The granules in cytoplasm of eosinophils stain red-orange, and the nucleus has only two lobes. Eosinophils detoxify foreign proteins and increase in allergies, skin infections, and parasitic infections.

Basophils (0%–1%)

Basophils are the least common of the leukocytes. The cytoplasm contains large granules that stain purple-black and release histamine in the inflammation process and heparin to prevent abnormal blood clotting.

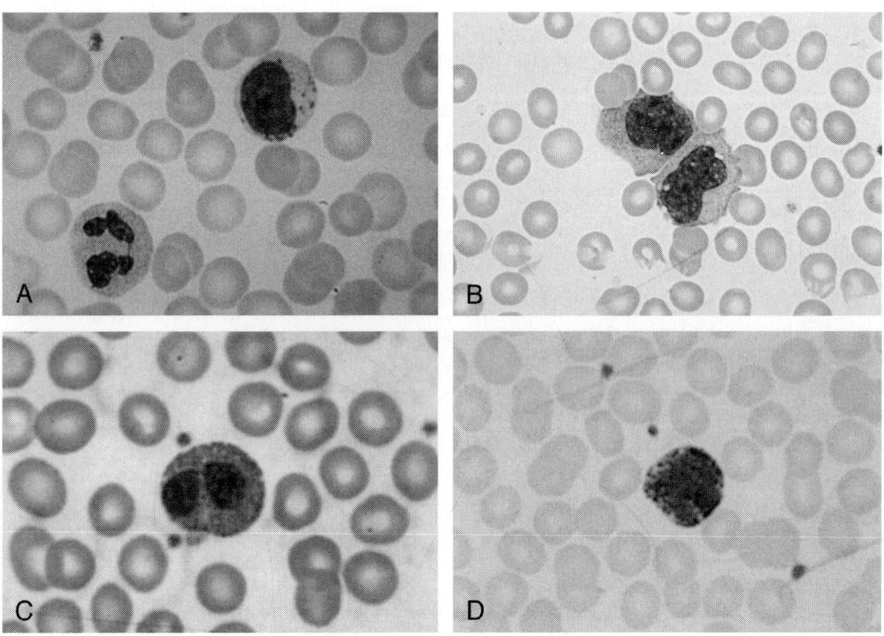

Figure 4–10 Normal white blood cells. (*A*) Neutrophil (left) and lymphocyte (right). (*B*) Monocyte. (*C*) Eosinophil. (*D*), Basophil. (From Harmening, DM: Clinical Hematology and Fundamentals of Hemostasis, ed. 4. FA Davis, Philadelphia, 2002, with permission.)

Thrombocytes

Thrombocytes or platelets are small, irregularly shaped disks formed from particles of a very large cell in the bone marrow called the megakaryocyte. Platelets have a life span of 9 to 12 days. The average number of platelets is between 140,000 and 440,000 per μL of blood. Platelets play a vital role in blood clotting in all stages of the coagulation mechanism.

Coagulation

A complex coagulation mechanism that involves blood vessels, platelets, and the coagulation factors maintains hemostasis. Hemostasis is the process of forming a blood clot to stop the leakage of blood when injury to a blood vessel occurs and lysing the clot when the injury has been repaired. A basic understanding of coagulation can be obtained by dividing the process into primary hemostasis, secondary hemostasis, and **fibrinolysis**.

Primary hemostasis forms a temporary platelet plug. It is the vascular platelet phase because blood vessels and platelets are the first to respond to an injury. Blood vessels constrict to slow the flow of blood to the injured area. Platelets become sticky, clump together (platelet aggregation), and adhere to the injured blood vessel wall (platelet adhesion) to stop bleeding. The bleeding time test evaluates formation of the platelet plug.

Secondary hemostasis involves the interaction of the coagulation factors to convert the primary platelet plug to a stable **fibrin** clot to stop bleeding more permanently. This interaction is the coagulation cascade. In this cascade, one factor becomes activated, which activates the next factor in a specific sequence. Substances released during an injury activate the coagulation factors, which in combination with calcium and platelet factor 3 (**PF3**), produce a tough fibrin clot. This clot stabilizes the platelet plug and stops bleeding. The coagulation cascade can be initiated by two pathways, the intrinsic and extrinsic, which come together in a common pathway (Fig. 4–11).

The intrinsic system is initiated when large molecules in the blood stream called contact factors activate factor XII and platelets release the phospholipid PF3. The release of tissue thromboplastin from an injured area activates factor VII, which initiates the extrinsic pathway. Both systems react with factors X and V to convert **prothrombin** (factor II) to **thrombin**. Thrombin converts fibrinogen (factor I) to the fibrin that forms the basis of the fibrin clot. Factor XIII stabilizes the fibrin clot.

The activated partial thromboplastin time and the activated clotting time tests evaluate the intrinsic pathway and monitor **heparin** therapy. The prothrombin time test evaluates the extrinsic pathway and monitors warfarin sodium (**Coumadin**) therapy.

Fibrinolysis is the process of breakdown and removal of a clot after healing has occurred. Fibrin in the clot is broken down into small fragments called fibrin degradation products (FDPs), which are cleared from the circulation by the liver. The measurement of FDPs or **D-dimers** monitors fibrinolysis.

Disorders

Blood Vessels

Aneurysm

A bulge formed by a weakness in the wall of a blood vessel, usually an artery, that can burst and cause severe hemorrhaging.

Arteriosclerosis

Hardening of the artery walls contributing to aneurysm or stroke.

Atherosclerosis

A form of arteriosclerosis characterized by the accumulation of lipids and other materials in the walls of arteries causing the lumen of the vessel to narrow and stimulate clot formation.

Embolism

Obstruction of a blood vessel by a moving blood clot or other foreign matter in the vascular system; tissue destruction or death occurs if the embolus lodges in an organ.

Phlebitis

Inflammation of the vein wall causing pain and tenderness.

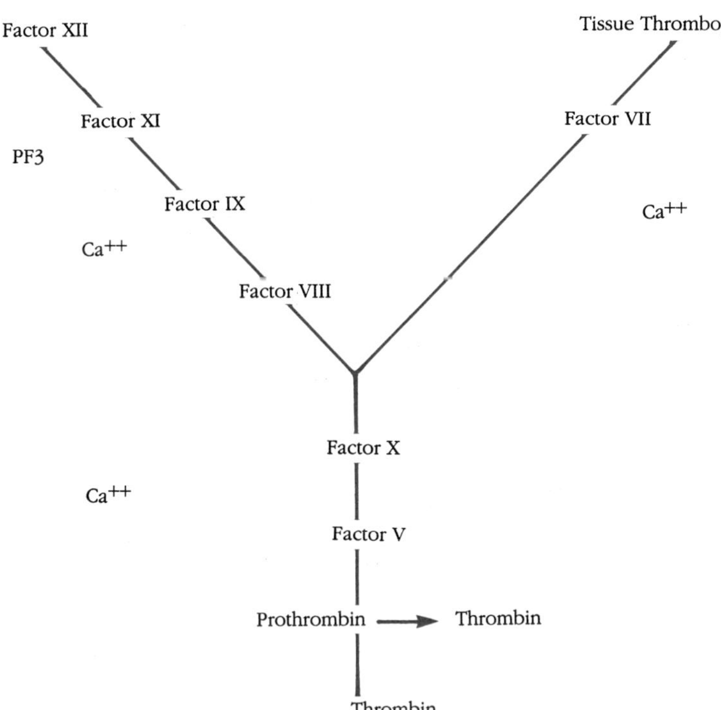

Figure 4–11 The coagulation cascade. (Ca^{++} = calcium; PF3 = platelet factor 3.) (From Strasinger, SK, and Di Lorenzo, MS: Skills for the Patient Care Technician. FA Davis, Philadelphia, 1999, p. 99, with permission.)

Thrombosis

Obstruction of a blood vessel by a stationary blood clot, causing an aching pain.

Varicose Veins

Swollen peripheral veins caused by damaged valves, allowing backflow of blood that causes swelling (**edema**) in the tissues.

Heart

Angina Pectoris (Angina)

Sharp chest pain caused by deceased blood flow to the heart, usually because of an obstruction in the coronary arteries.

Bacterial Endocarditis

Inflammation of the inner lining of the heart caused by a bacterial infection, usually streptococcal.

Congestive Heart Failure

A chronic disorder, congestive heart failure (CHF) impairs the ability of the heart to pump blood efficiently, causing fluid accumulation in the lungs and other tissues.

Myocardial Infarction

Death (**necrosis**) of the heart muscle caused by a lack of oxygen to the myocardium because of an occluded coronary artery, commonly known as a heart attack; symptoms of myocardial infarction are a feeling of pressure in the chest just inside the breast bone, pain in the jaw or down part of either arm (usually the left arm), nausea, sweating, dizziness, shortness of breath, or irregular pulse.

Pericarditis

Inflammation of the membrane surrounding the heart, the pericardium, induced by bacteria, viruses, trauma, or malignancy; a throbbing pain may occur with each heartbeat.

Rheumatic Heart Disease

An autoimmune disorder affecting heart tissue

following a streptococcal infection, generally seen in childhood; can result in painful swollen joints, unusual rashes, and heart damage.

Blood

Anemia

A decrease in the number of erythrocytes or the amount of hemoglobin in the circulating blood. A variety of anemias exist, including aplastic anemia, iron deficiency anemia, hemolytic anemia, pernicious anemia, sickle cell anemia, and thalassemia; symptoms are difficulty in breathing, rapid heartbeat, paleness, and low BP.

Leukemia

A marked increase in the number of WBCs in the bone marrow and circulating blood; leuke-mias are named for the particular type of leukocyte that is increased; an acute leukemia is characterized by the presence of immature cell forms and a rapidly progressing disease course. Chronic leukemia is characterized by mature cell forms and slower disease progression.

Leukocytosis

An abnormal increase in the number of normal leukocytes in the circulating blood, as seen in infections.

Leukopenia

A decrease below normal values in the number of leukocytes, often caused by exposure to radiation or chemotherapy.

Polycythemia

A consistent increase in the number of erythrocytes and other formed elements, causing the blood to have a viscous consistency; frequently treated by therapeutic phlebotomy.

Thrombocytopenia

A decrease in the number of circulating platelets, frequently seen in patients receiving chemotherapy; spontaneous bleeding can result.

Thrombocytosis

An increase in the number of circulating platelets.

Coagulation

Disseminated Intravascular Coagulation (DIC)

Spontaneous activation of the coagulation system by certain foreign substances entering the circulatory system causing a depletion of the platelets and coagulation factors and elevated FDPs resulting in hemorrhage.

Hemophilia

A hereditary disorder characterized by excessive bleeding because of the lack of a coagulation factor, usually factor VIII.

Diagnostic Tests

The most frequently ordered diagnostic tests associated with the circulatory system and their clinical correlations are presented in Table 4–2.

Medications

Table 4–3 lists the brand names of the most commonly used medications for the circulatory system and their purpose.

Bibliography

Scanlon, VC, and Sanders, T: Essentials of Anatomy and Physiology, ed. 3. FA Davis, Philadelphia, 1999.

Strasinger, SK, and Di Lorenzo, MS: Skills for the Patient Care Technician. FA Davis, Philadelphia, 1999.

Tamparo, CD, and Lewis, MA: Diseases of the Human Body, ed. 3. FA Davis, Philadelphia, 2000.

TABLE 4-2
Diagnostic Tests Associated with the Circulatory System

Test	Clinical Correlation
Activated clotting time (ACT)	Heparin therapy
Activated partial thromboplastin time [APTT(PTT)]	Heparin therapy or coagulation disorders
Angiogram	Blood vessel integrity
Antibody (Ab) screen	Blood transfusion
Antistreptolysin O (ASO) titer	Rheumatic fever
Antithrombin III	Coagulation disorders
Apo-A, Apo-B lipoprotein	Cardiac risk
Aspartate aminotransferase [AST(SGOT)]	Cardiac muscle damage
Bilirubin	Hemolytic disorders
Bleeding time (BT)	Platelet function
Blood culture	Microbial infection
Blood group and type	ABO group, type, and Rh factor
Bone marrow	Blood cell disorders
Brain natriuretic peptide (BNP)	Congestive heart failure
C-reactive protein (CRP)	Inflammatory disorders
Cardiac catheterization	Coronary artery examination
Cholesterol	Coronary artery disease
Complete blood count (CBC)	Bleeding disorders, anemia, or leukemia
Computerized axial tomography (CT scan)	Soft-tissue examination
Creatine kinase [CK(CPK)]	Myocardial infarction
Creatine kinase isoenzymes (CK-MB)	Myocardial infarction
Direct antihuman globulin test (DAT)	Anemia or hemolytic disease of the newborn
Echocardiogram	Cardiac abnormalities
Electrocardiogram (ECG)	Myocardial damage
Erythrocyte sedimentation rate (ESR)	Inflammatory disorders
Fibrin degradation products (FDP)	Disseminated intravascular coagulation
Fibrinogen	Coagulation disorders
Hematocrit (Hct)	Anemia
Hemoglobin (Hgb)	Anemia
Hemoglobin (Hgb) electrophoresis	Hemoglobin abnormalities
High-density lipoprotein (HDL)	Coronary risk
Iron	Anemia
Lactic dehydrogenase [LD(LDH)]	Myocardial infarction
Low-density lipoprotein (LDL)	Coronary risk
Myoglobin	Myocardial infarction
Platelet (plt) count	Bleeding tendencies
Prothrombin time (PT)	Coumadin therapy and coagulation disorders
Reticulocyte (retic) count	Bone marrow function
Sickle cell screening	Sickle cell anemia
Stress test	Cardiac function
Total iron binding capacity (TIBC)	Anemia
Triglycerides	Coronary artery disease
Troponin I and T	Myocardial infarction
Type and crossmatch (T & C)	Blood transfusion
Type and screen	Blood transfusion
Ultrasonogram	Organ examination
White blood cell (WBC) count	Infections or leukemia

TABLE 4-3
Commonly Used Medications for the Circulatory System

Type	Generic and Trade Names	Purpose
ACE inhibitors	Accupril, Capoten, Lotensin, Vasotec, and Zestril	Lower blood pressure
Angiotensin receptor blockers	Avapro, Cozaar, and Diovan	Lower blood pressure
Antiarrhythmic	Betapace, Cordarone, Inderal, Lanoxin, Mexitil, Norpace, Quinidex, Rythmol, Tambocor, and Tonocard	Treat cardiac arrhythmias
Anticoagulants	Aggrenox, Athrombin K, Coumadin, heparin sodium, Lovenox, Plavix, and Ticlid	Inhibit blood clotting
Antihypertensive agents	Aldomet, Capoten, Cardizem, Catapres, Isoptin, Lopressor, Norvasc, and Procardia	Lower blood pressure
Digitalis compounds	Cedilanid D and Crystodigin	Strengthen heart muscle and alter heart contractions
Hematinic agents	Feosol, ferrous fumarate, ferrous gluconate, ferrous sulfate, Niferex, and Trinsicon	Treat iron deficiency anemia
Hemostatic agents	Amicar, Humafac, Proplex, Protamine, Surgicel, and vitamin K	Stop bleeding
Hypolipidemics	Atromid-S, Lescol, Lipitor, Lopid, Mevacor, niacin, Pravachol, Questran, TriCor, WelChol, and Zocor	Lower lipid blood levels
Thrombolytic agents	Activase, Eminase, streptokinase, and urokinase	Dissolve clots
Vasodilators	Apresoline, Cardilate, nitroglycerin, and Sorbitrate	Lower blood pressure
Vasopressors	Aramine, Dopastat, and levorphanol tartrate	Raise blood pressure

Study Questions

1. State the function for each of the three major types of blood vessels.

   a. ____

   ____

   b. ____

   ____

   c. ____

   ____

2. The most common site to check a BP is the

   ____.

3. Where is the saphenous vein located?

   ____

4. Why do veins contain valves?

   ____

5. Name the three layers of the heart.

   a. ____

   b. ____

   c. ____

6. Name the vein that carries oxygenated blood.

   ____

7. The contraction phase of the heart is called the ______________________.

8. How does the heart muscle receive oxygen and nutrients?

   ____

9. The chamber of the heart that receives blood from the venae cavae is the ______________.

10. The pacemaker of the heart is the ______________________________.

11. Trace the flow of blood through the heart starting with the vena cava. The pathway should include four chambers, two veins, two arteries, four valves, and one accessory organ.

a. ______________________

b. ______________________

c. ______________________

d. ______________________

e. ______________________

f. ______________________

g. ______________________

h. ______________________

i. ______________________

j. ______________________

k. ______________________

l. ______________________

m. ______________________

12. What is the most common site used to take a pulse rate?

____

13. When using a sphygmomanometer and a stethoscope, what does the first heart sound represent and how is it reported?

____

____

14. Name the three formed elements of the blood and state their function.

	Element	Function
a.	______________	______________
b.	______________	______________
c.	______________	______________

15. Describe what will occur when a person with type B positive blood receives a unit of type A negative blood.

____

____

____

16. Name the leukocyte for each of the following functions.

    a. Recognizes foreign antigens ______________________

    b. Increased in allergies ______________________

    c. Phagocytizes bacteria ______________________

    d. Becomes a macrophage ______________________

    e. Produces antibodies ______________________

    f. Releases histamine ______________________

17. Define:

    a. Leukocytosis

    ____

    b. Leukemia

    ____

    c. Anemia

    ____

18. List three stages of blood coagulation and state the primary process taking place.

Stage	**Primary Process**
a. ______________	______________
b. ______________	______________
c. ______________	______________

19. Name a disorder in which FDPs are elevated.

    ____

20. Name the two coagulation pathways and a test used to monitor each pathway.

Pathway	**Test**
a. ______________	______________
b. ______________	______________

21. Label the indicated parts of the heart.

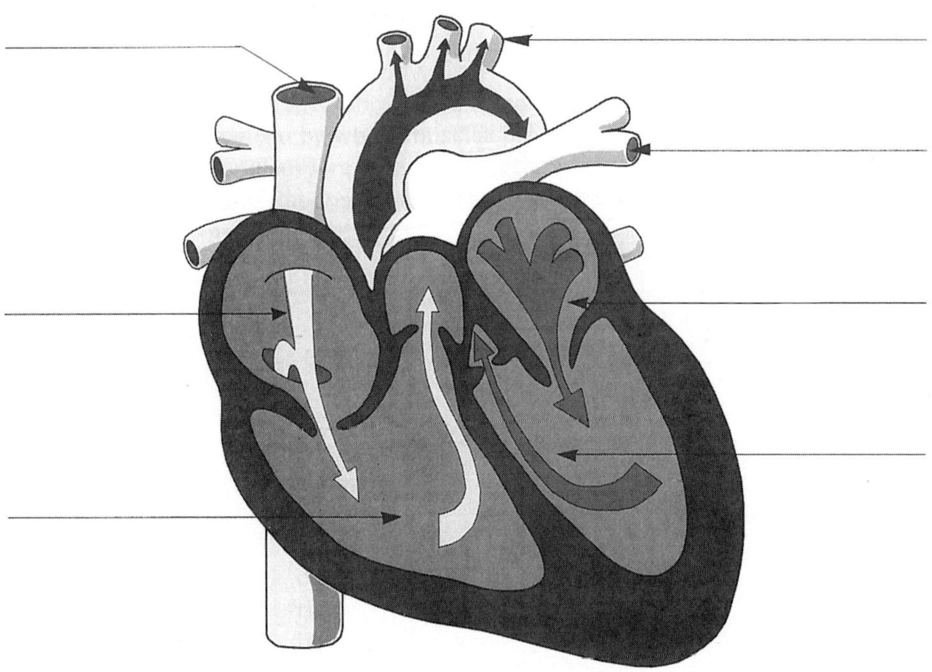

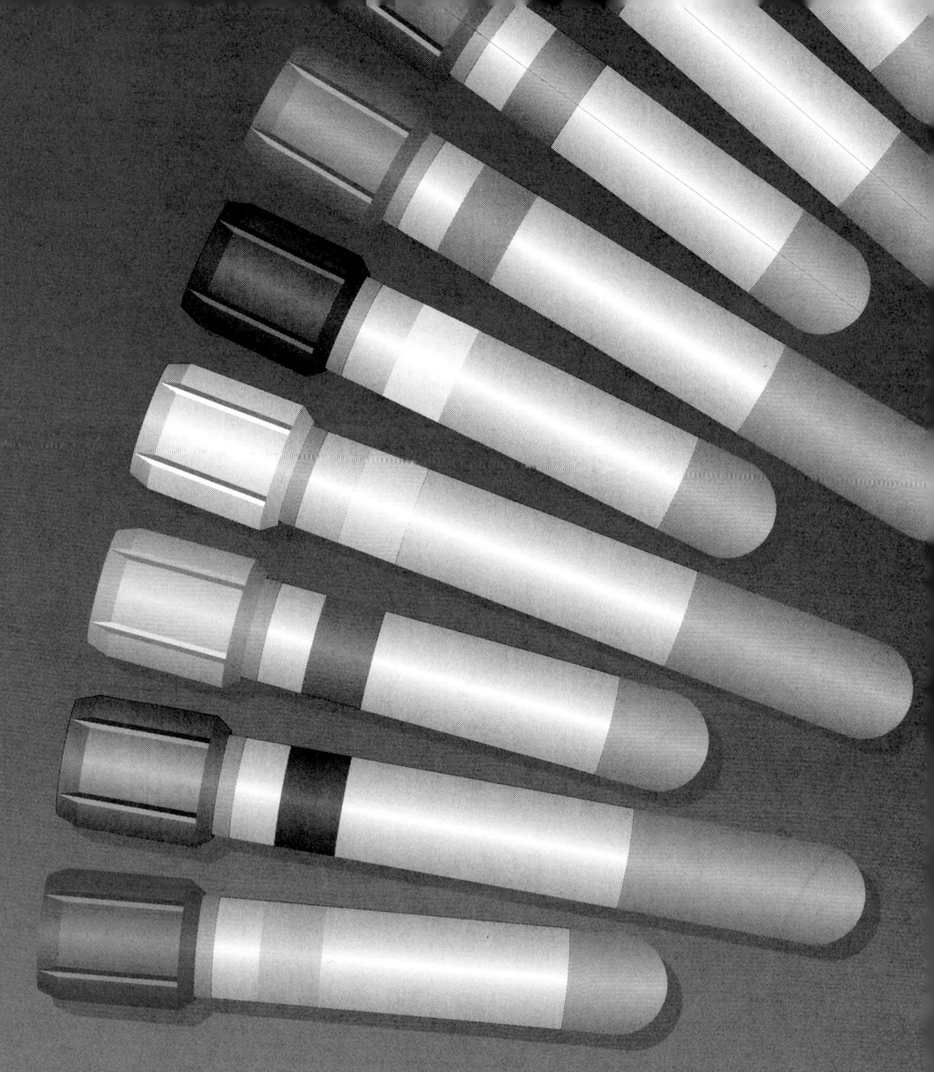

Section Two

Phlebotomy Techniques

Chapter 5

Venipuncture Equipment

Chapter Outline

Organization of Equipment

Evacuated Tube System

Needles

Needle Adapters

Needle Disposal Systems

Collection Tubes

- Principles and Use of Color-Coded Tubes
- Order of Draw

Syringes

Winged Infusion Sets

Tourniquets

Gloves

Puncture Site Protection Supplies

Additional Supplies

Quality Control

Learning Objectives

Upon completion of this chapter, the reader will be able to:

1. Discuss the use of a blood collection tray, transport carriers, and drawing stations.
2. List the items that may be carried on a phlebotomist's tray.
3. Differentiate among the various needle sizes as to gauge and purpose.
4. Describe the OSHA-required safety needles and equipment.
5. Discuss methods to dispose of contaminated needles safely.
6. Differentiate between an evacuated tube system, a syringe, and a winged infusion set, and state the advantages and disadvantages of each.
7. Identify the types of evacuated tubes by color code, and state the anticoagulants and additives present, any special characteristics, and the purpose of each.
8. State the mechanism of action, advantages, and disadvantages of the anticoagulants EDTA, sodium citrate, potassium oxalate, and heparin.
9. List the correct order of draw for the evacuated tube system, and the correct order of fill for tubes collected by syringe.
10. Describe the purpose and types of tourniquets.
11. Name the substances used to cleanse the skin before venipuncture.
12. Discuss the use of sterile gauze, bandages, gloves, and slides when performing venipuncture.
13. Describe the quality control of venipuncture equipment.
14. Correctly select and assemble venipuncture equipment when presented with a clinical situation.

Key Terms

Antiglycolytic agent
Clot activator
Evacuated tube
Thixotropic gel
Winged infusion set

The first step in learning to perform a venipuncture is knowledge of the needed equipment. Considering the many types of blood specimens that may be required for laboratory testing and the risks to both patients and healthcare personnel associated with blood collection, it is understandable that a considerable amount of equipment is required for the procedure. This chapter covers the latest types of equipment used when performing venipunctures with evacuated tube systems, syringes, and ***winged infusion sets***. Discussion includes the advantages and disadvantages of the various pieces of equipment, the situations in which they are used, and when appropriate, the mechanisms by which the equipment works.

Equipment necessary to perform venipunctures includes needles, safety needle disposal containers, needle holders (adapters), blood collection tubes, syringes, winged infusion sets, tourniquets, **antiseptic** cleansing solutions, gauze pads, bandages, and gloves.

Organization of Equipment

An important key to successful blood collection is making sure that all the required equipment is conveniently present in the collection area. Maintaining a well-equipped blood collection tray that the phlebotomist carries into the patient's room is the ideal way to prevent unnecessary errors during blood collection. Trays designed to organize and transport collection equipment are available from several manufacturers (Fig. 5–1). The phlebotomy tray provides a convenient way for the phlebotomist to carry equipment to the patients' rooms. Except in isolation situations, the tray is carried into the patient's room. It should be placed on a solid surface, such as a night stand, and not on the patient's bed, where it could be knocked off. Only the needed equipment should be brought directly to the patient's bed.

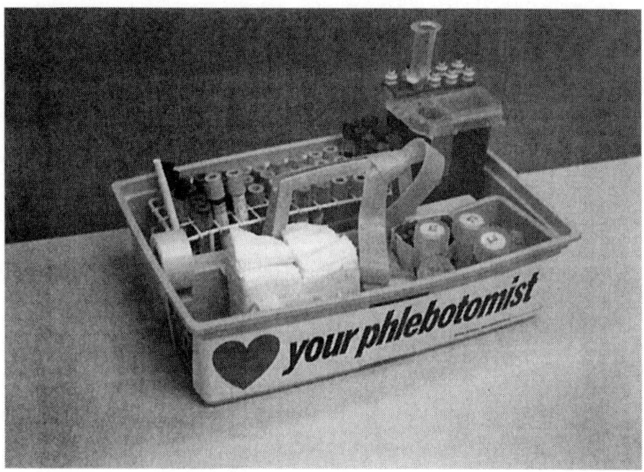

Figure 5–1. Phlebotomy collection tray.

technical tip A well-organized tray instills patient confidence.

Mobile phlebotomy workstations with swivel caster wheels have replaced the traditional phlebotomy tray in some institutions. With the increased amounts of required equipment necessary for safe phlebotomy, these versatile mobile workstations can be configured to accommodate phlebotomy trays, hazardous waste containers, sharps containers, and storage drawers and shelves. The cart is designed to be wheeled around the hospital and up to the patient's bedside to eliminate placing equipment or a phlebotomy tray on the patient's bed (Fig. 5–2).

In outpatient settings, a more permanent arrangement can be located at the drawing station (Fig. 5–3). A blood drawing chair has an attached or adjacently placed stand to hold equipment. Drawing chairs have an armrest that locks in place in front of the patient to provide arm support and protect the patient from falling out of the chair if he or she faints. A reclining chair or bed should be available for special procedures or for patients who feel faint or ill. Infant cradle pads are available for collection of blood from an infant (Fig. 5–4).

The duties of a phlebotomist include the cleaning, disinfecting, and restocking of the phlebotomy trays, work stations, and outpatient drawing stations. Trays should be totally emptied and disinfected on a weekly basis. Trays also contain equipment for performing the microcollection techniques to be discussed in Chapter 9.

Evacuated Tube System

The evacuated tube system (Fig. 5–5) is the most frequently used method for performing venipunc-

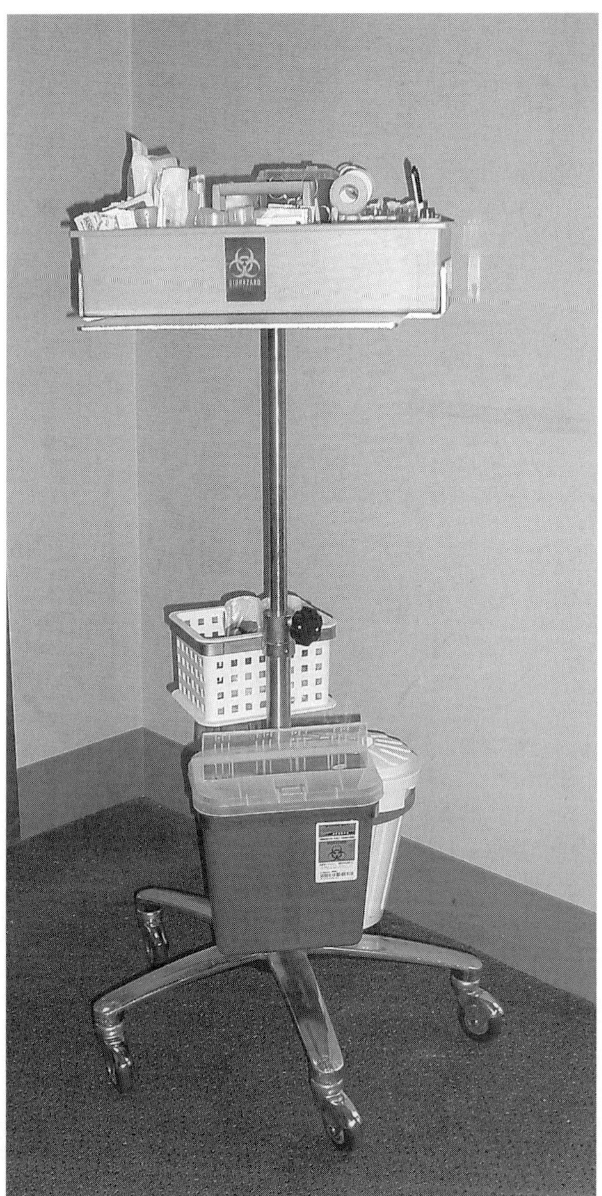

Figure 5–2. Mobile phlebotomy workstation.

ture. Blood is collected directly into the evacuated tube, eliminating the need for transfer of specimens and minimizing the risk of biohazard exposure. The evacuated tube system consists of a double-pointed needle to puncture the stopper of the collection tube, an adapter to hold the needle and blood collection tube, and color-coded evacuated tubes.

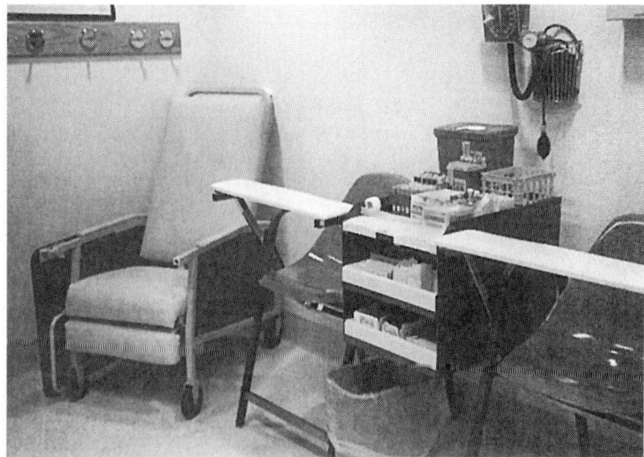

Figure 5–3. Phlebotomy drawing station, including a reclining chair.

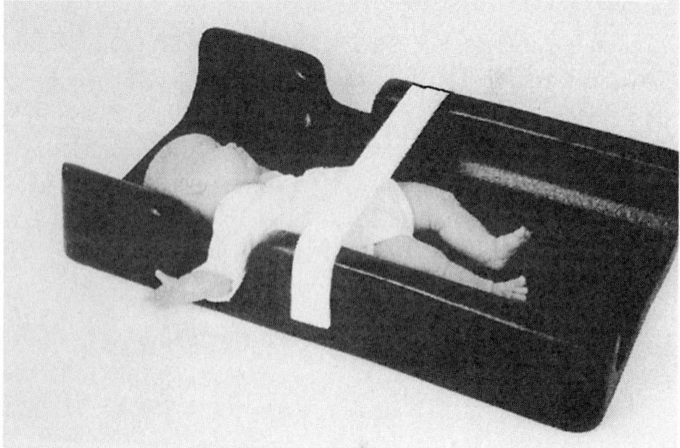

Figure 5–4. Infant cradle pad. (Courtesy of Innovative Laboratory Acrylics, Inc., Brighton, MI.)

Needles

All needles used in venipuncture are disposable and are used only once. Needle size varies by both length and gauge (diameter). For routine venipuncture 1-inch and 1.5-inch lengths are used.

Needle **gauge** refers to the diameter of the needle bore. Needles vary from large (16-gauge) needles used to collect units of blood for transfusion to much smaller (23-gauge) needles used for very small veins. Notice that the smaller the gauge number the bigger the diameter of the needle. Needles with gauges smaller than 23 are available, but they can cause hemolysis when used for drawing blood specimens. They are most frequently used for injections and intravenous (IV) infusions.

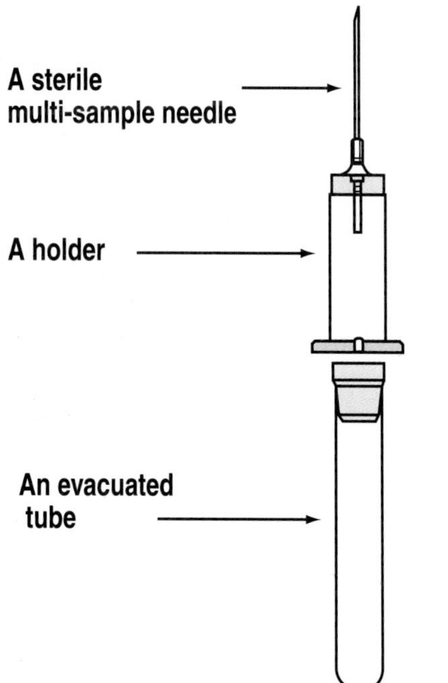

Figure 5–5. Evacuated tube system. (From Wedding, ME, and Toenjes, SA: Medical Laboratory Procedures, ed 2. FA Davis, Philadelphia, 1998, p. 95, with permission.)

technical tip Many phlebotomists believe that using a 1-inch needle gives better control and is less frightening to the patient.

Manufacturers package needles individually in sterile twist-apart sealed shields that are color coded by gauge for easy identification. Needles must not be used if the seal is broken.

As shown in Figure 5–6, needle structure varies to adapt to the type of collection equipment being used. All needles consist of a **beveled** point, shaft, **lumen**, and hub. Needles should be visually examined before use to determine if any structural defects, such as nonbeveled points or bent shafts, are present. Defective needles should not be used. Needles should never be recapped once the shield is removed regardless of whether they have or have not been used.

Evacuated tube system needles are threaded in the middle and have a beveled point at each end designed so that one end is for phlebotomy and the other end punctures the rubber stopper of the evacuated blood collection tube. Evacuated tube system

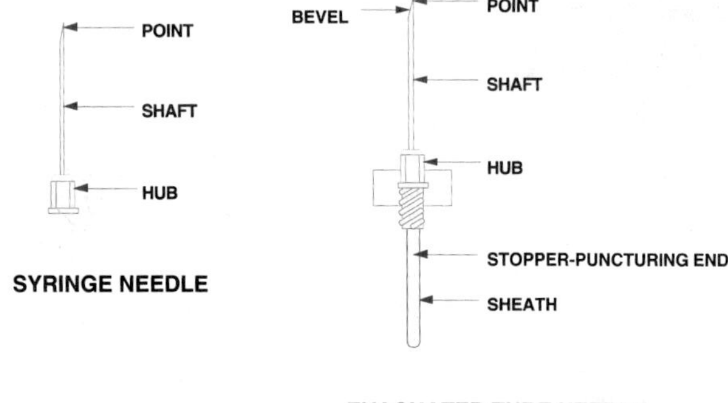

Figure 5–6. Needle structure.

needles are designated as multi-sample needles. Multi-sample needles have the puncturing needle covered by a rubber sheath that is pushed back when a tube is attached and returns to full needle coverage when the tube is removed. This prevents leakage of blood when tubes are being changed. The increased possibility of blood contamination when using single-sample needles, even when only one tube of blood is being drawn, has caused most institutions to use multi-sample needles for all venipunctures. However, phlebotomists should check the type of needle when working in an unfamiliar setting.

The Needlestick Prevention and Safety Act has mandated the evaluation and use of safety needle devices. State mandates also have been issued. Various safety shields and blunting devices are available from different manufacturers. The BD Vacutainer Eclipse™ blood collection needle (Becton, Dickinson, Franklin Lakes, NJ) uses a shield that the phlebotomist locks over the needle tip after completion of the venipuncture (Fig. 5–7).

Self-blunting needles (PUNCTUR-GUARD by ICU Medical Inc., San Clemente, CA) are available to provide additional protection against needlestick injuries by making the needles blunt before removal from the patient. A hollow, blunt inner needle is contained inside the standard needle. Before removing the needle from the patient's vein, an additional push on the final tube in the adapter advances the internal blunt cannula past the sharp tip of the outer needle. The blunt cannula is hollow, allowing blood to continue to flow into the tube (Fig. 5–8).

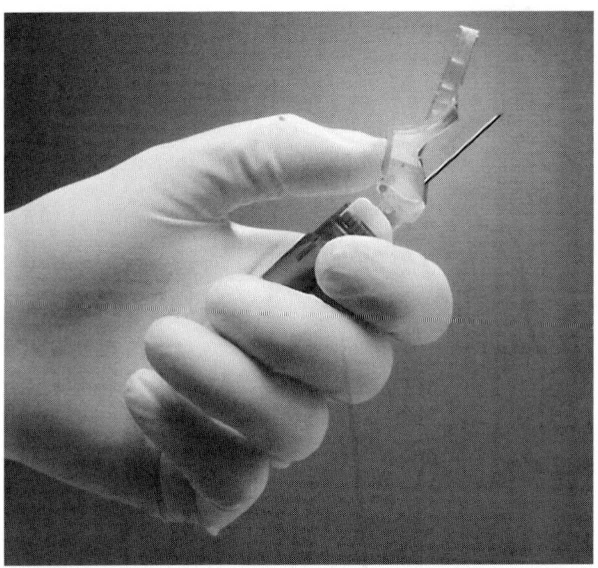

Figure 5–7. Eclipse™ blood collection needle. (Courtesy of Becton, Dickinson and Company © 2002 BD.)

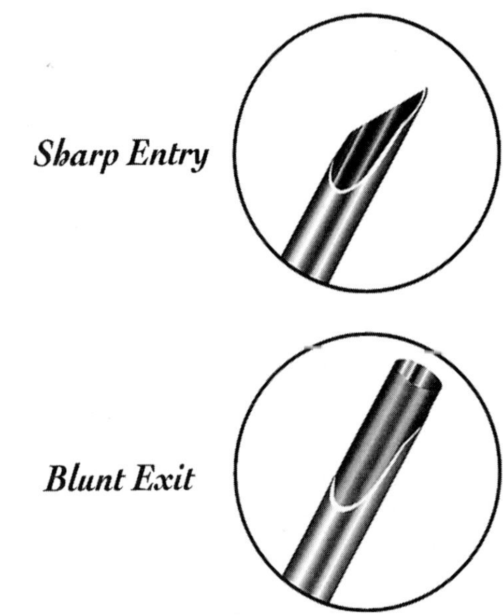

Figure 5–8. Blunting needle principle. (Courtesy of ICU Medical Inc., San Clemente, CA.)

Needle Adapters

Needles used in the evacuated tube collection systems attach to an adapter that holds the collection tube. Adapters are made of clear, rigid plastic and may be designed to act as a safety shield for the used needle. As discussed in Chapter 3, the Occupational Safety and Health Administration (OSHA) directs that adapters must be discarded with the used needle.

The One-Use Holder by Becton, Dickinson is available with a different threading to allow a needle to be threaded into the adapter only one time. The entire needle/adapter assembly is discarded in a sharps container after use. Another safety device is the Venipuncture Needle-Pro (Portex, Inc., Keene, NH), which consists of a plastic sheath attached by a hinge to the end of the evacuated tube adapter. The shield hangs free during the venipuncture and is engaged over the needle using a single-handed technique against a flat surface after the puncture is performed. The plastic shield can be rotated to provide the phlebotomist a better view of the venipuncture site and needle placement. The entire device is discarded in the sharps container. The ProGuard II safety needle holder (Kendall Healthcare, Manchester, MA) provides a one-handed method to retract the needle into the holder and a cover for the end that is open to the stopper-puncturing needle (Fig. 5–9).

Adapters are available to accommodate collection tubes of different sizes. To provide proper puncturing of the rubber stopper and maximum control, tubes should fit securely in the adapter. Adapters are

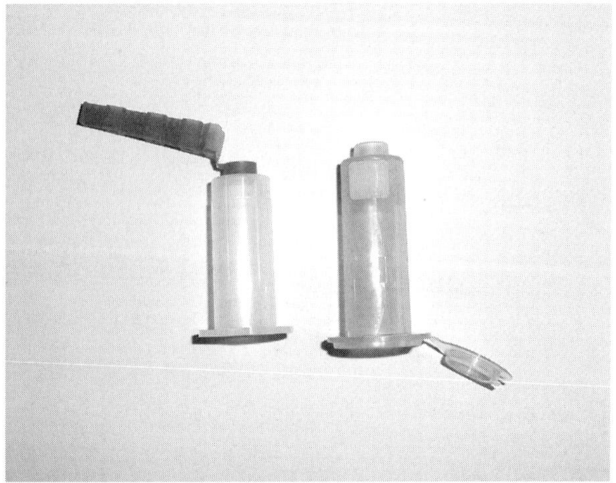

Figure 5–9. Portex Venipuncture Needle-Pro and Kendall ProGuard II safety needle holder.

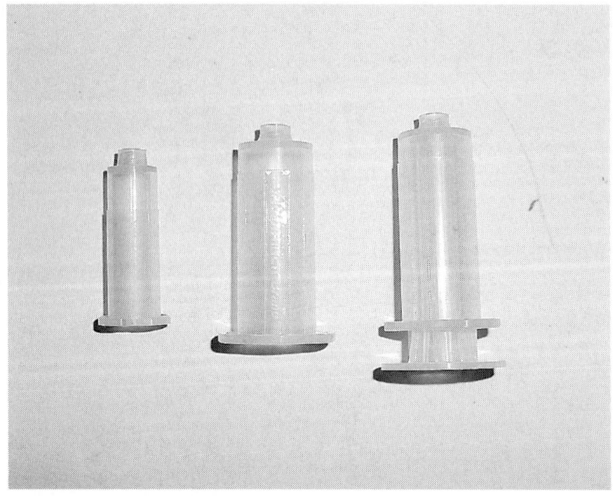

Figure 5–10. Pediatric tube adapter, regular size tube adapter, and regular size tube adapter with pediatric insert.

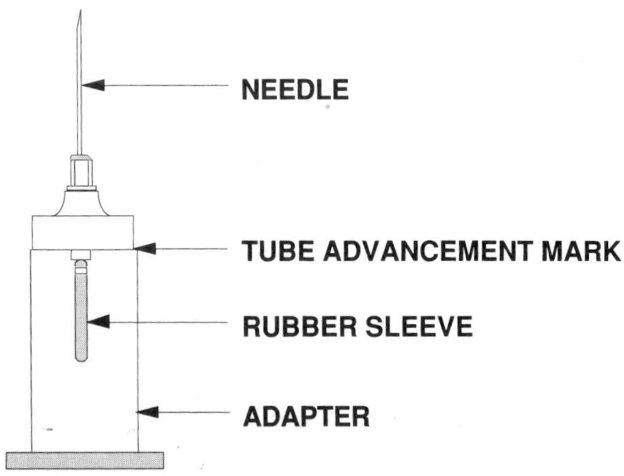

Figure 5–11. Diagram of a basic needle adapter.

available in two sizes to fit both regular and pediatric tubes. Ribbed pediatric adapter inserts can be inserted into the regular size adapter for pediatric tubes (Fig. 5–10).

The rubber-sheathed puncturing end of an evacuated tube system needle screws securely into the small opening at one end of the adapter, and the evacuated blood collection tube is placed into the large opening at the opposite end of the adapter. The first tube can be partially advanced onto the stopper-puncturing needle in the adapter. A marking near the top of the adapter indicates the distance an evacuated tube may be advanced into the stopper-puncturing needle without entering the tube and losing the vacuum (Fig. 5–11). The tube is fully advanced to the end of the adapter when the needle is in the vein. Blood will flow into the tube once the needle penetrates the stopper. The flared ends of the needle adapter aid the phlebotomist during the changing of tubes in multiple-sample situations. Tubes are removed with a slight twist to help disengage them from the needle.

technical tip Loss of tube vacuum is a primary cause of failure to obtain blood. The venipuncture can be performed before placing the tube on the needle. Practice both methods, and choose the one with which you are most comfortable.

Needle Disposal Systems

To protect phlebotomists from accidental needlesticks by contaminated needles, a means of safe disposal must be available whenever phlebotomy is performed. In recent years, owing to the increased concern over exposure to bloodborne pathogens and mandates by the OSHA, many disposal systems have been developed.

Needles must always be placed in rigid, puncture-resistant, leak-proof disposable containers labeled BIOHAZARD that are easily sealed when full. Syringes with the needles attached, winged infusion sets, and adapters with needles attached are disposed of directly into puncture-resistant containers (Fig. 5–12).

Under no circumstances should a needle be recapped.

technical tip To prevent accidental punctures from contaminated needles, become thoroughly familiar with the operation of your needle safety system before performing blood collection.

Collection Tubes

The collection tubes used with the evacuated system are often referred to as Vacutainers™ (Becton, Dickinson, Franklin Lakes, NJ), although they are also available from other manufacturers. Use of ***evacuated tubes*** with their corresponding needles

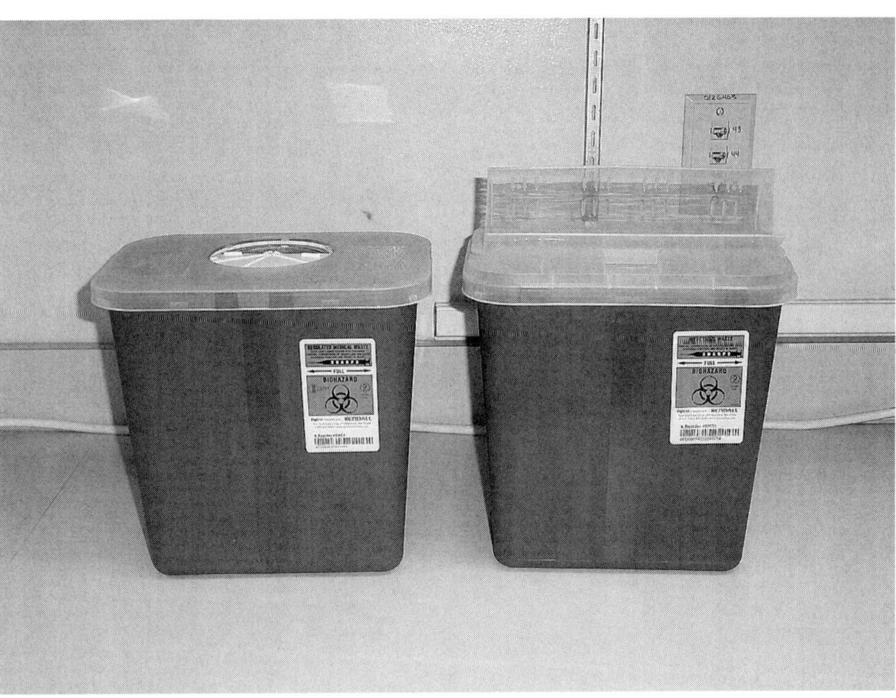

Figure 5–12. Sharps disposal containers.

and adapters provides a means of collecting blood directly into the tube. Laboratory instrumentation is also available for direct sampling from the evacuated tubes, providing additional protection for laboratory workers.

The amount of blood collected in an evacuated tube ranges from 1.8 to 15 mL and is determined by the size of the tube and the amount of vacuum present. As shown in Figure 5–13, a wide variety of sizes is available to accommodate adult, pediatric, and geriatric patients. When selecting the appropriate size tube, the phlebotomist must consider the amount of blood needed and the size and condition of the patient's veins. Using a 23-gauge needle with a large evacuated tube can produce hemolysis, because red blood cells are damaged when the large amount of vacuum causes them to be rapidly pulled through the small lumen of the needle. Therefore, if it is necessary to use a small-gauge needle, the phlebotomist should collect two small tubes instead of one large tube.

Evacuated tubes are available in glass and plastic (Plus tubes). Most tubes are sterile and many are silicone coated to prevent cells from adhering to the tube, or to prevent the activation of clotting factors in coagulation studies. Information about the characteristics of a tube is contained on the write-on label attached to the tube and should be verified by the phlebotomist when special collection procedures are needed. Tubes may also contain anticoagulants and additives. The tubes are labeled with the type of anticoagulant or additive, the draw volume, and the expiration date. The manufacturer guarantees the integrity of the anticoagulant and vacuum in the tube until the expiration date.

As shown in Figure 5–14, evacuated tubes have thick rubber stoppers with a thinner central area to allow puncture by the needle. To aid the phlebotomist in identifying the many types of evacuated tubes, the stoppers are color-coded. Color coding for routinely used tubes is uniform among manufacturers, and instructions for sample collection usually refer to the tube color. This reference to tube color is found on most computer-generated forms. Each laboratory department has specified specimen requirements for the analysis of particular blood constituents. Phlebotomists and phlebotomy students should also understand that testing methodologies and types of instrumentation vary among laboratories. Therefore, the type of tube collected for a particular test may not be the same in all facilities. Direct sampling instrumentation may also be designed to only accept a specific type of tube, such as a rubber stopper and not a Hemogard closure or vice versa.

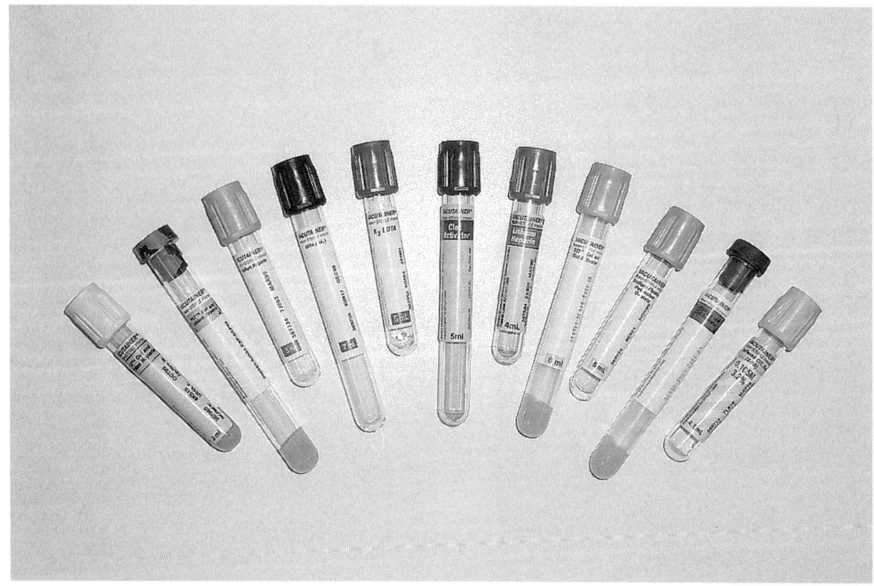

Figure 5–13. Examples of evacuated tubes.

EXAMPLE: Draw one red top, one light blue top, and one lavender top tube.

Two types of color-coded tops are available. Rubber stoppers may be colored, or a color-coded plastic shield may cover the stopper, as with the Hemogard Vacutainer System. Removing the rubber stoppers from evacuated tubes can be hazardous to laboratory personnel because an aerosol of blood can be produced if the stopper is quickly "popped off." Stoppers should be covered with a gauze pad and slowly loosened with the opening facing away from the body. Hemogard closures provide additional protection against blood splatter by allowing the stoppers to be easily twisted and pulled off and have a shield over the stopper. The plastic shield protects the phlebotomist from blood that remains on the stopper after the tubes are removed from the needle. The color of the Hemogard closures varies slightly from that of rubber stoppers.

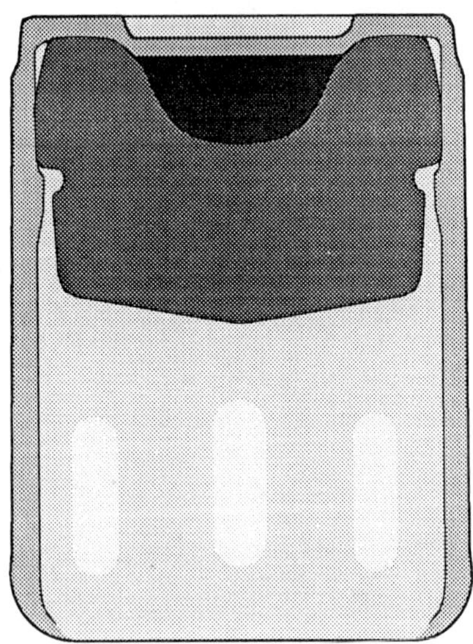

Figure 5–14. Cut-away view of a vacuum tube stopper (Hemogard closure). (Adapted from product literature, Becton, Dickinson, Franklin Lakes, NJ.)

Evacuated tubes fill automatically because a premeasured vacuum is present in the tube. This causes some tubes to fill almost to the top, whereas other tubes only partially fill. Partial-fill tubes are distinguished from regular-fill tubes by translucent colored Hemogard closures in the same color as regular-fill tubes.

Principles and Use of Color-Coded Tubes

Color coding indicates the type of specimen that will be obtained when a particular tube is used. As discussed in Chapter 2, tests may be run on plasma, serum, or whole blood. Tests may also require the presence of preservatives, inhibitors, clot activators, or barrier gels. To produce these necessary conditions, some tubes contain anticoagulants or additives, and others do not. Phlebotomists must be able to relate the color of the collection tubes to the types of specimens needed and to any special techniques, such as tube inversion, that may be required. This section discusses the routinely used tubes with regard to anticoagulants, additives, types of tests for which they are used, and special handling required.

Tests requiring whole blood or plasma are collected in tubes containing an anticoagulant to prevent clotting of the specimen. Anticoagulants prevent clotting by binding calcium or inhibiting thrombin in the coagulation cascade (Fig. 5–15). All tubes containing an anticoagulant must be gently inverted three to eight times immediately after collection to mix the contents and to avoid microclot formation. Before use, tubes with powdered anticoagulant should be gently tapped to loosen the powder from the tube for better mixing with the blood.

technical tip For anticoagulants to totally prevent clotting, specimens must be thoroughly mixed immediately following collection.

Lavender (Purple) Top

Lavender stopper tubes and Hemogard closures contain the anticoagulant ethylenediaminetetraacetic acid (EDTA) in the form of liquid tripotassium or spray-dried dipotassium ethylenediaminetetraacetic acid (**K_3EDTA** or **K_2EDTA**). Coagulation is prevented by the binding of calcium in the specimen to sites on the large EDTA molecule, thereby preventing the participation of the calcium in the coagulation cascade (see Fig. 5–15). Lavender stopper tubes should be gently inverted eight times.

For hematology procedures that require whole blood, such as the complete blood count (CBC), EDTA is the anticoagulant of choice because it maintains cellular integrity better than other anticoagulants, inhibits platelet clumping, and does not interfere with routine staining procedures. The lavender stopper tube should be completely filled to avoid excess EDTA that may shrink the red blood cells and decrease the hematocrit level, red blood cell indices, and erythrocyte sedimentation rate (ESR) results.

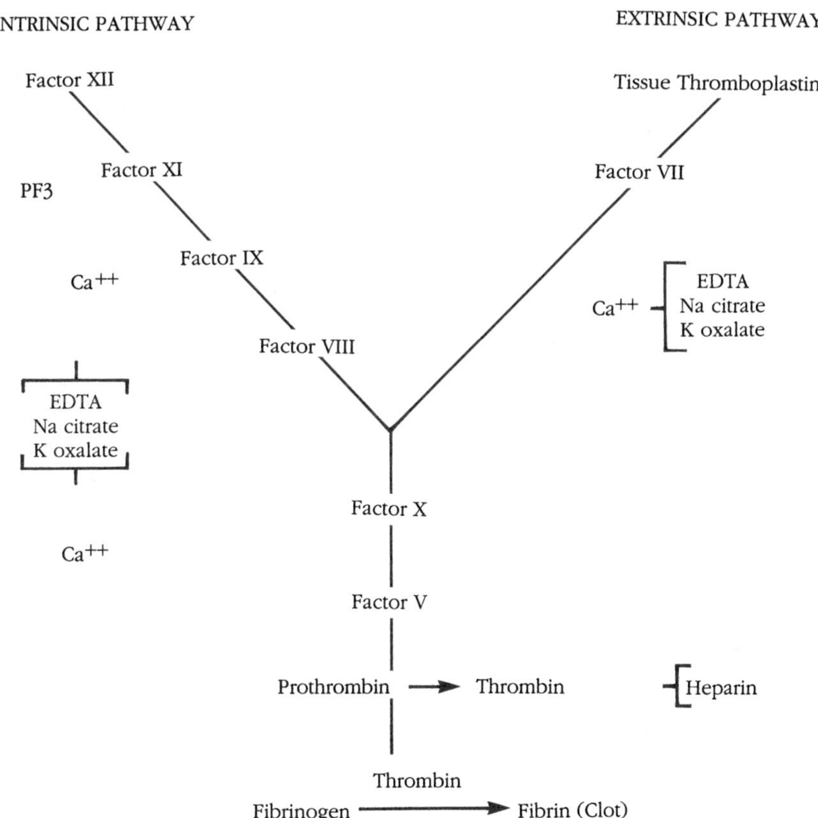

Figure 5–15. The role of anticoagulants in the coagulation cascade. (Ca^{++} = calcium; PF3 = platelet factor 3.)

Lavender stopper tubes cannot be used for coagulation studies because EDTA interferes with factor V and the thrombin-fibrinogen reaction.

Pink Top

Pink Hemogard closure tubes also contain a spray-dried K_2EDTA anticoagulant and are used specifically for blood bank in some facilities. Using a designated tube for blood bank is believed to help prevent testing of specimens from the wrong patient. The tubes are designed with special labels for patient information required by the American Association of Blood Banks (**AABB**). Tubes should be inverted eight times.

White Top

White Hemogard closure tubes containing a spray-dried K_2EDTA anticoagulant and a separation gel are called plasma preparation tubes (**PPTs**). This differentiates them from plasma separator tubes that contain heparin as the anticoagulant. White Hemogard closure tubes are primarily used for molecular diagnostics but can be used for myocardial infarction (MI) panels and ammonia levels, depending on the test methodology and instrumentation. Tubes should be inverted eight times.

Light Blue Top

Light blue stopper tubes and Hemogard closures contain the anticoagulant sodium citrate, which also prevents coagulation by binding calcium. Centrifugation of the anticoagulated light-blue stopper tubes provides the plasma used for coagulation tests. Sodium citrate (3.2% or 3.8%) is the required anticoagulant for coagulation studies because it preserves the **labile** coagulation factors. Tubes should be inverted three to four times. The ratio of blood to the liquid sodium citrate is critical and should be 9 to 1 (example: 4.5 mL blood and 0.5 mL sodium citrate). Therefore, light blue stopper tubes must be completely filled to ensure accurate results.

When collecting coagulation tests on patients with **polycythemia** or hematocrit readings greater than 55%, the amount of citrate anticoagulant should be decreased to prevent an increased amount of citrate in the plasma. The increased citrate in the specimen will interfere with the coagulation tests. The National Committee on Clinical Laboratory Standards (NCCLS) recommends the use of tubes containing 3.2% sodium citrate to prevent this problem. If necessary, tubes can also be specially prepared as described in the NCCLS guideline.

A special blue stopper tube containing thrombin and a soybean trypsin inhibitor is used when drawing blood for determinations of certain fibrin degradation products.

technical tip The laboratory always rejects incompletely filled light blue stopper tubes.

Black Top

Black stopper tubes containing buffered sodium citrate are used for Westergren sedimentation rates. They differ from light-blue top tubes in that they provide a ratio of blood to liquid anticoagulant of 4 to 1. Specially designed tubes for Westergren sedimentation rates are available.

Green Top

Green stopper tubes and Hemogard closures contain the anticoagulant heparin combined with sodium, lithium, or ammonium ion. Heparin prevents clotting by inhibiting thrombin in the coagulation cascade (see Fig. 5–15). Green stopper tubes are primarily used for chemistry tests performed on whole blood or plasma, particularly stat electrolytes. Interference by sodium and lithium heparin with their corresponding chemical tests and by ammonium heparin in blood urea nitrogen (BUN) determinations must be avoided. In general, lithium heparin has been shown to produce the least interference. Tubes should be inverted eight times. Green stopper tubes are not used for hematology because heparin interferes with the Wright's stained blood smear. Heparin causes the stain to have a blue background on the blood smear, making it difficult to interpret the differential cell identification.

Light Green Top

Light green Hemogard closure tubes and *green/black* stopper tubes containing lithium heparin and a separation gel are called plasma separator tubes (**PSTs**). PSTs are used for plasma determinations in chemistry. They are well suited for potassium determinations because heparin prevents the release of potassium by platelets during clotting, and the gel prevents contamination by red blood cell potassium. Tubes should be inverted eight times.

Gray Top

Gray stopper tubes and Hemogard closures are available with a variety of anticoagulants and additives for the primary purpose of preserving glucose. All gray stopper tubes contain a glucose preservative (***antiglycolytic agent***), either sodium fluoride or lithium iodoacetate. Sodium fluoride maintains glucose stability for 3 days and iodoacetate for 24 hours. Sodium fluoride and iodoacetate are not anticoagulants; therefore, if plasma is needed for analysis, an anticoagulant must also be present and the tubes must be inverted eight times. In gray stopper tubes the anticoagulant is potassium oxalate or K_2EDTA, which prevents clotting by binding calcium. When monitoring patient glucose levels, tubes for the collection of plasma and serum should not be interchanged. Sodium fluoride will interfere with some enzyme analyses; therefore, gray stopper tubes should not be used for other chemistry analyses. Gray stopper tubes are not used in hematology because oxalate distorts cellular morphology.

Blood alcohol levels are drawn in gray stopper tubes containing sodium fluoride to inhibit microbial growth, which could produce alcohol as a metabolic end product. Tubes with or without potassium oxalate can be used, depending on the need for plasma or serum in the test procedure.

Royal Blue Top

Royal blue stopper tubes and Hemogard closures are used for toxicology, trace metal, and nutritional analyses. Because many of the elements analyzed in these studies are significant at very low levels, the tubes must be chemically clean and the rubber stoppers are specially formulated to contain the lowest possible levels of metal. Royal blue stopper tubes are available plain or with sodium heparin to conform to a variety of testing requirements. Tubes with an anticoagulant present must be inverted eight times.

Tan Top

Tan Hemogard closure tubes are available for lead determinations. They are certified to contain less than 0.1 μg/mL of lead. The glass tubes contain the anticoagulant sodium heparin and the plastic tubes contain K_2EDTA; both types of tubes must be inverted eight times.

Yellow Top

Yellow stopper tubes are available for two different purposes and contain different additives. Yellow stopper tubes containing the red blood cell preservative acid citrate dextrose (**ACD**) are used for cellular studies in blood bank, human leukocyte antigen (**HLA**) phenotyping, and paternity testing.

Sterile yellow stopper tubes containing the anticoagulant sodium polyanetholesulfonate (**SPS**) are used to collect specimens to be cultured for the presence of microorganisms. SPS aids in the recovery of microorganisms by inhibiting the actions of complement, phagocytes, and certain antibiotics. Yellow stopper tubes should be inverted eight times.

Yellow/Gray and Orange Top

Yellow/gray stopper tubes and *orange* Hemogard closures are found on tubes containing the ***clot activator*** thrombin. Notice in Figure 5–15 that thrombin is generated near the end of the coagulation cascade; addition of thrombin to the tube results in faster clot formation, usually within 5 minutes. Tubes should be inverted eight times. Tubes containing thrombin are used for stat serum chemistry determinations and on samples from patients receiving anticoagulant therapy.

Red/Gray and Gold Top

Red/gray stopper tubes and *gold Hemogard closures* are found on tubes containing a clot activator and a separation gel. They are frequently referred to as serum separator tubes (**SSTs**). Clot activators such as glass particles, silica, and celite increase platelet activation, thereby shortening the time required for clot formation. Tubes should be inverted five times to expose the blood to the clot activator. A nonreactive ***thixotropic gel*** that undergoes a temporary change in viscosity during centrifugation is located at the bottom of the tube. As shown in Figure 5–16, when the tube is centrifuged, the gel forms a barrier between the cells and serum to prevent contamination of the serum with cellular materials. To produce a solid separation barrier, specimens must be allowed to clot completely before centrifuging. Clotting time is approximately 30 minutes.

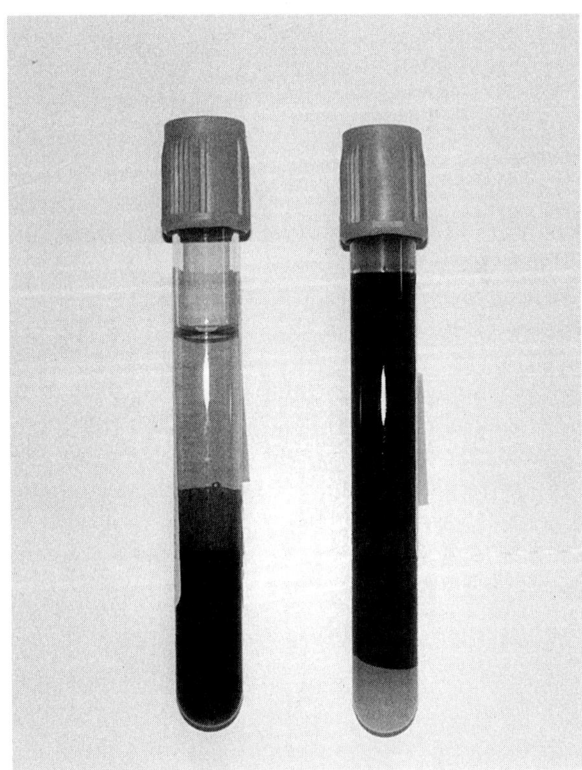

Figure 5–16. Centrifuged and uncentrifuged SSTs. (From Strasinger, SK, and Di Lorenzo, MS: Skills for the Patient Care Technician. FA Davis, Philadelphia, 1999, p. 119, with permission.)

Specimens should be centrifuged as soon as clot formation is complete.

technical tip Centrifugation of incompletely clotted SST tubes can produce a nonintact gel barrier and possible cellular contamination of the serum.

SSTs are used for most chemistry tests and prevent contamination of the serum by cellular chemicals and products of cellular metabolism. They are not suitable for use in the blood bank and certain immunology and serology tests because the gel may interfere with the immunologic reactions. SSTs are also not recommended for therapeutic drug testing.

Red Top

Red stopper glass tubes and Hemogard closures are often referred to as "plain" or "clot" tubes because they contain no anticoagulants or additives. Blood drawn in red stopper tubes clots by the normal coagulation process in about 60 minutes. Centrifuging then yields serum as the liquid portion. Red stopper tubes are used for serum chemistry tests, serology tests, and in blood bank, where both serum and red blood cells are used. There is no need to invert red stopper tubes.

Notice the emphasis placed on glass red stopper tubes. Plastic with red Hemogard closure tubes are also available, and these tubes contain silica as a clot activator. They are used for the same purpose as the glass tubes except that they are not recommended for blood banking. Red stopper plastic tubes are inverted five times to initiate the clotting process.

Evacuated tubes are summarized in Table 5–1. Appendix I lists laboratory tests and the required types of anticoagulants and volume of blood required.

Order of Draw

When collecting multiple specimens and specimens for coagulation tests, the order in which tubes are drawn can affect some test results. Tubes must be collected in a specific order to prevent invalid test results caused by bacterial contamination, tissue fluid contamination, or carry-over of additives or anticoagulants between tubes.

technical tip Following the correct order of draw is essential to ensure accurate test results.

As shown in Figure 5–15, the extrinsic pathway of the coagulation cascade is initiated by the presence of tissue thromboplastin. Release of tissue thromboplastin from the skin as it is punctured can result in its presence in the first tube collected, and this could interfere with coagulation tests. Therefore, a light blue stopper tube should not be drawn first. If only a coagulation test is ordered, it is recommended that a small red stopper tube be drawn first; it can be discarded if it is not needed. Recent studies suggest that the discard tube may no longer be necessary for routine coagulation tests (activated partial thromboplastin time [APTT] and prothrombin time [PT]), but it is still required for special coagulation tests. It is important that the phlebotomist follow the blood collection protocol of the facility.

TABLE 5-1
Summary of Evacuated Tubes

Stopper Color	Anticoagulant/Additive	Specimen Type	Laboratory Use
Lavender	Ethylenediaminetetraacetic acid (EDTA)	Whole blood/plasma	Hematology
Pink	EDTA	Whole blood/plasma	Blood bank
White	EDTA and gel	Plasma	Molecular diagnostics
Light blue	Sodium citrate	Plasma	Coagulation
Red/gray, gold	Clot activator and gel	Serum	Chemistry
Green	Ammonium heparin Lithium heparin Sodium heparin	Whole blood/plasma	Chemistry
Light green, green/black	Lithium heparin and gel	Plasma	Chemistry
Red (glass)	None	Serum	Blood bank, chemistry, serology
Red (plastic)	Clot activator	Serum	Chemistry, serology
Yellow/gray, orange	Thrombin	Serum	Chemistry
Gray	Potassium oxalate/sodium fluoride Sodium fluoride Sodium fluoride/K_2EDTA Lithium iodoacetate Lithium heparin/iodoacetate	Plasma Serum Plasma Serum Plasma	Chemistry glucose tests
Tan	Sodium heparin K_2EDTA	Plasma Plasma	Chemistry lead tests
Royal blue	Sodium heparin Na_2EDTA None	Plasma Plasma Serum	Chemistry trace elements, toxicology, and nutrient analyses
Yellow	Sodium polyanetholesulfonate (SPS)	Whole blood	Microbiology blood cultures
	Acid citrate dextrose (ACD)	Whole blood	Blood bank
Black	Sodium citrate	Whole blood	Hematology sedimentation rates

Transfer of anticoagulants among tubes because of possible contamination of the stopper-puncturing needle must be avoided. This is why the red stopper tube is drawn before the coagulation tube and why tubes containing other anticoagulants are drawn after the light blue stopper tube. EDTA and heparin can cause falsely increased PT and APTT time results. Also, tubes containing EDTA, which can bind calcium and iron, should not be drawn before a tube for chemistry tests on these substances. Contamination of a green or red stopper tube designated for sodium, potassium, and calcium determinations with EDTA, sodium citrate, or potassium oxalate would falsely decrease the calcium and elevate the sodium or potassium results. Holding blood collection tubes in a downward position so that the tube fills from the bottom up helps avoid the transfer of anticoagulants from tube to tube.

When sterile specimens, such as blood cultures, are to be collected, they must be considered in the order of draw. Such specimens are always drawn first to prevent microbial contamination. The order of draw as recommended by the NCCLS is:

1 Sterile specimens (yellow stopper tubes, culture bottles)
2 Glass red stopper tubes (plain, nonadditive)
3 Light blue stopper tubes (sodium citrate)
4 Plastic red stopper tubes (clot activator)
5 Red/gray, gold stopper tubes (serum separator tubes)
6 Green stopper tubes (heparin)

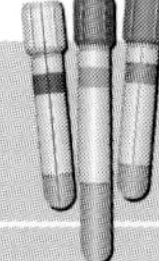

Tests Affected by Anticoagulant Contamination

- EDTA
  - Calcium
  - Activated partial thromboplastin time
  - Potassium
  - Prothrombin time
  - Iron
  - Sodium
- Heparin
  - Activated clotting time
  - Activated partial thromboplastin time
  - Prothrombin time
  - Sodium (Na heparin)
  - Lithium (Li heparin)
  - BUN (ammonium heparin)
  - Ammonia (ammonium heparin)
- Potassium Oxalate
  - Potassium
  - Red blood cell morphology

7 Light green stopper tubes (plasma separator tube)
8 Lavender stopper tubes (EDTA)
9 Gray stopper tubes (oxalate/fluoride)
10 Yellow/gray or orange stopper tubes (thrombin clot activator)

Other colored stopper tubes that contain EDTA such as the pink, white, and tan should be drawn in the same order as the lavender stopper tube. If the royal blue or tan stopper tube contains the anticoagulant sodium heparin, it should be drawn in the same order as the green stopper tubes. When the royal blue stopper tube does not contain an anticoagulant, it should be drawn in the same order as nonadditive tubes.

Syringes

Syringes are often preferred over an evacuated tube system when drawing blood from patients with small or fragile veins. The advantage of this system is that the phlebotomist is able to control the suction pressure on the vein by slowly withdrawing the syringe plunger.

Syringes consist of a barrel graduated in milliliters (mL) or cubic centimeters (cc) and a plunger that fits tightly within the barrel, creating a vacuum

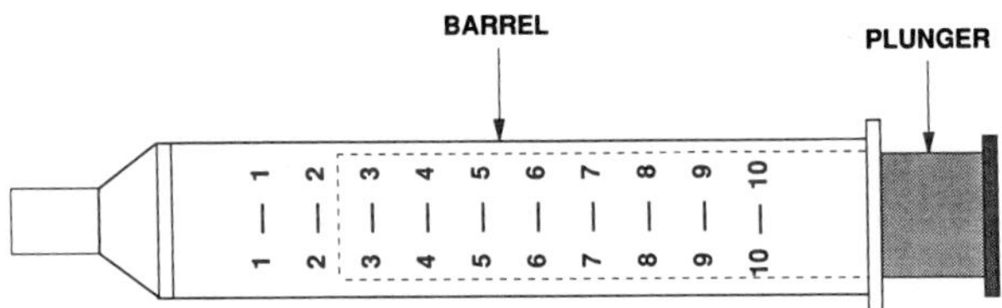

Figure 5–17. Diagram of a syringe. (From Di Lorenzo, MS, and Strasinger, SK: Blood Collection in Healthcare. FA Davis, Philadelphia, 2002, p. 20, with permission.)

when retracted (Fig. 5–17). Syringes routinely used for venipuncture range from 2 to 20 mL, and a size corresponding to the amount of blood needed should be used.

Needles used with syringes are attached to a plastic hub designed to fit onto the barrel of the syringe. They are also individually packaged, sterile, and color coded as to gauge size. Routinely used syringe needles range from 20- to 25-gauge with 1-inch and 1.5-inch lengths. An advantage when using syringe needles is that blood will appear in the hub of the needle when the vein has been successfully entered. Needle protection devices are available for **hypodermic** syringe needles similar to evacuated tube needles. Portex Inc, Keene, NH makes the Blood Draw Hypodermic Needle-Pro device, a nonlatex hypodermic needle with a disposable plastic sheath attached by a hinge (Fig. 5–18). The sheath hangs free during the venipuncture and is engaged over the needle by pressing the sheath against a flat surface after the procedure is complete. The SafetyGlide hypodermic needle by Becton, Dickinson (Fig. 5–19) has a movable shield that the phlebotomist pushes along the cannula with the thumb to enclose the needle tip after the venipuncture. Becton, Dickinson also has an Eclipse™ hypodermic needle that employs a shield that the phlebotomist locks over the needle tip after completion of the venipuncture procedure. The entire needle and syringe assembly is discarded in the designated sharps container. The technique for use of syringes is discussed in Chapter 7.

Blood drawn in a syringe is immediately transferred to appropriate evacuated tubes to prevent the formation of clots. It is acceptable to puncture the rubber stopper with the syringe needle and allow the blood to be drawn, but not forced, into the tube. Care must be taken to avoid hemolysis and needle punctures. As shown in Figure 5–20, the tube should

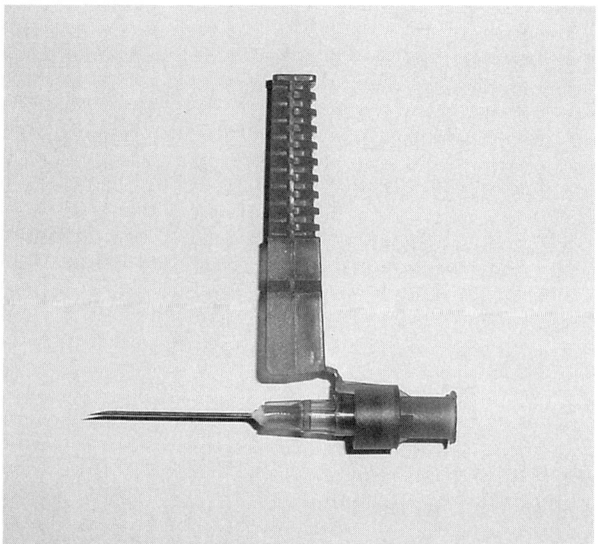

Figure 5-18. Portex Blood Draw Hypodermic Needle-Pro. (Courtesy of Portex, Inc., Keene, NH.)

be placed in a rack, not held in the free hand, and the needle should be angled toward the side of the tube for gentler transfer of the blood. The BD blood transfer device (Becton, Dickinson, Franklin Lakes, NJ) provides a safer means for blood transfer. It is an evacuated tube adapter with a rubber-sheathed needle inside. After blood collection, the syringe tip is inserted into the hub of the device and evacuated tubes are filled by pushing them onto the rubber-sheathed needle in the holder as in an evacuated tube system. The entire syringe/adapter assembly is

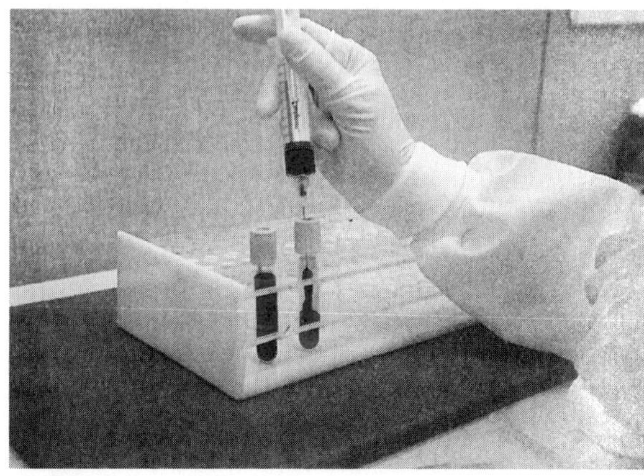

Figure 5-20. Transfer of blood from a syringe to an evacuated tube. (Note how the phlebotomist directs the blood against the side of the tube.)

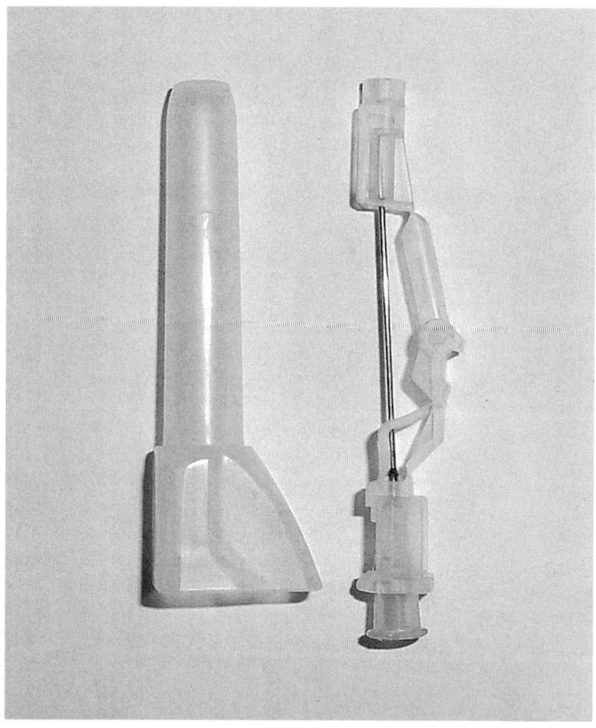

Figure 5-19. BD SafetyGlide™ hypodermic needle (safety device activated). (Courtesy of Becton, Dickinson and Company © 2002 BD.)

technical tip Never hold the evacuated tube in your hand when transferring blood from a syringe.

technical tip Let the vacuum in the evacuated tube draw the appropriate amount of blood into the tube. Discard any extra blood left in the syringe; do not force it into the tube.

technical tip Do not unthread the syringe from the blood transfer device. .Place the entire assembly in a sharps container. Use a safety needle device with this system.

discarded in the sharps container after use. Only syringes with built-in needle protection shields should be used with this system. The shield must be activated immediately when the needle is removed from the vein to avoid accidental needle sticks (Fig. 5-21).

When tubes are filled from a syringe, NCCLS recommends the tubes be filled in the same order

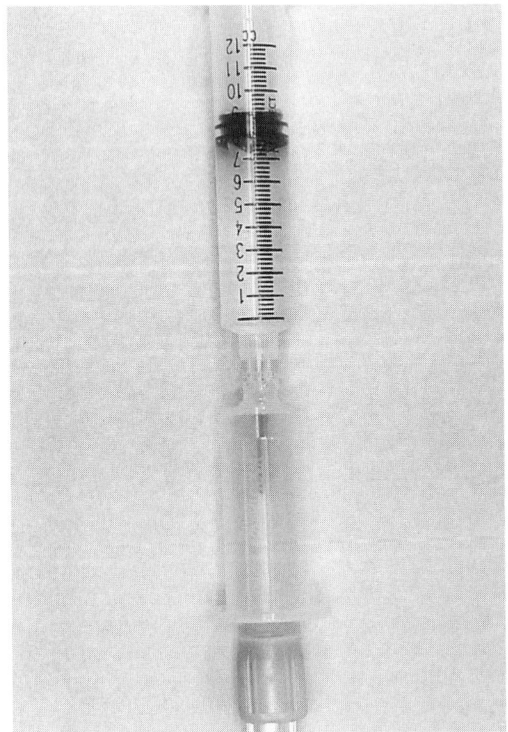

Figure 5–21. BD blood transfer device. (Courtesy of Becton, Dickinson and Company © 2002 BD.)

as recommended for the order of draw. However, the personnel in some institutions believe that, because the portion of blood possibly contaminated by tissue thromboplastin is the first portion to enter the syringe, it is the last to be expelled. At the same time, the possible transfer of anticoagulants and additives among tubes must also be considered and will be minimized by using the NCCLS protocol. Institutional protocol should be followed.

Winged Infusion Sets

Winged infusion sets, or **"butterflies"** as they are routinely called, are used for the infusion of IV fluids and for performing venipuncture from very small veins often seen in children and in the geriatric population. Butterfly needles used for phlebotomy are usually 21-, 23-, or 25-gauge with lengths of 1/2 to 3/4 inch. Plastic attachments to the needle that resemble butterfly wings are used for holding the needle during insertion and to secure the apparatus during IV therapy. They also provide the ability to lower the needle insertion angle when working with very small veins. To accommodate the dual purpose of venipuncture and infusion, the needle is attached to a flexible plastic tubing that can then be attached to an IV setup, syringe, or specially designed evacuated tube adapters (Fig. 5–22).

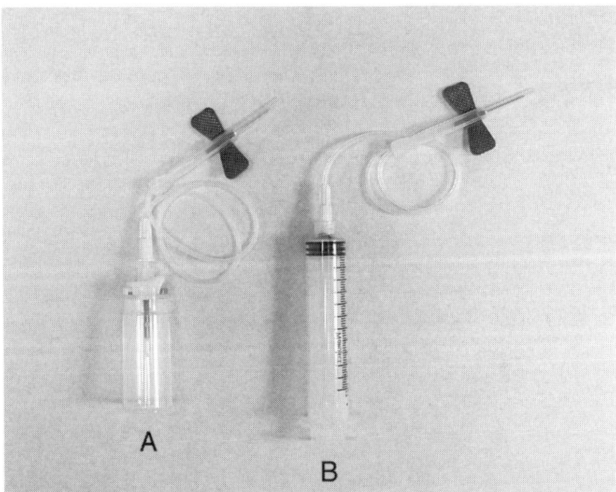

Figure 5–22. Winged infusion sets. *A*, Attached to an evacuated tube holder. *B*, Attached to a syringe.

technical tip In the interest of cost containment, phlebotomists should not become dependent on the use of butterflies for patients with veins than can be accessed with a standard evacuated tube system.

The flexible tubing can make the butterfly apparatus more difficult to manage. The length of the tubing also results in approximately 0.5 mL less blood entering the first collection tube, which could interfere with coagulation tests. It is more expensive to use the butterfly apparatus than the standard evacuated tube system, and phlebotomists should avoid becoming overly dependent on the butterfly for specimen collection.

There are several winged needle sets with safety devices built into the system. The BD Vacutainer Safety-Lok blood collection set (Becton, Dickinson, Franklin Lakes, NJ) uses a translucent protective shield that covers the needle immediately after removal from the vein. After use, the needle is completely retracted into the shield and locked in place by pushing the shield forward (Fig. 5–23). Another needle set is the Angel Wing safety needle

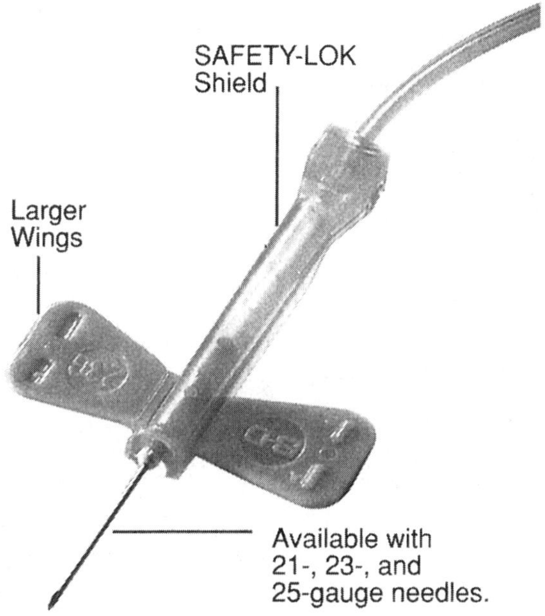

Figure 5–23. Safety-Lok™ blood collection set. (Courtesy of Becton, Dickinson and Company © 2002 BD.)

(Kendall, Mansfield, MA) (Fig. 5–24). When the needle is withdrawn from the vein, a stainless steel safety shield is activated and locks in place to cover the needle.

The technique for use of winged infusion sets is covered in Chapter 7.

Tourniquets

Tourniquets are used during venipuncture to make it easier to locate patients' veins. They do this by impeding venous but not arterial blood flow in the area just below where the tourniquet is applied. The distended vein then becomes more visible or palpable. Tourniquets are available in both adult and pediatric sizes.

The most frequently used tourniquets are flat latex strips (Fig. 5–25). They are inexpensive and may be disposed of between patients, or reused if disinfected. Flat nonlatex strips are available for patients or phlebotomists allergic to latex.

Tourniquets with Velcro and buckle closures are easier to apply but are more difficult to decontaminate. The advantage of the buckle closure is that it stays on the patient's arm after release and can be retightened if necessary.

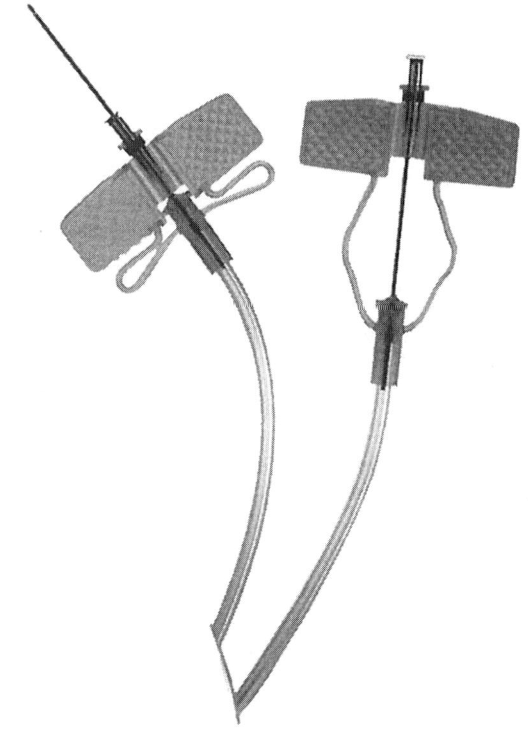

Figure 5–24. Angel Wing safety needles. (Courtesy of Kendall, Mansfield, MA.)

technical tip Latex-free tourniquets are available on a roll that is perforated and should always be carried on the phlebotomist's tray. The stretch tourniquet is used and discarded.

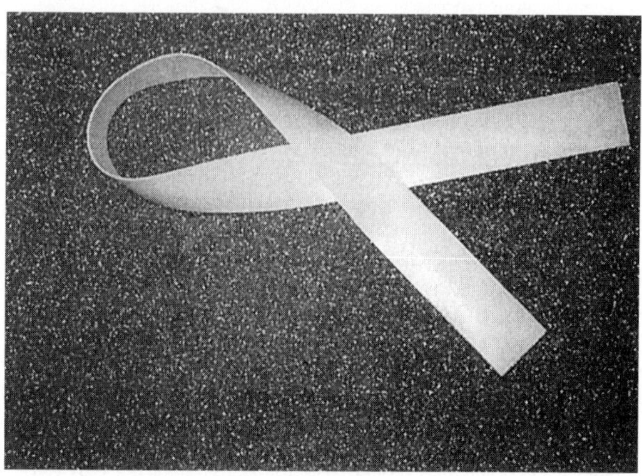

Figure 5–25. Latex strip tourniquet.

Blood pressure cuffs can be used as tourniquets. They are used primarily for veins that are difficult to locate. The cuff should be inflated to a pressure below the patient's systolic blood pressure reading and above the diastolic reading. This allows blood to flow into but not out of the affected veins.

The application of tourniquets and their effects on blood tests are discussed in Chapters 6 and 7.

Gloves

OSHA mandates that gloves must be worn when collecting blood and must be changed after each patient. Under routine circumstances, gloves do not need to be sterile. To provide maximal manual dexterity, they should fit securely.

Gloves are available in several varieties, including powdered and powder-free, and latex and nonlatex (vinyl). Gloves with powder are not recommended because the powder can contaminate patient specimens and cause falsely elevated calcium values. The glove powder can also cause a sensitization to latex. Allergenic latex proteins are absorbed on the glove powder, which become airborne and can be inhaled when the gloves are put on and taken off. As discussed in Chapter 3, allergy to latex is increasing among healthcare workers. Persons who develop symptoms of allergy to latex should avoid latex gloves and other latex products, such as tourniquets, at all times. Cotton glove liners can be worn under latex gloves for persons that develop an allergic dermatitis to gloves. Hands must be washed after removing gloves to prevent the transmission of bloodborne pathogens and to decrease the time of latex exposure and transmission of latex proteins to other parts of the body.

technical tip To avoid specimen contamination and latex allergy, do not use powdered gloves.

Puncture Site Protection Supplies

The primary antiseptic used for cleansing the skin in routine phlebotomy is 70% isopropyl alcohol. This is a **bacteriostatic** antiseptic used to prevent contamination by normal skin bacteria during the short period required to perform collection of the specimen.

For collections that require additional sterility, such as blood cultures and arterial punctures, the stronger antiseptics such as iodine or chlorhexidene gluconate (for patients allergic to iodine) are used to cleanse the area. To prevent skin discomfort, iodine should always be removed from the patient's skin with alcohol after a phlebotomy procedure.

Sterile 2 × 2 inch gauze pads are used for applying pressure to the puncture site after the needle has been removed. Gauze pads can also serve as additional protection when folded in quarters and placed under a bandage. A bandage or adhesive tape is placed over the puncture site when the bleeding has stopped. Latex-free tape should be used for persons who are allergic to adhesive bandages. Self-adhering Ace-type bandages are available for elderly patients. It is not recommended to use cotton balls to apply pressure because the cotton ball fibers can stick to the venipuncture site and may cause bleeding to begin again when the cotton is removed. Patients should be instructed to remove the bandage in about an hour.

Additional Supplies

Clean glass slides may be needed to prepare blood films for certain hematology tests. This procedure is discussed in Chapter 10. Biohazard bags should be available for transport of specimens based on institutional protocol.

The final piece of equipment needed by the phlebotomist is a pen for labeling tubes, initialing computer-generated labels, or noting unusual circumstances on the requisition form.

Quality Control

Ensuring the sterility of needles and puncture devices and the stability of evacuated tubes, anticoagulants, and additives is essential to patient safety and specimen quality. Disposable needles and puncture devices are individually packaged in tightly sealed sterile containers. Phlebotomists should not use puncture equipment if the seal has been broken.

Visual inspection for nonpointed or barbed needles may detect manufacturing defects. Manufacturers of evacuated tubes must ensure that tubes, anticoagulants, and additives meet the standards established by the NCCLS. Evacuated tubes produced at the same time are referred to as a **lot** and have a distinguishing lot number printed on the packages. There is also an expiration date printed on each package. The expiration date represents the last day the manufacturer guarantees the stability of the specified amount of vacuum in the tube and the reactivity of the anticoagulants and additives. The expiration date should be checked each time a new package of tubes is opened, and outdated tubes should not be used. Use of expired tubes may cause incompletely filled tubes (short draws), clotted anticoagulated specimens, improperly preserved specimens, and insecure gel barriers.

technical tip Consider giving outdated tubes to a local phlebotomy program for student practice on artificial arms.

Failure to completely fill tubes (short draws) containing anticoagulants and additives affects specimen quality because the amount of anticoagulant or additive present in the tube is based on the assumption that the tube will be completely filled. Possible errors include excessive dilution of the specimen by liquid anticoagulants and distortion of cellular structures by increased chemical concentrations.

Bibliography

Becton, Dickinson Safety Blood Collection and Culture Products. Website: http://bd.com/dadfety/ products/bcollect/index.asp

Bush, VJ, Leonard, L, and Szamosi, DI: Advancements in Blood Collection Devices. Lab Med 29:616–622, 1998.

National Committee for Clinical Laboratory Standards. Procedure for the Collection of Diagnostic Blood Specimens by Venipuncture. Approved Standard H3-A4. NCCLS, Wayne, PA, 1998.

National Committee for Clinical Laboratory Standards. Procedure for the Handling and Processing of Blood Specimens. Approved Guideline, H18-A2. NCCLS, Wayne, PA, 1999.

National Committee for Clinical Laboratory Standards. Collection, Transport and Processing of Blood Specimens For Coagulation Testing and Performance of Coagulation Assays. Approved Guideline H21-A3. NCCLS, Wayne, PA, 1998.

Study Questions

1. State a purpose for which a phlebotomist would use each of the following:
   a. 16-gauge needle

   ____

   b. 21-gauge needle

   ____

   c. 23-gauge needle

   ____

2. Using a 25-gauge needle with a 10-mL evacuated tube to perform phlebotomy may cause

   ______________________________.

3. List three parts common to all needles.
   a. ______________________________
   b. ______________________________
   c. ______________________________

4. How does the anticoagulant in a green stopper tube work?

   ____

5. Name three anticoagulants that prevent clotting by binding calcium and the color-coded stopper associated with them.

Anticoagulant	**Color-Coded Stopper**
a. ______________	______________
b. ______________	______________
c. ______________	______________

6 What is the purpose of sodium fluoride in a gray stopper tube?

   ____

7. Why is EDTA the anticoagulant of choice for the CBC?

   ____

8. The stopper color of the tube that must always be completely filled is

   ______________________________.

9. What is the purpose of tapping an evacuated tube containing dried anticoagulant before using it?

____

10. Which of the following tubes will clot first: red, gold, or orange?

____

11. Using the numbers 1 through 5, list the order of draw using an evacuated tube system for the following tests.

a. ________ CBC

b. ________ Blood culture

c. ________ Plasma glucose

d. ________ Cholesterol

e. ________ Coagulation studies

12. List two possible orders of tube fill from a syringe for the tests in study question 11.

a. _______________

b. _______________

c. _______________

d. _______________

e. _______________

13. Under what circumstances should the amount of anticoagulant in a light blue stopper tube be decreased?

____

14. Why are royal blue stopper tubes used for collecting trace metal analyses?

____

15. List an advantage and a disadvantage of syringe use.

____

____

16. When are winged infusion sets used in phlebotomy?

____

17. Syringes are graduated in _______________.

18. When a blood pressure cuff is used as a tourniquet, how should the pressure be adjusted?

____

19. List two precautions a phlebotomist would take when collecting a blood specimen from a patient with a latex allergy.

    a. ______________________________

    b. ______________________________

20. List two antiseptics used in venipuncture and state a situation when each is used.

Antiseptic	**Used For**
a. ______________	______________
b. ______________	______________

21. Fill in the blanks in the following chart.

Tube Color	**Anticoagulant/Additive**	**Test**	**Department**
Red	None	RPR	Serology
	EDTA		
		Prothrombin	
Pink			
		Ammonia	
	Sodium fluoride		
Tan			

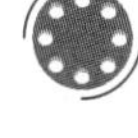

Clinical Situations

1. Information on a requisition form requesting a liver panel, an amylase, and a theophylline level tells the phlebotomist to collect a red/gray SST, gold Hemogard tube, and a red stopper tube.

    a. State a reason why this laboratory cannot perform both the liver panel and the amylase on the red/gray SST.

    ____

    b. Which test must be performed on the red stopper tube?

    ____

    c. Serum from which tube could be used by the serology department if an additional test was requested?

    ____

d. Why is a red/gray SST preferred over a red stopper tube for most chemistry tests?

____

2. The phlebotomy supervisor is investigating the following complaints. State a technical phlebotomy error that could be the cause of each problem.

   a. Patient Smith's calcium and prothrombin time results are noticeably decreased.

   ____

   b. The coagulation laboratory rejects a light blue stopper tube for a prothrombin time.

   ____

   c. The chemistry laboratory rejects an SST into which blood from a syringe has been transferred.

   ____

   d. A phlebotomist complains about getting short draws with lavender stopper tubes, but not red stopper tubes during morning collections.

   ____

3. Can a lavender stopper tube be used to perform a prothrombin time? Why or why not?

   ____

4. Can a green stopper tube be used to perform a CBC? Why or why not?

   ____

5. Can a glucose and a cardiac risk profile be performed on a gray stopper tube? Why or why not?

   ____

6. Can a white Hemogard closure tube be used to perform a crossmatch? Why or why not?

   ____

   ____

Venipuncture Equipment Exercise

INSTRUCTIONS

State or assemble (if requested) the appropriate equipment for the situations described in this exercise. Include the number and stopper color of evacuated tubes, needle size, syringe size, or butterfly, if appropriate. Instructors may specify the inclusion of other supplies.

1. Collection of a CBC from a 35-year-old woman.

   ____

2. Collection of a CBC from a 3-year-old boy.

   ____

3. Collection of a stat CBC and stat electrolytes from a 40-year-old man.

   ____

4. Collection of a stat amylase from the hand of an obese patient who is taking anticoagulants.

   ____

5. Collection of a PT from an elderly patient.

   ____

6. Collection of a chemistry profile from a patient with a latex allergy.

   ____

7. Assemble the equipment to collect a type and crossmatch on a 50-year-old man.

   ____

8. Assemble the equipment to collect a cardiac risk profile and ESR from a patient with fragile veins.

   ____

9. Assemble the equipment to collect a lead level from a 2-year-old patient.

   ____

10. Assemble the tubes in the order they would be drawn for a CBC, APTT, and a glucose using an evacuated tube system.

    ____

NAME ______________________

Evaluation of Equipment Selection and Assembly

RATING SYSTEM 2 = SATISFACTORILY PERFORMED 1 = NEEDS IMPROVEMENT 0 = INCORRECT/ DID NOT PERFORM

__________ 1. Collects all necessary equipment and supplies

__________ 2. Selects appropriate tubes for requested tests

__________ 3. Selects correct number of tubes or syringe size

__________ 4. Correctly attaches needle to adapter or syringe

__________ 5. Does not uncap needle prematurely

__________ 6. Advances tube correctly into adapter or checks plunger movement

__________ 7. Arranges supplies and extra tubes conveniently

TOTAL POINTS __________

MAXIMUM POINTS = 14

Comments:

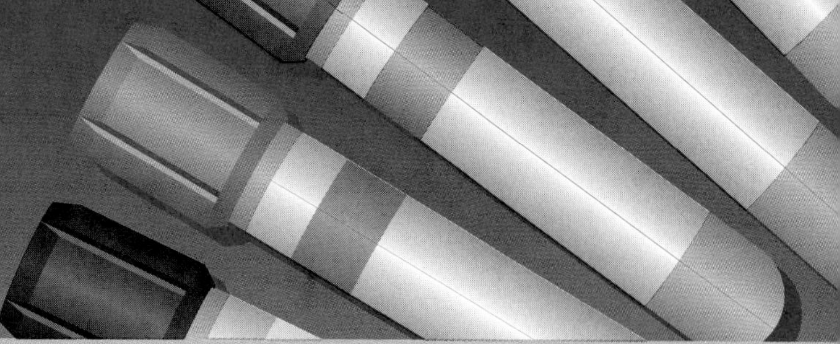

Chapter 6

Routine Venipuncture

Chapter Outline

Requisitions
Greeting the Patient
Patient Identification
Patient Preparation and Patient Positioning
Equipment Selection
Wash Hands and Apply Gloves
Tourniquet Application
Site Selection
Cleansing the Site
Assembly of Puncture Equipment
Performing the Venipuncture
Removal of the Needle
Disposal of the Needle
Labeling the Tubes
Bandaging the Patient's Arm
Leaving the Patient
Completing the Venipuncture Procedure
Summary of Venipuncture Technique with an Evacuated Tube System

Learning Objectives

Upon completion of this chapter, the reader will be able to:

1 List the required information on a requisition form.
2 Discuss the appropriate procedure to follow when greeting and reassuring a patient.
3 Describe correct patient identification procedures for inpatients and outpatients.
4 Describe patient preparation and positioning.
5 Correctly assemble venipuncture equipment and supplies.
6 Name and locate the three most frequently used veins for venipuncture.
7 Correctly apply a tourniquet.
8 Describe vein palpation.
9 Discuss the venipuncture site cleansing procedure.
10 Correctly perform a routine venipuncture using an evacuated tube system.
11 Safely dispose of contaminated needles and supplies.
12 List the information required on a specimen tube label.
13 Explain the importance of delivering specimens to the laboratory in a timely manner.

Key Terms

Antecubital fossa
Bar codes
Basilic vein
Cephalic vein
Hematoma
Hemoconcentration
Identification band
Median cubital vein
Palpation
Requisition

The most frequently performed procedure in phlebotomy is the venipuncture. The ability to perform this technique in an organized, patient-considerate manner is the key to success as a phlebotomist. Each phlebotomist develops his or her own style for dealing with patients and performing the actual venipuncture. Administrative protocols vary among institutions and, of course, every patient is different; however, many basic rules are the same in all situations. These basic rules must be followed to ensure the safety of the patient and the phlebotomist, produce specimens that are representative of the patient's condition, and create an efficient phlebotomy service for the institution.

In this chapter, the routine venipuncture technique is presented for the beginning phlebotomist in the recommended step-by-step procedure. The procedure is outlined again in Chapter 7 with a presentation of the complications that may occur at each step.

Requisitions

All phlebotomy procedures begin with the receipt of a test ***requisition*** form that is generated by or at the request of a healthcare provider. The requisition is essential to provide the phlebotomist with the information needed to correctly identify the patient, organize the necessary equipment, collect the appropriate specimens, and provide legal protection. Phlebotomists should not collect a specimen without a requisition form, and this form must accompany the specimen to the laboratory.

The method by which a phlebotomist receives a requisition varies with the setting. Requisitions from outpatients may be hand carried by the patient, or requests may be telephoned to the central processing or accessioning area by the healthcare provider's office staff, where the laboratory staff generates a requisition form. Inpatient requisitions may be delivered to the laboratory, sent by pneumatic tube system, or entered into the hospital computer at the nursing station and printed out by the laboratory computer. In emergency situations, the phlebotomy request may be telephoned to the laboratory and the requisition form picked up by the phlebotomist at the patient site.

Phlebotomists should carefully examine all requisitions for which they are responsible before leaving the laboratory. They should check to be sure that all requisitions for a particular patient are together so that all tests are collected with one venipuncture. They must be sure they have all the necessary equipment.

The actual format of a requisition form may vary. Patient information may be handwritten or imprinted by an imprinter on color-coded forms with test check off lists for different departments. There may be multiple copies for purposes of record keeping and billing. Computer-generated forms can include not only the patient information and tests requested but also tube labels and ***bar codes*** for specimen processing, the number and type of collection tubes needed, and special collection instructions. Figure 6–1 shows a sample computer-generated requisition form with accompanying labels.

Requisitions must contain certain basic information to ensure that the specimen drawn and the test results are correlated with the appropriate patient and that these can be correctly interpreted with regard to any special conditions, such as the time of collection. This information includes the following:

1 *Patient's Name and Identification Number* (The identification number may be a hospital-generated number that is also present on the patient's wrist ***identification*** [ID] ***band*** and in

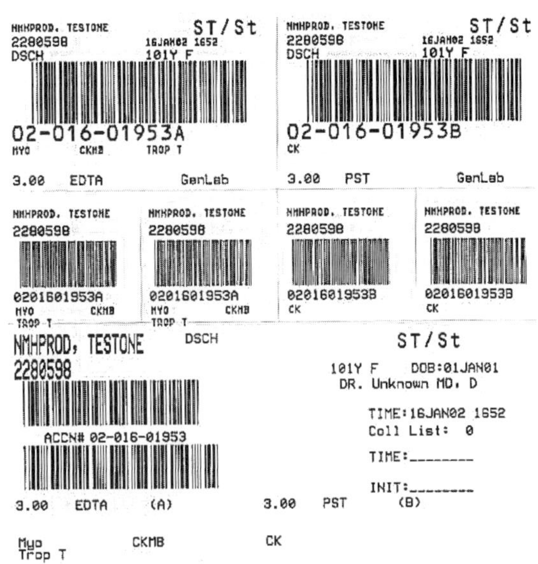
NMHPROD. TESTONE ST/St
2280598 16JAN02 1652
DSCH 101Y F
02-016-01953A
MYO CKMB TROP T
3.00 EDTA GenLab

NMHPROD. TESTONE ST/St
2280598 16JAN02 1652
DSCH 101Y F
02-016-01953B
CK
3.00 PST GenLab

NMHPROD. TESTONE
2280598
0201601953A
MYO CKMB
TROP T

NMHPROD. TESTONE
2280598
0201601953A
MYO CKMB
TROP T

NMHPROD. TESTONE
2280598
0201601953B
CK

NMHPROD. TESTONE
2280598
0201601953B
CK

NMHPROD, TESTONE DSCH ST/St
2280598
101Y F DOB:01JAN01
DR. Unknown MD, D
TIME:16JAN02 1652
Coll List: 0
ACCN# 02-016-01953
TIME:________
INIT:________
3.00 EDTA (A) 3.00 PST (B)
Myo CKMB CK
Trop T

Figure 6–1 Sample requisition form and labels. (Courtesy of Diane Wolff, MLT [ASCP], Phlebotomy Team Leader, Nebraska Methodist Hospital, Omaha, NE.)

all hospital documents; in an outpatient setting it may be a laboratory-assigned number or the patient's Social Security number.)

2 *Patient's Location*
3 *Ordering Healthcare Provider's Name*
4 *Tests Requested*
5 *Requested Date and Time of Specimen Collection* (When the specimen is collected, the phlebotomist must write the actual date and time on the requisition and the specimen label. Most hospitals have adopted the military time system because they operate continuously for 24 hours.)
6 *Status of Specimen* (stat, timed, routine)

Other information that may be present includes the following:

- *Patient's Date of Birth*
- *Special Collection Information* (such as fasting specimen)
- *Special Patient Information* (such as areas that should not be used for venipuncture)
- *Number and Type of Collection Tubes*

technical tip Phlebotomists should never collect samples before receiving or generating the requisition form.

Greeting the Patient

A phlebotomist's professional demeanor instills confidence and trust in the patient, which can effectively ease patient apprehension about the procedure. When approaching patients, phlebotomists should introduce themselves, say that they are from the laboratory, and explain that they will be collecting a blood specimen. In the outpatient setting, the patient usually knows what is about to occur (Fig. 6–2).

technical tip The more relaxed and trusting your patient, the greater chance of a successful atraumatic venipuncture.

Observe any signs on the patient's door or in the patient's room relaying special instructions, such as "allergic to latex," nothing by mouth (**NPO**), do not resuscitate (**DNR**), "do not draw blood from [a particular] arm" or "patient expired." When entering a patient's room, it is polite to knock lightly on the open or closed door. If the curtain is closed around the bed, speak to the patient first through the curtain. This will avoid any embarrassment if the patient happens to be bathing or using the bedpan. In the hospital setting, a variety of other circumstances may be present that require additional consideration when greeting the patient. These circumstances are discussed in Chapter 7 ☞.

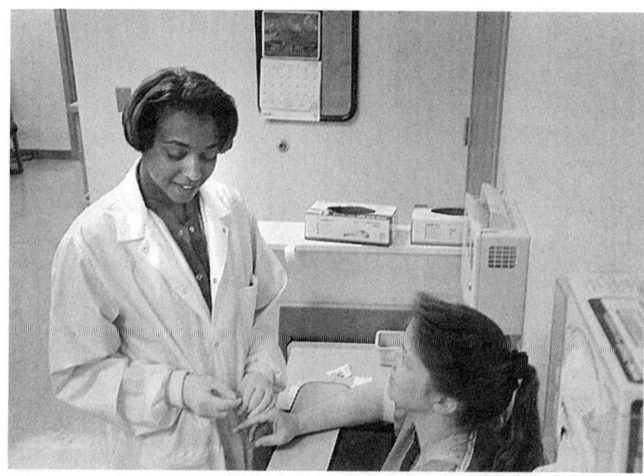

Figure 6–2 A phlebotomist greeting a patient in an outpatient setting.

Patient Identification

The most important procedure in phlebotomy is correct identification of the patient. Serious diagnostic or treatment errors and even death can occur when blood is drawn from the wrong patient. Ideally, identification is made by comparing information obtained verbally and from the patient's wrist ID band with the information on the requisition form (Fig. 6–3).

Verbal identification is made after the patient greeting by asking the patient to state his or her full name. Always have patients state their names. Do not ask, "Are you John Jones?" because many patients have a tendency to say "yes" to anything. In an outpatient setting, comparison of verbal information with the requisition form may be the only means of verifying identification. Asking the patient's date of birth or for the spelling of his or her last name may be helpful in this situation.

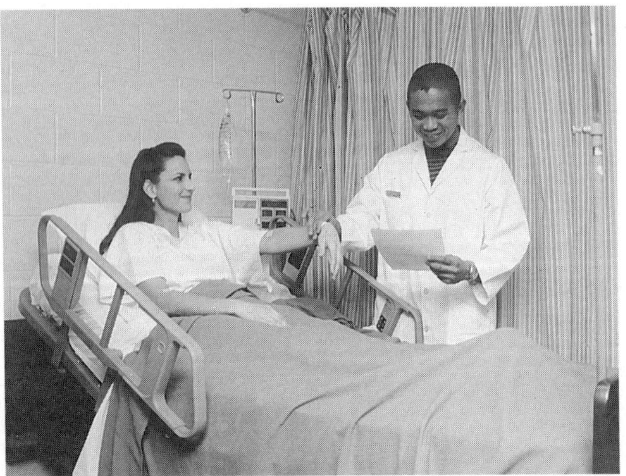

Figure 6–3 Phlebotomist checking a wristband. (From Strasinger, SK, and Di Lorenzo, MS: Skills for the Patient Care Technician. FA Davis, Philadelphia, 1999, p. 137, with permission.)

Examining the information on the patient's wrist ID band, which should always be present on hospitalized patients, follows verbal identification. Information on the wrist ID band should include patient's name, hospital identification number, date of birth, and physician. All information on the wrist ID band should match the information on the requisition form. Particular attention should be paid to the hospital identification number, because it is possible for two patients to have the same name, date of birth, and physician; however, they could not have the same identification number.

It is essential that identification of hospitalized patients be made from an ID band attached to the patient. Wristbands are sometimes removed when intravenous (**IV**) fluids are being administered in the wrist or when fluids have infiltrated the area. They should be reattached to the patient's ankle. Ankle bands are frequently used with pediatric patients and newborns. A wristband lying on the bedside table cannot be used for identification—it could belong to anyone. Likewise, a sign over the patient's bed or on the door cannot be relied on because the patient could be in the wrong bed.

Positive patient identification can be made using barcode technology. Using a hand-held computer, the phlebotomist positively identifies the patient by scanning the bar code on the patient's hospital ID band (Fig. 6–4). A visual and audible signal confirms that the identification is correct. The

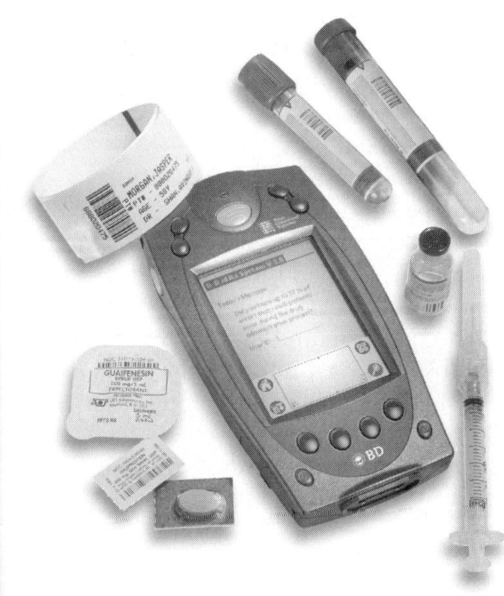

Figure 6–4 Becton, Dickinson Dx System for patient identification. (Courtesy of Becton, Dickinson and Company © 2002 BD.)

system, which is interfaced with the laboratory information management system (**LIMS**), specifies which kind of tube should be used, the correct order of draw, and special handling instructions. Following collection a lightweight hand-held printer creates a bar code label that can be affixed to the tube.

technical tip A hospitalized patient must always be correctly identified by an ID band that is attached to the patient.

Patient Preparation and Patient Positioning

Reassurance of the patient actually begins with the greeting and continues throughout the procedure. Phlebotomists should demonstrate both concern for the patient's comfort and confidence in their ability to perform the procedure. Patients should be given a brief explanation of the procedure, including any nonroutine techniques that will be used, such as the additional site preparation performed when collecting blood cultures. They should not be told that the procedure will be painless.

Patients often question the phlebotomist about what tests are being performed or why their blood is being drawn so frequently. The best policy is to politely suggest that they ask their healthcare provider these questions. Even listing the names of tests can cause problems, because many medical books and Internet sites are available to the general public. The patient may reach erroneous conclusions, because many tests have several diagnostic purposes; or the patient may misunderstand the test name and look up an inappropriate test associated with a very severe condition.

The phlebotomist's conversation with the patient should include verifying that the appropriate pretest preparation such as fasting or abstaining from medications has occurred. When these procedures have not been followed, this problem should be reported to the nursing station before drawing the blood. If the specimen is still required, the irregular condition, such as "not fasting," should be written on the requisition form and the specimen.

technical tip Good verbal, listening, and nonverbal skills are very important for patient reassurance.

When patient identification is completed, the patient must be positioned conveniently and safely for the procedure. Always ask the patient if he or she is allergic to latex.

Blood should never be drawn from a patient who is in a standing position. Outpatients are seated or reclined at a drawing station as shown in Figure 5–3. In some drawing stations, the movable arm serves the dual purposes of providing a solid surface for the patient's arm and preventing a patient who faints from falling out of the chair. The patient's arm should be firmly supported and extended downward in a straight line, allowing the tubes to fill from the bottom up to prevent reflux and anticoagulant carry-over between tubes. Asking the patient to make a fist with the hand of the arm not being used and placing it behind the elbow will provide support and make the vein easier to locate (Fig. 6–5). Phlebotomists should always be alert for any changes in the patient's condition while the procedure is being performed. Some patients know that they experience difficulties during venipuncture, and provisions should be made to allow them to lie down for the procedure.

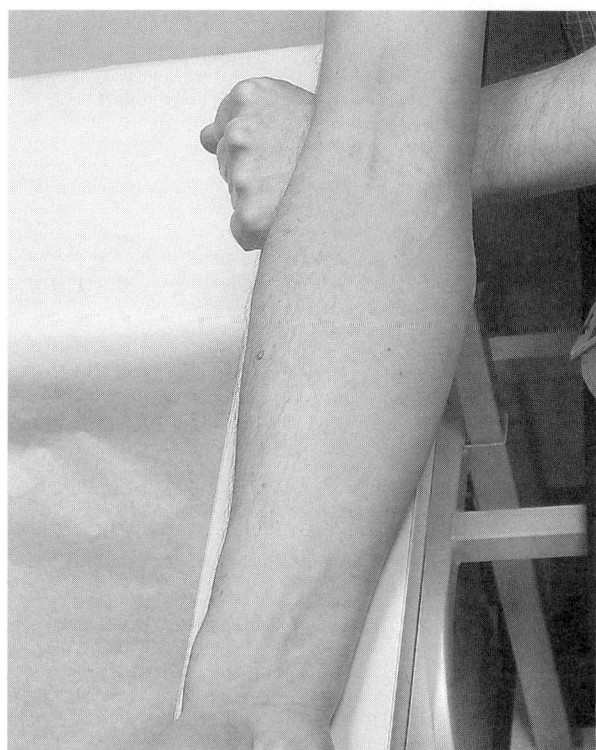

Figure 6–5 Positioning the patient's arm.

technical tip When supporting the patient's arm, do not hyperextend the elbow. This may make vein palpation difficult. Sometimes bending the elbow very slightly may aid in vein palpation.

It may be necessary to move a hospitalized patient slightly to make the arm more accessible, or to place a pillow or towel under the patient's arm for better support and to position the arm in a straight line downward. If bed rails are lowered, they must always be returned to the raised position before the phlebotomist leaves the room.

Patients should remove any objects such as food, drink, gum, or a thermometer from their mouths before performance of the venipuncture. Any foreign object in the mouth could cause choking.

Equipment Selection

Before approaching the patient for the actual venipuncture, the phlebotomist should collect all

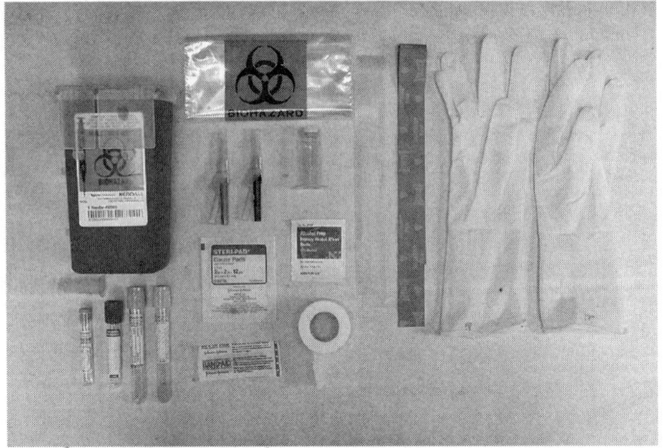

Figure 6–6 Venipuncture collection equipment.

necessary supplies (including collection equipment, antiseptic pads, sterile gauze, bandages, and needle disposal system) and place them close to the patient (Fig. 6–6). The requisition form is re-examined, and the appropriate number and type of collection tubes are selected.

Place the tubes in the correct order for specimen collection, and have additional tubes readily available for possible use during the procedure. It is not uncommon to find an evacuated tube that does not contain the necessary amount of vacuum to collect a full tube of blood. Accidentally pushing a tube past the indicator mark on the adapter before the vein is entered also results in loss of vacuum.

Wash Hands and Apply Gloves

In front of the patient, the phlebotomist should wash his or her hands using the procedure described in Chapter 3 (Fig. 3–2) and apply clean gloves. The gloves are pulled over the cuffs of protective clothing. Gloves are changed between each patient.

technical tip Patients are often reassured that proper safety measures are being followed when gloves are donned in their presence.

Tourniquet Application

The tourniquet serves two functions in the venipuncture procedure. By impeding venous, but not arterial, blood flow, the tourniquet causes blood to accumulate in the veins making them more easily located and provides a larger amount of blood for collection. Use of a tourniquet can alter some test results by increasing the ratio of cellular elements to plasma (***hemoconcentration***) and by causing hemolysis. Therefore, the maximum amount of time the tourniquet should remain in place is 1 minute. This requires that the tourniquet be applied twice during the venipuncture procedure, first when vein selection is being made and then immediately before the puncture is performed. When the tourniquet is used during vein selection, it should be released for 2 minutes before being reapplied.

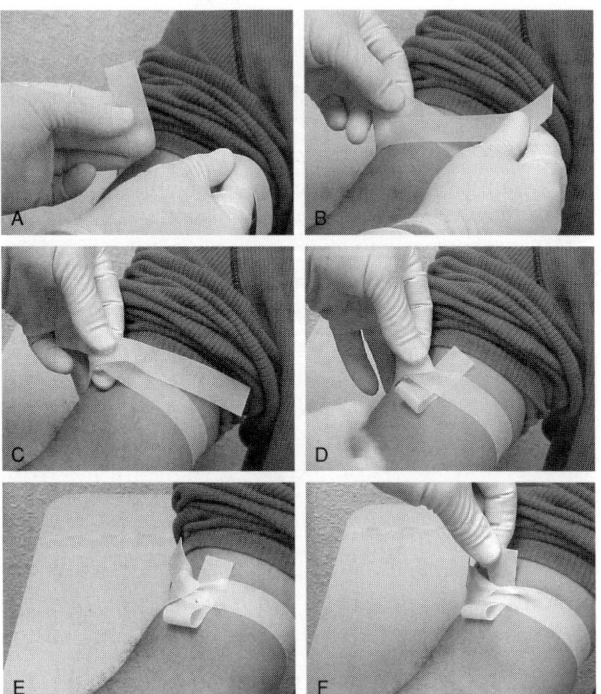

Figure 6–7 Tourniquet application. *(A)* Position the latex strip 3 to 4 inches above the venipuncture site. *(B)* Cross the tourniquet over the patient's arm. *(C)* Hold the tourniquet in one hand close to the arm. *(D)* Tuck a portion of one end under the opposite end to form a loop. *(E)* Properly applied tourniquet. *(F)* Pull end of loop to release tourniquet. (From Di Lorenzo, MS, and Strasinger, SK: Blood Collection in Healthcare. FA Davis, Philadelphia, 2002, p 32, with permission.)

The tourniquet should be placed on the arm 3 to 4 inches above the venipuncture site. Application of the commonly used latex strip requires practice to develop a smooth technique and can be difficult if properly fitting gloves are not worn. Figure 6–7 shows the technique used with latex strip tourniquets. To achieve adequate pressure, both sides of the tourniquet must be grasped near the patient's arm, and while maintaining tension, the left side is tucked under the right side. The loop formed should face downward toward the patient's antecubital area, and the free end should be away from the venipuncture area but in a position that allows it to be easily pulled to release the pressure. Left-handed persons would reverse this procedure.

Tourniquets that are folded or applied too tightly are uncomfortable for the patient and may obstruct blood flow to the area. The appearance of small, reddish discolorations (**petechiae**) on the patient's arm, blanching of the skin around the tourniquet, and the inability to feel a radial pulse are indications of a tourniquet that is tied too tightly.

Site Selection

The preferred site for venipuncture is the ***antecubital fossa*** located anterior to the elbow. As shown in Figure 6–8 three major ***veins***—the ***median cubital***, the ***cephalic***, and the ***basilic***—are located in this area, and in most patients, at least one of these veins can be easily located. Notice that the veins continue down the forearm to the wrist area; however, in these areas, they become smaller and less well anchored, and punctures are more painful to the patient. Small prominent veins are also located in the back of the hand. When necessary, these veins can be used for venipuncture, but they may require a smaller needle or butterfly apparatus. The veins of the lower arm and hand are also the preferred site for administering intravenous fluids because they allow the patient more arm flexibility. Frequent venipuncture in these veins could make them unsuitable for IV use. Some institutions have special ID bands that indicate the restricted use of veins being used for other procedures.

Of the three veins located in the antecubital area, the median cubital is the vein of choice because it is large and does not tend to move when the needle is inserted. It is often closer to the surface of the skin, more isolated from underlying structures, and the least painful to puncture. The cephalic vein located on the thumb side of the arm is usually more difficult to locate, except possibly in obese patients, and has more tendency to move. The cephalic vein

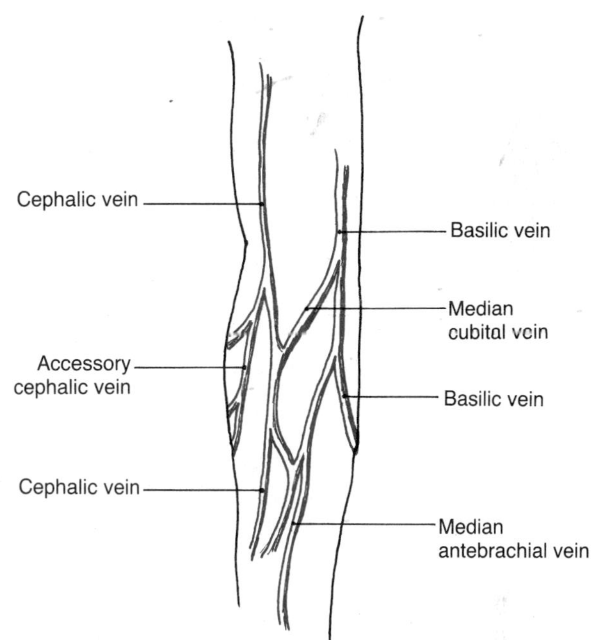

Figure 6–8 The veins in the arm most often chosen for venipuncture. (From Di Lorenzo, MS, and Strasinger, SK: Blood Collection in Healthcare. FA Davis, Philadelphia, 2002, p 33, with permission.)

should be the second choice if the median cubital is inaccessible in both arms. The basilic vein is the least firmly anchored and is located near the median nerve and the brachial artery. Care must be taken not to puncture the artery accidentally. The basilic vein should be used as the last choice because the median nerve and brachial artery are in close proximity to it, increasing the risk of permanent injury.

Two routine steps in the venipuncture procedure aid the phlebotomist in locating a suitable vein. These steps are applying a tourniquet and asking the patients to clench their fists. Continuous clenching or pumping of the fist should not be encouraged because it will result in hemoconcentration and alter some test results. The difference in vein prominence before and after these procedures are used is usually remarkable, and phlebotomists examining an arm before they have been done should not become overly concerned about finding a vein. Most phlebotomists prefer to apply the tourniquet before examining the arm. As discussed earlier, the tourniquet can only be applied for 1 minute; therefore, after the vein is located, the tourniquet is removed while the site is being cleansed and is reapplied immediately before the venipuncture.

technical tip Patients often think they are helping by pumping their fists, because this is an acceptable practice when donating blood. In contrast to laboratory specimens, a donated unit of blood is even better when it is hemoconcentrated.

Veins are located by sight and by touch (referred to as ***palpation***). The ability to feel a vein is much more important than the ability to see a vein—a concept that is often difficult for beginning phlebotomists to accept. Palpation is usually performed using the index and second fingers of the nondominant hand to probe the antecubital area with a pushing motion rather than a stroking motion. The pressure applied by palpating locates deep veins; distinguishes veins, which feel like spongy cords, from rigid tendon cords; and differentiates veins from arteries, which produce a pulse (Fig. 6–9). The thumb should not be used to palpate because it has a pulse beat. Select a vein that is easily palpated and large enough to support good blood flow. Once an acceptable vein is located, palpation is used to determine the direction and depth of the vein to aid the phlebotomist during needle insertion. It is often helpful to find a visual reference for the selected vein, such as its location near a mole, freckle, or skin crease, to assist in relocating the vein after cleansing the site.

technical tip Using the nondominant hand routinely for palpation may be helpful when additional palpation is required immediately before performing the puncture.

technical tip To increase the sensitivity of the palpating finger when wearing gloves, swab the finger with alcohol. Do not make a hole in the glove finger.

technical tip Often, a patient has veins that are more prominent in the dominant arm.

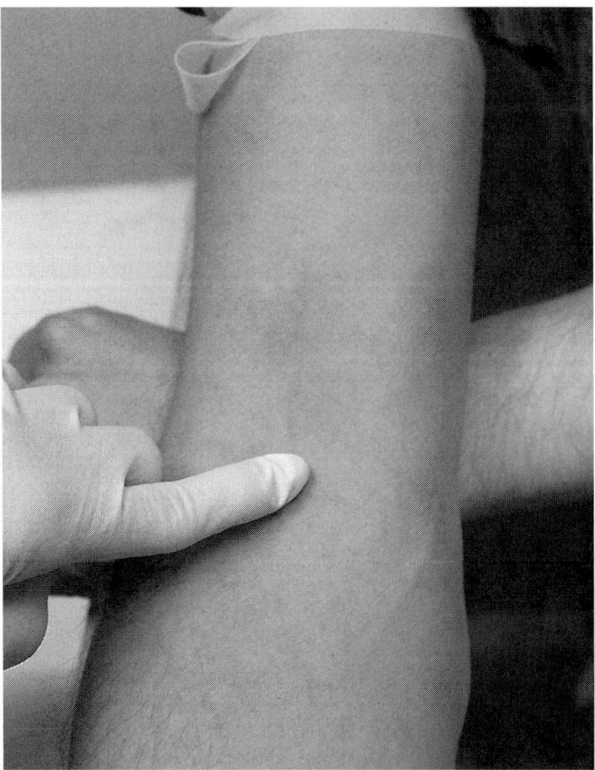

Figure 6–9 Palpating for a vein using the fingers, not the thumb.

Cleansing the Site

When an appropriate vein has been located, the tourniquet is released and the area cleansed using a 70% isopropyl alcohol prep pad. Cleansing is performed with a circular motion, starting at the inside of the venipuncture site and working outward in widening concentric circles (Fig. 6–10). Repeat this procedure for particularly dirty skin.

For maximum bacteriostatic action to occur, the alcohol should be allowed to dry for 30 to 60 seconds on the patient's arm rather than being wiped off with a gauze pad. Performing a venipuncture before the alcohol has dried will cause a stinging sensation for the patient and may hemolyze the specimen. Do not reintroduce microbial contaminants by blowing on the site, fanning the area, or drying the area with nonsterile gauze.

If additional palpation of the vein is needed after the cleansing process, the phlebotomist should use alcohol to cleanse the gloved end of the finger to be used.

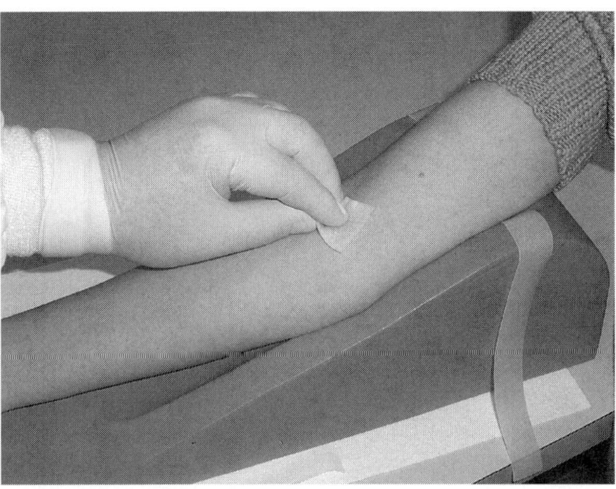

Figure 6–10 Cleansing the site.

technical tip Patients are quick to complain about a painful venipuncture. The stinging sensation caused by undry alcohol is a frequent, yet easily avoided, cause of complaints.

Assembly of Puncture Equipment

While the alcohol is drying, the phlebotomist can make a final survey of the supplies at hand to be sure everything required for the procedure is present and can then assemble the equipment.

The stopper-puncturing end of the double-ended evacuated tube needle is screwed into the needle adapter. The sterile cap is not removed from the other end of the needle. The first tube to be collected can be inserted into the needle adapter up to the designated mark. After the tube is pushed up to the mark, it may retract slightly when pressure is released. This is acceptable.

Visual examination cannot detect defective evacuated tubes; therefore, extra tubes should be near at hand. It is not uncommon for the vacuum in a tube to be lost.

technical tip Place assembled venipuncture equipment within easy reach; however, do not place the collection tray on the patient's bed.

Performing the Venipuncture

Reapply the tourniquet, and confirm the puncture site. If necessary, cleanse the gloved palpating finger for additional vein palpation. Again, ask the patient to make a fist.

Immediately before entering the vein, the plastic cap of the needle is removed and the point of the needle is visually examined for any defects such as a nonpointed or rough (barbed) end. The needle is then positioned for entry into the vein with the bevel facing up.

The evacuated tube holder/adapter or syringe is held securely in the dominant hand with the thumb on top and the remaining fingers below. After insertion is made, the fingers can be braced against the patient's arm to provide stability while tubes are being changed in the holder, or the plunger of the syringe is being pulled back. Figures 6–11 and 6–12 demonstrate the venipuncture procedure. Refer to these pictures during the following discussion.

Use the thumb of the nondominant hand to anchor the selected vein while inserting the needle (Fig. 6–11*A*). Place the thumb 1 or 2 inches below the insertion site and the four fingers on the back of the arm and pull the skin taut. Anchoring the vein above and below the site using the thumb and index finger is not an acceptable technique, because sudden patient movement could cause the index finger to be punctured. A vein that moves to the side is said to have "rolled." Patients often state that they have "rolling veins"; however, all veins will roll if they are not properly anchored. These patients are really saying that they have had blood drawn by phlebotomists who were not anchoring the veins well enough. As mentioned previously, the median cubital vein is the easiest to anchor and the basilic vein the most difficult. In general, the closer a vein is to the surface, the more likely it is to roll.

When the vein is securely anchored, align the needle with the vein and insert it, bevel up, at an angle of 15 to 30 degrees depending on the depth of the vein (Fig. 6–11*B*). This should be done in a smooth movement so the patient feels the stick only briefly. The phlebotomist will notice a feeling of lessening of resistance to the needle movement when the vein has been entered.

Once the vein has been entered, the hand anchoring the vein can be moved and used to push the evacuated tube completely into the holder/adapter

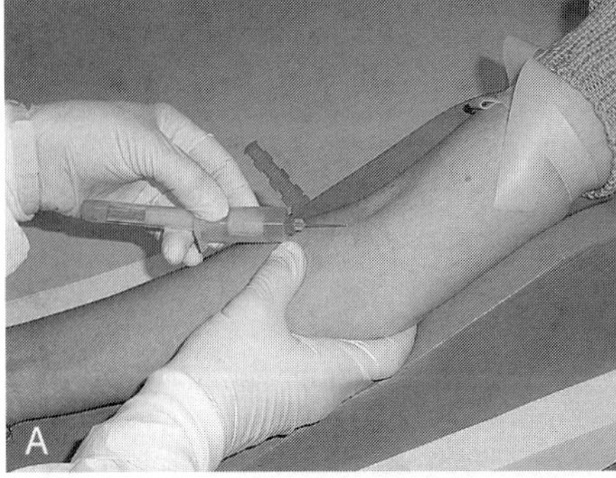

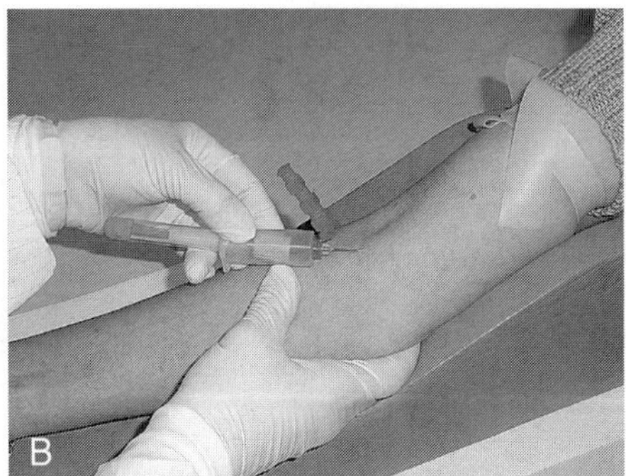

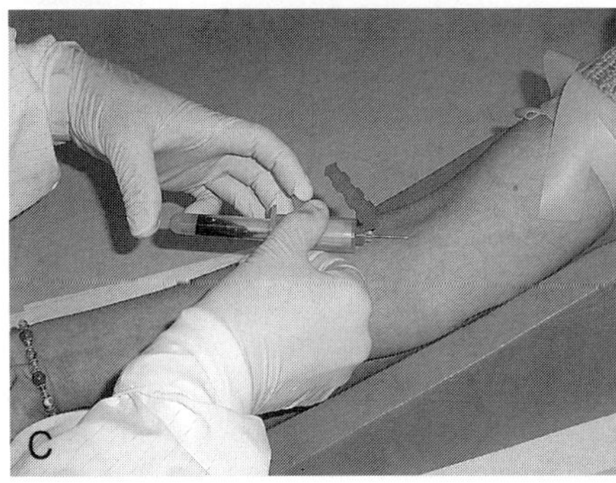

Figure 6–11 Venipuncture technique. *(A)* Anchoring the vein. *(B)* Inserting the needle. *(C)* Advancing the tube onto the needle. (Notice that this phlebotomist is left-handed and has switched hands during the procedure.)

or to pull back on the syringe plunger (Fig. 6–11*C*). Use the thumb to push the tube onto the back of the evacuated tube needle, while the index and middle fingers grasp the flared ends of the adapter. Blood should begin to flow into the tube, and the fist and tourniquet can be released, although if the procedure does not last more than 1 minute, the tourniquet can be left on until the last tube is filled. Some phlebotomists prefer to change hands at this point so that the dominant hand is free for performing the remaining tasks. This method of operating is usually better suited for use by experienced phlebotomists because holding the needle steady in the patient's vein is often difficult for beginners.

The hand used to hold the needle assembly should remain braced on the patient's arm. This is of particular importance when evacuated tubes are being inserted or removed from the holder/adapter, because a certain amount of resistance is encountered and can cause the needle to be pushed through or pulled out of the vein. Tubes should be gently twisted on and off the puncturing needle using the flared ends of the adapter as an additional brace (Fig. 6–12*A* and *B*).

To prevent any chance of blood refluxing back into the needle, tubes should be held at a downward angle while they are being filled and have slight pressure applied to them. Be sure to follow the prescribed order of draw when multiple tubes are being collected, and allow the tubes to fill completely before removing them. Mixing of evacuated tubes should be done as soon as the tube is removed, before another tube is placed in the assembly. The few seconds that this procedure requires does not cause additional discomfort to the patient and ensures that the specimen will be acceptable.

technical tip Pulling up or pressing down on the needle while it is in the vein can cause pain to the patient or a hematoma formation if blood leaks from the enlarged hole.

When the last tube has been filled, it is removed from the assembly and mixed before completing the procedure (Fig. 6–12*C*). Failure to remove the evacuated tube before removing the needle causes blood to drip from the end of the needle, resulting in unnecessary contamination and possible damage to the patient's clothes.

technical tip Allow tubes to fill until the vacuum is exhausted to ensure the correct blood to anticoagulant ratio.

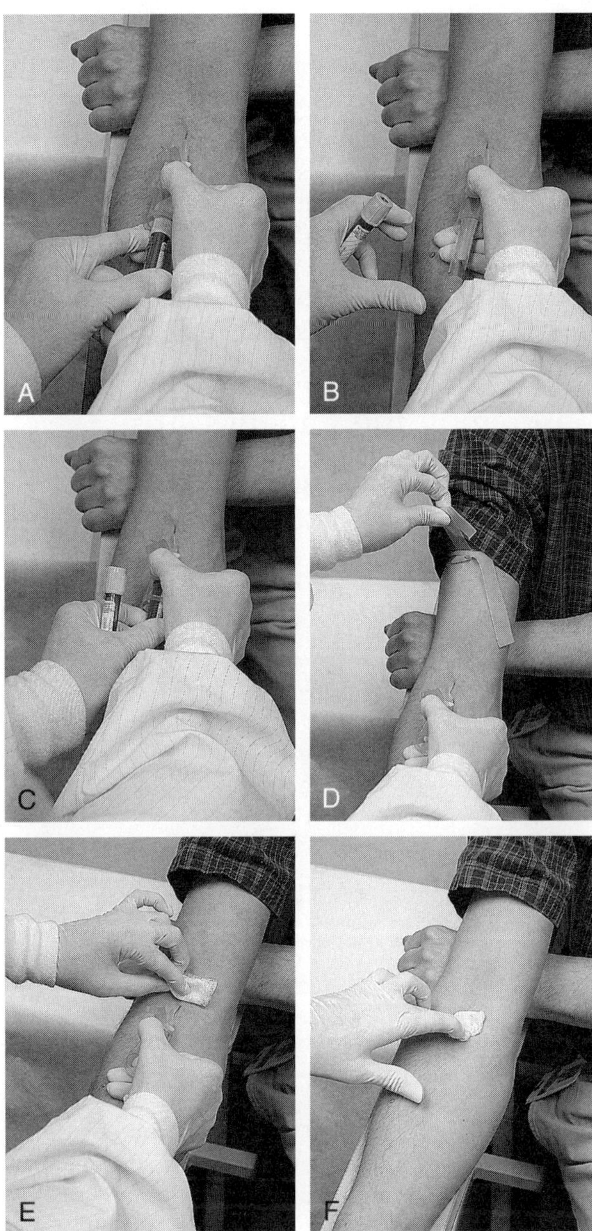

Figure 6–12 Venipuncture technique. *(A)* Sample collection. *(B)* Additional tube collection. *(C)* Removing the last tube. *(D)* Removing the tourniquet. *(E)* Removing the needle. *(F)* Applying pressure.

Removal of the Needle

Before removing the needle, remove the tourniquet by pulling on the free end and tell the patient to relax his or her hand (Fig. 6–12*D*). Failure to remove the tourniquet before removing the needle may produce a bruise (***hematoma***).

Place folded sterile gauze over the venipuncture site and withdraw the needle; apply pressure to the site as soon as the needle is withdrawn (Figs. 6–12*E* and *F*). Do not apply pressure while the needle is still in the vein. To prevent blood from leaking into the surrounding tissue and producing a hematoma, pressure must be applied until the bleeding has stopped. The arm should be held in a raised, outstretched position. Bending the elbow to apply pressure allows blood to leak more easily into the tissue, causing a hematoma. A capable patient can be asked to apply the pressure, thereby freeing the phlebotomist to dispose of the used needle and label the specimen tubes. If this is not possible, the phlebotomist must apply the pressure and perform the other tasks after the bleeding has stopped.

Disposal of the Needle

On completion of the venipuncture, the first thing the phlebotomist must do is dispose of the contaminated needle in an acceptable sharps container conveniently located near the patient (Fig. 6–13*A* to *C*). As discussed in Chapter 5, the method by which this is done will depend on the type of disposal equipment selected by the institution. Under no circumstance should the needle be bent, cut, placed on a counter or bed, or manually recapped.

technical tip Needle safety devices must be activated immediately upon removal of the needle from the vein following the manufacturer's guidelines.

Labeling the Tubes

Tubes are labeled by writing with an indelible pen on the attached label or by applying a computer-generated label that may also contain a designated bar code (Fig. 6–14*A* and *B*). Tubes must be labeled at the time of collection, before leaving the patient's room or before accepting another outpatient requisition. Traditionally, tubes have been labeled after the specimen has been collected to prevent confusion of specimens when additional tubes are needed because of lost vacuum or a restick is necessary. In

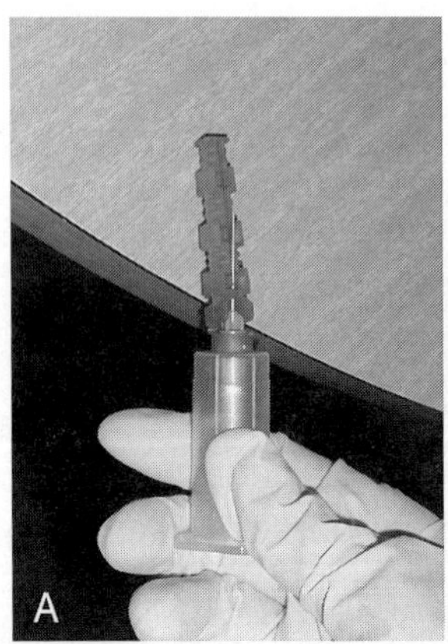

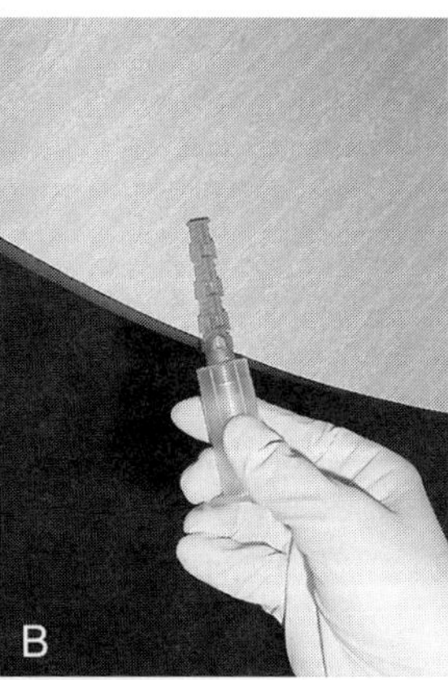

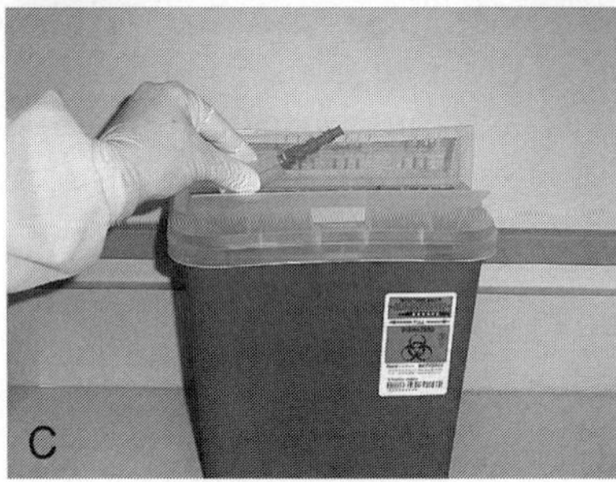

Figure 6–13 Needle disposal. *(A)* Activating safety shield. *(B)* Safety shield activated. *(C)* Disposal of safety needle and adapter.

the outpatient setting, some institutions attach computer-generated labels to the tubes before collection, and this is considered acceptable by the National Committee for Clinical Laboratory Standards (NCCLS). All preprinted labels must be carefully checked with the patient's identification before being attached to the specimen. Mislabeled specimens, just like misidentified patients, can result in serious patient harm.

Information on the specimen label must include the following:

- Patient's name and identification number
- Date and time of collection
- Phlebotomist's initials

Additional information may be present on computer-generated labels. Specimens for the blood bank may require an additional label obtained from the patient's blood bank ID band.

Specimens requiring special handling, such as cooling or warming, are placed in the appropriate container when labeling is complete.

Bandaging the Patient's Arm

Bleeding at the venipuncture site should stop within 5 minutes. Before applying the adhesive bandage, the phlebotomist should examine the patient's arm to be sure the bleeding has stopped. Paper tape should be used for patients allergic to adhesive bandages. For additional pressure, an adhesive bandage or tape is applied over a folded gauze square (Fig. 6–15). The patient should be instructed to remove the bandage within an hour and to avoid using the arm to carry heavy objects during that period.

technical tip The practice of quickly applying tape over the gauze without checking the puncture site frequently produces a hematoma.

Leaving the Patient

Before leaving the patient's room, the phlebotomist disposes of all contaminated supplies such as alcohol pads and gauze in a biohazard container, re-

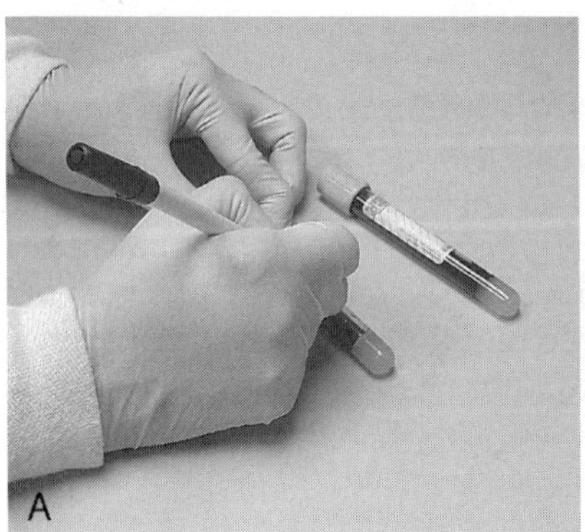

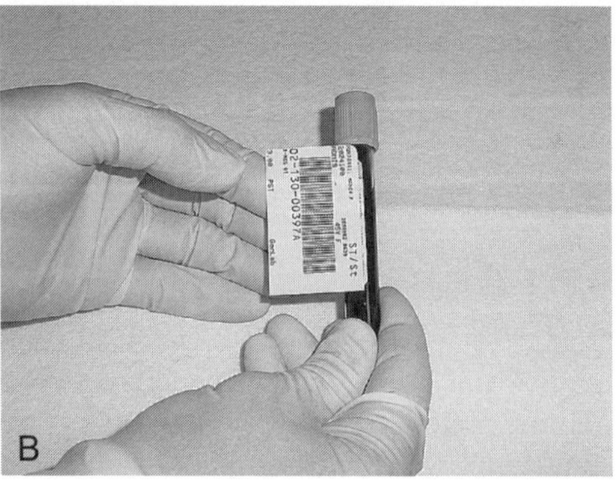

Figure 6–14 Labeling the tube. *(A)* Handwriting a label. *(B)* Applying computer label to a tube.

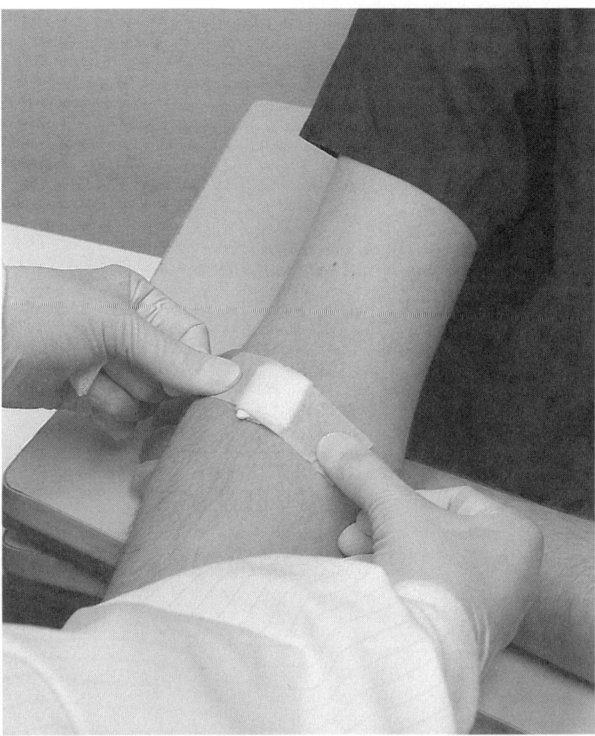

Figure 6–15 Bandaging the patient's arm.

moves gloves and disposes of them in the biohazard container, and washes the hands. Return the bed and bedrails to the original position if they have been moved. Failure to replace bedrails that results in patient injury can result in legal action.

In the outpatient setting, patients can be excused when the arm is bandaged. If patients have been fasting and no more procedures are scheduled, they should be instructed to eat. Before calling the next patient, the phlebotomist cleans up the area as described earlier. In both the inpatient and outpatient settings, patients should be thanked for their cooperation.

Completing the Venipuncture Procedure

The venipuncture procedure is complete when the specimen is delivered to the laboratory in satisfactory condition and all appropriate paperwork has been completed. These procedures vary depending on institutional protocol and the types of specimens collected. The phlebotomist needs to be familiar with procedures such as verifying collection in the computer system, making entries in the logbook, stamping the time of specimen arrival in the laboratory on the requisition form, and informing the nursing station that the procedure has been completed.

Delivering each specimen to the laboratory as soon as it is collected would not be efficient. However, this may be necessary for specimens requiring special handling, which is covered in the following chapters, and in stat situations. When possible, the phlebotomist should try to schedule patients so that a specimen requiring special handling is collected last.

Use designated containers for transport, and securely attach the requisitions with the specimen when using the pneumatic tube system.

Blood specimens should be transported to the laboratory for processing in a timely manner. The stability of analytes varies greatly, as do the accepted methods of preservation. This is why delivery to the laboratory or following laboratory prescribed specimen-handling protocols is essential. Common protocols include separation of the plasma or serum from the cells (either manually or by gel), storage temperature, and protecting the specimen from exposure to light. Gel separation tubes must always be stored in an upright position.

NCCLS recommends centrifugation of clotted tubes and separation of the serum from the cells within 2 hours. Ideally, the specimen should reach the laboratory within 45 minutes and be centrifuged on arrival. Tests most frequently affected by improper processing include glucose, potassium, and coagulation tests. **Glycolysis** caused by the use of glucose in cellular metabolism causes falsely lower glucose values. Hemolysis and leakage of intracellular potassium into the serum or plasma falsely elevates potassium results. Coagulation factors are destroyed in specimens remaining at room temperature for extended periods of time. Appendix I summarizes the requirements of some routinely encountered analytes.

technical tip Verification of the specimen collection either into the computer or recorded in a log book completes the collection process.

Summary of Venipuncture Technique with an Evacuated Tube System

1. Obtain and examine the requisition form.
2. Greet the patient.
3. Identify the patient.
4. Reassure the patient and explain the procedure.
5. Prepare the patient.
6. Select equipment and supplies.
7. Wash hands and apply gloves.
8. Apply the tourniquet.
9. Select the venipuncture site.
10. Release the tourniquet.
11. Cleanse the site.
12. Survey the supplies and assemble equipment.
13. Reapply the tourniquet.
14. Confirm the venipuncture site.
15. Examine the needle.
16. Anchor the vein.
17. Insert the needle.
18. Push the evacuated tube completely into adapter.
19. Gently invert the specimens, as they are collected.
20. Remove the last tube from the adapter.
21. Release the tourniquet.
22. Place sterile gauze over the needle.
23. Remove the needle, and apply pressure.
24. Activate needle safety device.
25. Dispose of the needle.
26. Label the tubes.
27. Perform appropriate specimen handling.
28. Examine the patient's arm.
29. Bandage the patient's arm.
30. Dispose of used supplies.
31. Remove and dispose of gloves.
32. Wash hands.
33. Complete any required paperwork.
34. Thank the patient.
35. Deliver specimens to appropriate locations.

Bibliography

National Committee for Clinical Laboratory Standards Approved Standard H3-A4: Procedure for Collection of Diagnostic Blood Specimens by Venipuncture. NCCLS, Wayne, PA, 1998.

National Committee for Clinical Laboratory Standards, Approved Guideline H18-A2: Procedure for the Handling and Processing of Blood Specimens. NCCLS, Wayne, PA, 1999.

Study Questions

1. List three reasons for requiring a requisition form before performing a venipuncture.
   a. ______________________
   b. ______________________
   c. ______________________
2. List five pieces of information that must be present on a requisition form.
   a. ______________________
   b. ______________________
   c. ______________________
   d. ______________________
   e. ______________________
3. List four pieces of information that must be present on a patient's ID band.
   a. ______________________
   b. ______________________
   c. ______________________
   d. ______________________
4. If no ID band is found on the patient's wrist, where should the phlebotomist look next?

   ____
5. What is the most serious error a phlebotomist can make?

   ____
6. List two reasons why an evacuated tube must be filled from the bottom up.
   a. ______________________
   b. ______________________
7. How does a phlebotomist prepare for the possibility of encountering a defective evacuated tube?

   ____
8. How does a properly applied tourniquet affect blood flow?

   ____
9. The maximum length of time a tourniquet should be applied is ______________________ .

10. List the three major veins located in the antecubital fossa.

    a. ______________________________

    b. ______________________________

    c. ______________________________

11. The preferred vein for venipuncture is the ______________________________.

12. The vein located on the thumb side of the arm is the ______________________________.

13. List three reasons for vein palpation.

    a. ______________________________

    b. ______________________________

    c. ______________________________

14. What might cause a patient to complain about a stinging sensation during a venipuncture?

    ____

15. The cause of "rolling veins" is ______________________________.

16. The angle of the needle during insertion is ______________________________.

17. Place the following steps in the venipuncture technique in the correct order by numbering them 1 through 10.

    a. ______________ Release the tourniquet

    b. ______________ Identify the patient

    c. ______________ Anchor the vein

    d. ______________ Cleanse the site

    e. ______________ Obtain a requisition form

    f. ______________ Label the tubes

    g. ______________ Bandage the puncture site

    h. ______________ Insert the needle

    i. ______________ Remove the needle and apply pressure

    j. ______________ Select equipment

18. When should a specimen collected in a lavender stopper tube be mixed?

    ____

19. List five pieces of information that should be present on the specimen label.

    a. ______________________________

    b. ______________________________

c. ______________________________

d. ______________________________

e. ______________________________

20. What should phlebotomists do immediately after removing their gloves?

____

Clinical Situations

1. A phlebotomist enters a patient's room. The phlebotomist asks "Are you Sandra Jones?" The patient answers "Yes." The phlebotomist applies the tourniquet, selects a vein, assembles the equipment, labels the tubes, cleanses the site, blows on the site to dry the alcohol, and performs the venipuncture.

   a. What is wrong with this situation?

   ____

   ____

   ____

   b. State three ways the patient in this scenario could be affected.

      1. ______________________________
      2. ______________________________
      3. ______________________________

2. Determine if the following are acceptable or not acceptable when performing a venipuncture, and explain your reason in one sentence.

   a. An outpatient with a sore back wishes to stand during the procedure.

   ____

   b. Assembling equipment prior to applying the tourniquet.

   ____

   c. Explaining the procedure to the patient.

   ____

   d. Requesting patients to pump their fists during sample collection.

   ____

   e. Palpating with the thumb.

   ____

   f. Cleansing the site in a circular motion from inside to outside.

   ____

g. Bending the patient's elbow while applying pressure to the puncture site.

____

h. Bracing the hand holding the needle against the patient's arm during specimen collection.

____

3. State an error in routine venipuncture technique that may cause:

a. a hematoma

____

b. petechiae

____

c. a patient to choke

____

d. blood to stop flowing when a tube is changed

____

e. blood drops on a patient's slacks when the needle is removed

____

f. a patient falling out of bed

____

4. A phlebotomist fails to deliver a light blue tube and an SST to the laboratory within the recommended time.

a. Name two tests that will have falsely decreased values.

____

____

b. Name a test that will have a falsely increased value.

____

NAME ______________________________

Evaluation of Tourniquet Application and Vein Selection

RATING SYSTEM 2 = SATISFACTORILY PERFORMED 1 = NEEDS IMPROVEMENT 0 = INCORRECT/DID NOT PERFORM

__________ 1. Positions arm correctly for vein selection

__________ 2. Selects appropriate tourniquet application site

__________ 3. Places tourniquet in flat position behind arm

__________ 4. Smoothly positions hands when crossing and tucking tourniquet

__________ 5. Fastens tourniquet at appropriate tightness

__________ 6. Tourniquet is not folded into arm

__________ 7. Loop and loose end do not interfere with puncture site

__________ 8. Asks patient to clench fist

__________ 9. Selects antecubital area to palpate

__________ 10. Performs palpation using correct fingers

__________ 11. Palpates entire area or both arms if necessary

__________ 12. Checks depth and direction of veins

__________ 13. Removes tourniquet smoothly

__________ 14. Removes tourniquet in a timely manner

TOTAL POINTS __________

MAXIMUM POINTS = 28

Comments:

NAME ____________________

Evaluation of Venipuncture Technique Using an Evacuated Tube

RATING SYSTEM 2 = SATISFACTORILY PERFORMED 1 = NEEDS IMPROVEMENT 0 = INCORRECT/DID NOT PERFORM

_______ 1. Examines requisition form

_______ 2. Greets patient and states procedure to be done

_______ 3. Identifies patient verbally

_______ 4. Examines patient's ID band

_______ 5. Compares requisition information with ID band

_______ 6. ~~Selects correct tubes and equipment for~~ procedure

_______ 7. Washes hands

_______ 8. Puts on gloves

_______ 9. Positions patient's arm

_______ 10. Applies tourniquet

_______ 11. Identifies vein by palpation

_______ 12. Releases tourniquet

_______ 13. Cleanses site and allows it to air dry 16

_______ 14. Assembles equipment

_______ 15. Reapplies tourniquet. 15

_______ 16. Does not touch puncture site with unclean finger

_______ 17. Anchors vein below puncture site

_______ 18. Smoothly enters vein at appropriate angle with bevel up

_______ 19. Does not move needle when changing tubes

_______ 20. Collects tubes in correct order

_______ 21. Mixes anticoagulated tubes promptly

_______ 22. Fills tubes completely

__________ 23. Removes last tube collected from adapter

__________ 24. Releases tourniquet within 1 minute

__________ 25. Covers puncture site with gauze

__________ 26. Removes the needle smoothly and applies pressure

__________ 27. Disposes of the needle in sharps container

__________ 28. Labels tubes

__________ 29. Examines puncture site

__________ 30. Applies bandage

__________ 31. Disposes of used supplies

__________ 32. Removes gloves and washes hands

__________ 33. Thanks patient

__________ 34. Converses appropriately with patient during procedure

TOTAL POINTS __________

MAXIMUM POINTS = 68

Comments:

Chapter 7

Venipuncture Complications

Chapter Outline

Requisitions

Greeting the Patient

Patient Identification

Patient Preparation
- Diet
- Posture
- Exercise
- Stress
- Smoking
- Diurnal Variation
- Medications
- Patient Complications

Equipment Assembly

Tourniquet Application

Site Selection
- Areas to be Avoided
- Cannulas and Fistulas

Cleansing the Site

Examination of Puncture Equipment

Performing the Venipuncture
- Using a Syringe
- Using a Winged Infusion Set
- Using Central Venous Access Devices
- Failure to Obtain Blood
- Hemolyzed Specimens

Removal of the Needle

Disposal of the Needle

Labeling the Tubes

Bandaging the Patient's Arm

Leaving the Patient

Completing the Venipuncture Procedure

Learning Objectives

Upon completion of this chapter, the reader will be able to:

1. State the procedure for coordinating requisition forms, patient identification, and labeling of tubes for unidentified patients.
2. Discuss the procedures to follow when patients are asleep, not in their rooms, or being visited by a physician, member of the clergy, or friend.
3. Describe the preanalytical variables that affect laboratory tests.
4. Discuss the procedure to follow when a patient develops syncope during the venipuncture procedure.
5. State the policy regarding patients who refuse to have their blood drawn.
6. State the reasons why the tourniquet can only be applied for 1 minute.
7. List four methods used to locate veins that are not prominent.
8. List three conditions when it is not advisable to draw from veins in the legs or feet.
9. State reasons why blood should not be drawn from a hematoma, burned or scarred area, or an arm adjacent to a mastectomy.
10. State three methods for obtaining blood from a patient with an intravenous device.
11. Discuss blood collection from central venous access devices.
12. State the procedure to follow when drawing blood from a patient with a fistula.
13. Describe the venipuncture procedure using a syringe, including equipment examination, technique for exchanging syringes, transfer of blood to evacuated tubes, and disposal of the equipment.
14. Describe the venipuncture procedure using a winged infusion set (butterfly), the technique involved, and disposal of equipment.
15. List six reasons why blood may not be immediately obtained from a venipuncture and the procedures to follow to obtain blood.
16. List 10 tests affected by hemolysis.
17. List 10 venipuncture errors that may produce hemolysis.
18. List six causes of hematomas.
19. List nine reasons for rejecting a specimen.

Key Terms

Basal state	*Heparin lock*	*Occluded*
Central venous access device	*Lymphostasis*	*Preanalytical variable*
Fistula	*Mastectomy*	*Syncope*

The venipuncture procedure discussed in Chapter 6 describes the procedure under normal circumstances; however, complications to the routine procedure can occur at any step. In this chapter, the procedure is reviewed in the same order with emphasis on the complications that may be encountered.

Requisitions

In the emergency room or other emergency situations, the request for phlebotomy may be telephoned to the laboratory and the requisition picked up by the phlebotomist at the patient site. A requisition picked up in an emergency situation must still contain all pertinent information for patient identification. The patient ID number from the patient's wristband may have to be written on the requisition form when a temporary identification system has been used.

Greeting the Patient

Patients are frequently asleep and should be gently awakened and given time to become oriented before the venipuncture is performed. Unconscious patients should be greeted in the same manner as conscious patients, because they may be capable of hearing and understanding even though they cannot respond. In this circumstance, nursing personnel are often present and can assist with the patient, if necessary.

It is usually preferable to have a nurse assist with patients on the psychiatric unit. These patients are often anxious about the venipuncture procedure and feel more comfortable when a caregiver with whom they are familiar is present. Be sure to place blood collection equipment away from the patient.

Physicians, members of the clergy, and visitors may be present when the phlebotomist enters the room. When the physician or clergy member is with the patient, it is preferable to return at another time, unless the request is for a stat or timed specimen. When this occurs, the phlebotomist should explain the situation and request permission to perform the procedure at that time. Visitors should be greeted in the same manner as the patient and given the option to step outside. If they choose to stay, the phlebotomist should assess their possible reactions and may elect to pull the curtain around the bed. Visitors can sometimes be helpful in the case of pediatric or very apprehensive patients.

Patients are not always in the room when the phlebotomist arrives. The phlebotomist should attempt to locate the patient by checking with the nursing station. The patient may be in the lounge or walking in the hall, or may have been taken to another department. If the specimen must be collected at a particular time, it may be possible to draw the patient in the area to which he or she has been taken. If this is not possible, the nursing station must be notified and the appropriate forms completed so that the test can be rescheduled. The requisition form is usually left at the nursing station. Message boards in the patient's room can be used to alert the nurse to call the lab for blood collection when the patient returns to the room.

Patient Identification

The phlebotomist will occasionally encounter a patient who has no ID band on either the wrist or the ankle. In this circumstance, the phlebotomist must contact the nursing station and request that the patient be banded before the drawing of blood. The nurse's signature on the requisition form verifying identification should be accepted in only emergency situations or according to hospital policy. Patients in psychiatric units often do not wear an identification band. Positive identification by the nursing staff is required with these patients. Follow strict institutional protocol in all special situations.

Unidentified patients are sometimes brought into the emergency room, and a system must be in place to ensure that they are correctly matched with their laboratory work. The American Association of Blood Banks (AABB) requires that the patient be positively identified with a temporary but clear designation attached to the body. Some hospitals generate identification bands with an identification number and a tentative name, such as John Doe or Patient X. Commercial identification systems are particularly useful when blood transfusions are required. In these systems, the identification band that is attached to the patient comes with matching identification stickers. The stickers are placed on the specimen tubes, requisition form, and any units of blood designated for the patient. Many hospitals use this type of system, in addition to the routine identification system, for all patients receiving transfusions. In some institutions, patients are required to wear the blood bank identification band for 48 hours during their inpatient stay to indicate how long the specimen that has been drawn can be used.

Patient Preparation

Numerous ***preanalytical variables*** associated with the patient's activities before specimen collection can affect the quality of the specimen. These variables can include diet, posture, exercise, stress, alcohol, smoking, time of day, and medications. The ideal time to collect blood from a patient is when the patient is in a ***basal state*** (has refrained from strenuous exercise and has not ingested food or beverages except water for 12 hours [**fasting**]). Normal values (reference ranges) for laboratory tests are determined from a normal, representative sample of volunteers who are in a basal state. Not all tests are affected by fasting and exercise, as evidenced by the collection and testing of specimens throughout the day, and many diagnostic results can be obtained at any time. However, the best comparison of a patient's results with the normal values can be made while the patient is in the basal state. This explains why phlebotomists begin blood collection in the hospital very early in the morning while the patient is in a basal state and why the majority of outpatients arrive in the laboratory as soon as the drawing station opens. Table 7–1 summarizes the major tests affected by variables that change the basal state. Phlebotomists should be aware of the effects these conditions have on test results and document them to help avoid a misdiagnosis.

Diet

The ingestion of food and beverages alters the level of certain blood components. The tests most affected are glucose and triglycerides. However, some laboratory tests require the patient to refrain from certain foods for a number of days before having blood collected. This is done to avoid interference with the interpretation of the test caused by substances present in the food.

Serum or plasma collected from patients shortly after a meal may appear cloudy or turbid (lipemic) owing to the presence of fatty compounds such as meat, cheese, butter, and cream. Lipemia will interfere with many test procedures.

TABLE 7–1
Major Tests Affected by Patient Preanalytical Variables

Variable	Increased Results	Decreased Results
Nonfasting	Glucose and triglycerides	
Prolonged fasting	Bilirubin and triglycerides	Glucose
Posture	Albumin, bilirubin, calcium, enzymes, cholesterol, total protein, triglycerides, RBCs, and WBCs	
Short-term exercise	Creatinine, fatty acids, lactate, AST, CK, LD, and WBCs	
Long-term exercise	Aldolase, creatinine, sex hormones, AST, CK, and LD	
Stress	Adrenal hormones, pO_2, and WBCs	Serum iron and pCO_2
Alcohol	Glucose and triglycerides	
Caffeine	Fatty acids and hormone levels	pH
Tobacco	Catecholamines, cortisol, hemoglobin, MCV, and WBCs	Eosinophil counts
Diurnal variation (a.m.)	Cortisol, testosterone and serum iron	Eosinophils, WBCs

AST = aspartate aminotransferase; CK = creatine phosphokinase; LD = lactic dehydrogenase

Certain beverages can also affect laboratory tests. Alcohol consumption can cause a transient elevation in glucose levels, and chronic alcohol consumption affects tests associated with the liver. Caffeine has been found to affect hormone levels, whereas hemoglobin levels and electrolyte balance can be altered by drinking too much liquid.

Because of these dietary interferences in laboratory testing, fasting specimens are often requested. When a fasting specimen is requested, it is the responsibility of the phlebotomist to determine whether the patient has been fasting for the required length of time. If the patient has not, this must be reported to a supervisor or the nurse and noted on the requisition form. For most tests, the patient is required to fast for 8 to 12 hours. As shown in Table 7–1, prolonged fasting, however, can also alter certain blood tests.

Posture

Changes in patient posture from a **supine** to an erect position cause variations in some blood constituents, such as cellular elements, plasma proteins, compounds bound to plasma proteins, and large-molecular-weight substances. The large size of these substances prevents their movement between the plasma and tissue fluid when body position changes. Therefore, when a person moves from a supine to an erect position and water leaves the plasma, the concentration of these substances increases in the plasma. Tests most noticeably elevated by the decreased plasma volume are cell counts, protein, albumin, bilirubin, cholesterol, triglycerides, calcium, and enzymes. The increase is most noticeable in patients with disorders such as congestive heart failure and liver diseases that cause increased fluid to remain in the tissue. When inpatient and outpatient results are being compared, the physician may request that an outpatient lie down before specimen collection.

Exercise

Moderate or strenuous exercise affects laboratory test results by increasing the blood levels of creatinine, fatty acids, lactic acid, aspartate aminotransferase (AST), creatine phosphokinase (CK), lactic dehydrogenase (LD), aldolase, sex hormones, and white blood cell (WBC) count. Transient short-term exercise and prolonged exercise or weight training affect test results differently. Short-term exercise elevates the enzymes associated with muscles (AST, CK, LD) and the WBC count because WBCs attached to the venous walls are released into the circulation. The values usually return to normal within several hours of relaxation in a healthy person. Prolonged exercise also increases the muscle-related waste products (AST, CK, and LD) and sex hormones, and they will remain more consistently elevated.

Stress

Failure to calm a frightened, nervous patient before specimen collection may increase levels of adrenal hormones (cortisol and catecholamines), increase WBC counts, decrease serum iron, and markedly affect arterial blood gas (ABG) results. It has been shown that WBC counts collected from a crying child may be noticeably elevated. This is also caused by the release of WBCs attached to the blood vessel walls into the circulation. In contrast, WBC counts on early morning specimens collected from patients in a basal state will be decreased until normal activity is resumed. Elevated WBC counts return to normal within 1 hour. For an accurate WBC count, discontinue blood collection from a crying child until after the child has been calm for at least 1 hour.

Severe anxiety that results in hyperventilation may cause acid-base imbalances and increased lactate and fatty acid levels.

Smoking

The immediate effects of tobacco include increases in plasma catecholamines and cortisol, with a resulting decrease in eosinophils and increase in neutrophils. Chronic smoking increases hemoglobin, red blood cell (RBC) counts, and the mean corpuscular volume (MCV) because the body is not receiving enough oxygen. This finding will also be seen in persons living in high altitude areas (i.e., the mountains).

Diurnal Variation

The concentration of some blood constituents is affected by the time of day. Diurnal rhythm is the normal fluctuation in blood levels at different times of the day based on a 24-hour cycle of eating and sleeping. Cortisol and serum iron levels are highest in the morning, whereas WBC counts and eosinophil counts are lower.

Medications

Administration of medication prior to specimen collection may affect tests results, either by changing a metabolic process within the patient or by producing interference with the testing procedure. Intravenous administration of dyes used in diagnostic procedures, including radiographic contrast media for kidney disorders and fluorescein used to evaluate cardiac blood vessels, can interfere with testing procedures. In general, understanding the affect of medications and diagnostic procedures on laboratory test results is the responsibility of the healthcare provider, pathologist, or clinical laboratory testing personnel. Phlebotomists, however, should be aware of any procedures being performed at the time they are collecting a specimen and note this on the requisition form. For example, specimens collected while a patient is receiving a blood transfusion may not represent the patient's true condition.

A variety of medications, both prescription and over-the-counter, can influence laboratory test results. Physicians frequently order tests to evaluate the effect of certain prescribed medications on body systems. In other cases, test results may be affected by over-the-counter medications not reported to the physician by the patient. An extensive list of drugs that can interfere with laboratory test results can be found in Effects of Drugs on Clinical Laboratory Tests, 5th Edition, by D.S. Young (AACC Press, Washington, D.C., 2000).

Medications that are toxic to the liver can cause an increase in blood liver enzymes and abnormal coagulation tests. Elevated blood urea nitrogen (BUN) levels or imbalanced electrolytes may be noted in patients taking medications that impair renal function. Patients taking corticosteroids, estrogens, or diuretics can develop pancreatitis and would have elevated serum amylase and lipase levels. Chemotherapy drugs cause a decrease in WBCs and platelets. Patients on diuretics may have elevated calcium, glucose, and uric acid levels, and decreased potassium levels. Aspirin, medications that contain salicylate, and certain herb use can interfere with platelet function or Coumadin anticoagulant therapy and may cause increased risk of bleeding. Herbs that have been reported to have effects on coagulation are chamomile, clove, echinacea, evening primrose oil, fever few, garlic, ginger, ginkgo biloba, ginseng, goldenseal, horse chestnut, kava kava, licorice, meadowsweet, poplar, and white willow (Table 7–2).

The College of American Pathologists recommends that drugs known to interfere with blood tests should be discontinued 4 to 24 hours before blood tests, and 48 to 72 hours before urine tests.

technical tip Patients taking herbs often do not realize the side effect of bleeding that can occur. When excessive post venipuncture bleeding occurs, question the patient about herbal medications and document this on the requisition.

TABLE 7–2
Common Medications Affecting Laboratory Tests

Medication	Affected Tests/Systems
Acetaminophen and certain antibiotics	Elevated liver enzymes and bilirubin
Cholesterol-lowering drugs	Prolonged PT and APTT
Certain antibiotics	Elevated BUN, creatinine, and electrolyte imbalance
Corticosteroids and estrogen diuretics	Elevated amylase, and lipase
Diuretics	Increased calcium, glucose, and uric acid
Chemotherapy	Decreased RBCs, WBCs, and platelets
Aspirin, salicylates, and herbal supplements	Prolonged PT and bleeding time
Radiographic contrast media	Routine urinalysis
Fluorescein dye	Increased creatinine, cortisol, and digoxin

APTT = activated partial thromboplastin time; BUN = blood urea nitrogen; PT = prothrombin time; RBCs =red blood cells; WBCs = white blood cells.

Patient Complications

It is common to encounter extremely apprehensive patients. Enlisting the help of the nurse who has been caring for the patient may help to calm the person's fears. It may also be necessary to ask for assistance from the nurse to hold the patient's arm steady during the procedure. Assistance from a nurse or parent is frequently required when working with children. Phlebotomists also may require nursing assistance when encountering patients in fixed positions, such as those in traction or body casts.

Apprehensive patients may be prone to fainting (*syncope*), and the phlebotomist should be alert to this possibility. It is sometimes possible to detect such patients during vein palpation because their skin feels cold and damp. Keeping their minds off the procedure through conversation can be helpful. If a patient begins to faint during the procedure, immediately remove the tourniquet and needle, and apply pressure to the venipuncture site. In the inpatient setting, notify the nursing station as soon as possible. In the outpatient area, make sure the patient is supported and that the patient lowers his or her head. Cold compresses applied to the forehead and back of the neck will help to revive the patient. Outpatients who have been fasting for prolonged periods should be given something sweet to drink and required to remain in the area for 15 to 30 minutes. All incidents of syncope should be documented following institutional policy.

technical tip Patients frequently mention previous adverse reactions. If these patients are sitting up, it may be wise to have them lie down before collection. It is not uncommon for patients with a history of fainting to faint again.

It is rare for patients to develop seizures during venipuncture. If this situation occurs, the tourniquet and needle should be removed, pressure applied to the site, and help summoned. Restrain the patient only to the extent that injury is prevented. Do not attempt to place anything in the patient's mouth. Any very deep puncture caused by sudden movement by the patient should be reported to the physician. Document the seizure following institutional policy.

Patients who present with small, nonraised red hemorrhagic spots (petechiae) may have prolonged bleeding following venipuncture. Petechiae can be an indication of a coagulation disorder, such as a low platelet count or abnormal platelet function. Additional pressure should be applied to the puncture site following needle removal.

Phlebotomists must be alert for changes in a patient's condition and notify the nursing station. Such changes could include the presence of vomitus, urine, or feces; infiltrated or removed intravenous fluid lines; extreme breathing difficulty; and possibly a patient who has expired.

Patient Refusal

Some patients may refuse to have their blood drawn, and they have the right to do this. The phlebotomist can stress to the patient that the results are needed by the healthcare provider for treatment and discuss the problem with the nurse, who may be able to convince the patient to agree to have the test performed. If the patient continues to refuse, this decision should be written on the requisition form and the form should be left at the nursing station or the area stated in the institution policy.

Equipment Assembly

When positioning the needed equipment and supplies within easy reach, the phlebotomist should include extra evacuated collection tubes. Occasionally, an evacuated tube does not contain the proper amount of vacuum necessary to collect a full tube of blood. Accidentally pushing a tube past the indicator mark on the needle holder before the vein is entered will also result in loss of vacuum.

As discussed in Chapter 3, remember that only the necessary amount of equipment is brought into isolation rooms. For patients on the psychiatric unit, leave the phlebotomy tray at the nursing station and take only the necessary equipment into the room. Do not leave any type of equipment in the patients' room.

Tourniquet Application

As discussed in Chapter 5, a blood pressure cuff is sometimes used to locate veins that are difficult to find. The cuff should be inflated to a pressure below the systolic and above the diastolic blood pressure readings. Too much pressure affects the flow of arterial blood.

When dealing with patients with skin conditions, it may be necessary to place the tourniquet over the patient's gown or to cover the area with gauze before application. If possible, another area should be selected for the venipuncture. Consideration should be given to using a disposable tourniquet.

Application of the tourniquet for more than 1 minute will interfere with some test results, which is why the National Committee for Clinical Laboratory Standards (NCCLS) set the limit on tourniquet application time to be 1 minute and states that the tourniquet should be released as soon as the vein is accessed. Prolonged tourniquet time causes hemoconcentration because the plasma portion of the blood passes into the tissue. Tests most likely to be affected are those measuring large molecules, such as plasma proteins and lipids, RBCs, and substances bound to protein such as iron, calcium, magnesium; or analytes affected by hemolysis, including potassium, lactic acid, and enzymes. Tourniquet application and fist clenching are not recommended when drawing specimens for lactic acid determinations.

Releasing the tourniquet as soon as blood begins to flow into the first tube can sometimes result in the inability to fill multiple collection tubes. Phlebotomists may have to make a decision regarding immediately removing the tourniquet based on the size of the patients' veins or the difficulty of the puncture. Regardless of the situation, the tourniquet should not remain in place for longer than 1 minute.

Other causes of hemoconcentration are excessive squeezing or probing a site, long-term intravenous (IV) therapy, sclerosed or occluded veins, and vigorous fist clenching.

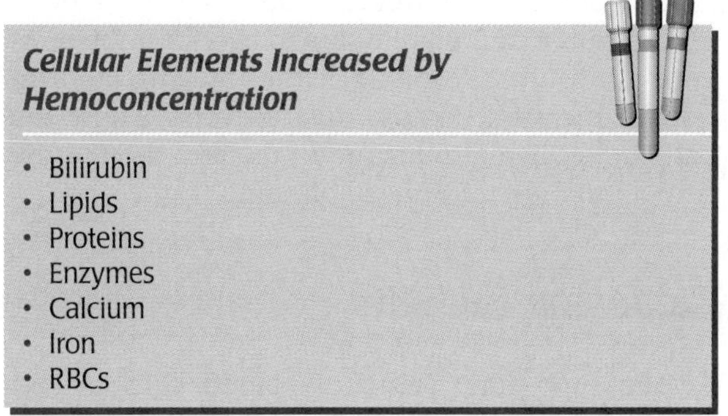

Cellular Elements Increased by Hemoconcentration

- Bilirubin
- Lipids
- Proteins
- Enzymes
- Calcium
- Iron
- RBCs

Site Selection

Not all patients have a median cubital, cephalic, or basilic vein that becomes immediately prominent when the tourniquet is applied. In fact, a high percentage of patients have veins that are not easily located, and the phlebotomist may have to use a variety of techniques to locate a suitable puncture site. Many patients have prominent veins in one arm and not in the other; therefore, checking the patient's other arm should be the first thing done when a site is not easily located. Patients with veins that are difficult to locate often point out areas where they remember previous successful phlebotomies. Palpation of these areas may prove beneficial and is also good for patient relations.

technical tip Never be reluctant to check both arms and to listen to the patient's suggestions.

Other techniques used by phlebotomists to enhance the prominence of veins include tapping the antecubital area with the index finger, massaging the arm upward from the wrist to the elbow, briefly hanging the arm down, and applying heat to the site for 3 to 5 minutes. Remember that when performing these techniques, the tourniquet should not remain tied for more than 1 minute at a time.

If no palpable veins are found in the antecubital area, the wrist and hand should be examined. The tourniquet is retied on the forearm. Because the veins in these areas are smaller, it may be necessary to change equipment and use a smaller needle with a syringe or winged infusion set or a smaller evacuated tube.

Veins in the legs and feet are sometimes used as venipuncture sites. They should be used only with physician approval. Leg veins are more susceptible to infection and the formation of thrombi (clots), particularly in patients with diabetes, cardiac problems, and coagulation disorders.

Areas to Be Avoided

Veins that contain thrombi or have been subjected to numerous venipunctures often feel hard (**sclerosed**) and should be avoided as they may be blocked (***occluded***) and have impaired circulation. Areas that appear blue or are cold may also have impaired circulation.

The presence of a hematoma indicates that blood has accumulated in the tissue surrounding a vein. Puncturing into a hematoma is not only painful for the patient but will result in the collection of old, hemolyzed blood from the hematoma rather than circulating venous blood that is representative of the patient's current condition. If a vein containing a hematoma must be used, blood should be collected below the hematoma to ensure sampling of free flowing blood. Drawing from areas containing excess tissue fluid (**edema**) is also not recommended because the sample will be contaminated with tissue fluid.

Extensively burned and scarred areas, including tattoos, are more susceptible to infection; they also have decreased circulation and veins that are difficult to palpate.

Applying a tourniquet to or drawing blood from an arm located on the same side of the body as a recent ***mastectomy*** can be harmful to the patient and produce erroneous test results. Removal of lymph nodes in the mastectomy procedure interferes with the flow of lymph fluid (***lymphostasis***) and increases the blood level of lymphocytes and waste products normally contained in the lymph fluid. Patients are in danger of developing **lymphedema** in the affected area, and this could be increased by application of a tourniquet. The protective functions of the lymphatic system are also lost, so that the area becomes more prone to infection. For these reasons, blood should be drawn from the other arm. In the case of a double mastectomy, the physician should be consulted as to an appropriate site, such as the hand. It may be possible to perform the tests from a fingerstick.

technical tip Most mastectomy patients have been told never to have blood drawn from the affected side. Make sure they receive appropriate reassurance in cases of a double mastectomy.

Frequently, the phlebotomist encounters patients receiving IV fluids in an arm vein. Whenever possible, blood should then be drawn from the other arm. If an arm containing an IV must be used for specimen collection, the site selected must be below the IV insertion point and preferably in a different vein. If blood is collected from the IV needle, the nurse should be asked to turn off the IV drip for at least 2 minutes. The first 5 mL of blood drawn must be discarded, because it may be contaminated with IV fluid. A new syringe is then used for the specimen collection. If a coagulation test is ordered, an additional 5 mL of blood should be drawn before collecting the coagulation test specimen because intravenous lines are frequently flushed with heparin. This additional blood can be used for other tests if they have been requested. Collections from an IV site are usually performed by the nursing staff to ensure proper care of the site. Whenever blood is collected from an arm containing an IV needle, this procedure must be noted on the requisition form.

Heparin or saline ***locks*** are winged infusion sets that can be left in a vein for up to 48 hours to provide a means for administering frequently required medications and for obtaining blood specimens. The devices must be flushed with heparin or saline periodically and after use to prevent blood clots from developing in the line.

technical tip Inappropriate collection of blood from an arm containing an IV is a major cause of erroneous test results. Unless the specimen is highly contaminated, the error may not be detected.

Cannulas and Fistulas

Patients receiving renal dialysis have a permanent surgical fusion of an artery and a vein called a ***fistula*** in one arm, and this arm should be avoided for venipuncture owing to the possibility of infection. The dialysis patient may also have a temporary external connection between the artery and a vein formed by a **cannula** that contains a special T-tube connector with a diaphragm for drawing blood. Only specifically trained personnel are authorized to draw blood from a cannula. Be sure to check for the presence of a fistula or cannula before applying a tourniquet to the arm, because this can compromise the patient. Accidental puncture of the area around the fistula can cause prolonged bleeding.

Cleansing the Site

Certain procedures, primarily blood cultures and ABGs, require that the site be cleansed with a stronger antiseptic than isopropyl alcohol (see Chapter 8). The most frequently used solutions are povidone-iodine and tincture of iodine or chlorhexidene gluconate for persons who are allergic to iodine.

Alcohol should not be used to cleanse the site before drawing a blood alcohol level. Thoroughly cleansing the site with soap and water will ensure the least amount of interference. Some institutions use benzalkonium chloride (Zephiran Chloride) to cleanse the site or find iodine to be acceptable.

Examination of Puncture Equipment

When using a syringe, the plunger is pulled back and pushed forward while the protective cap is still on the needle to ensure that it will move freely when the vein has been entered. The protective cap on the needle is then removed, and the needle point is examined for imperfections just before insertion. Syringe and butterfly needles should be examined for flaws in the same manner as evacuated tube needles.

Performing the Venipuncture

Although venipuncture is most frequently performed using an evacuated tube system, it may be necessary to use a syringe or butterfly apparatus to better control the pressure applied to the delicate veins found in pediatric and elderly patients, or when drawing from hand veins.

Using a Syringe

Except for a few minor differences, the procedure for drawing blood using a syringe is the same as when using an evacuated tube system. Blood is withdrawn from the vein by slowly pulling on the plunger of the syringe, using the hand that is free after the anchored vein is entered, as shown in Figure 7–1. The advantage of using a syringe is that when the vein is entered, blood will appear in the hub of the needle and the plunger can then be pulled back at a speed that corresponds to the rate of blood flow into the syringe. Pulling the plunger back faster than the rate of blood flow may cause the walls of the vein to collapse (see Fig. 7–5F) and can cause hemolysis. It is important to anchor the hand holding the syringe firmly on the patient's arm so that the needle will not move when the plunger is pulled.

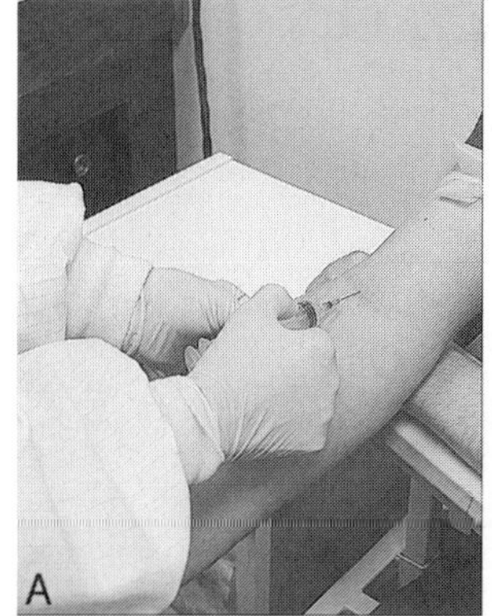

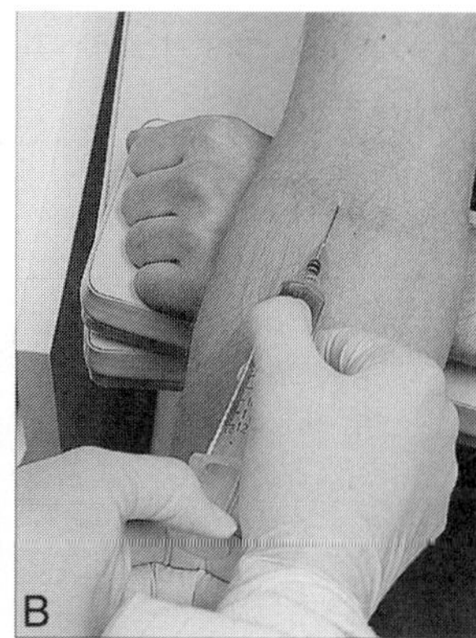

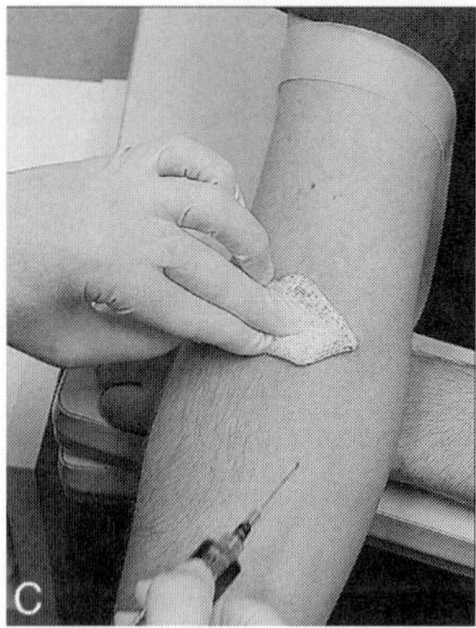

Figure 7–1 Venipuncture using a syringe. *(A)* Inserting the syringe needle into the vein. *(B)* Pulling back on the syringe plunger. *(C)* Removing the needle.

Ideally, the size of the syringe used should correspond with the amount of blood needed. However, with small veins that easily collapse, it may be necessary to fill two or more smaller syringes. This procedure will require assistance, because blood from the filled syringe must be transferred to the appropriate tubes while the second syringe is being filled. Before exchanging syringes, gauze must be placed on the patient's arm under the needle because blood will leak from the hub of the needle during the exchange.

technical tip In many circumstances, the use of small evacuated tubes instead of a syringe can prevent the need to change syringes.

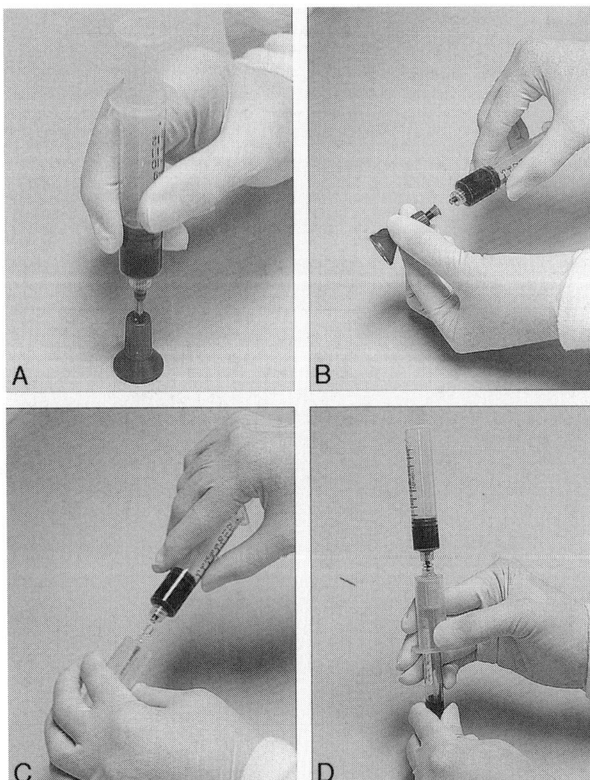

Figure 7–2 Transfer of blood from a syringe to an evacuated tube. *(A)* Inserting the syringe needle into the Portex Point-Lok device. *(B)* Removing needle from syringe. *(C)* Attaching the BD blood transfer device. *(D)* Advancing the tube onto the needle in the blood transfer device.

As discussed in Chapter 5, blood is transferred from the syringe to evacuated tubes, following the prescribed order of fill. Puncture the rubber tube stopper using a one-handed technique to avoid an accidental needlestick and allow the blood to flow slowly down the side of the tube to prevent hemolysis. A better alternative is to insert the needle into a Portex Point-Lok device and remove the needle. Then, using the BD blood transfer device, the sample is placed into tubes (Fig. 7–2). After transferring the sample, the needle, Point-Lok device, syringe, and transfer device are discarded into a sharps container (Fig. 7–3).

Using a Winged Infusion Set

All routine venipuncture procedures used with evacuated tubes and syringes also apply to blood collection using a winged infusion set (butterfly). This method is used for difficult venipuncture and is often less painful to patients. By folding the plastic needle attachments ("wings") upward while inserting the needle, the angle of insertion can be lowered to 10 to 15 degrees, thereby facilitating entry into small veins. Blood will appear in the tubing when the vein is entered. The needle can then be threaded securely into the vein and kept in place by holding the plastic wings against the patient's arm. Depending on the type of winged infusion set used, blood can be collected into evacuated tubes or into a syringe. The tubing contains a small amount of air that will cause

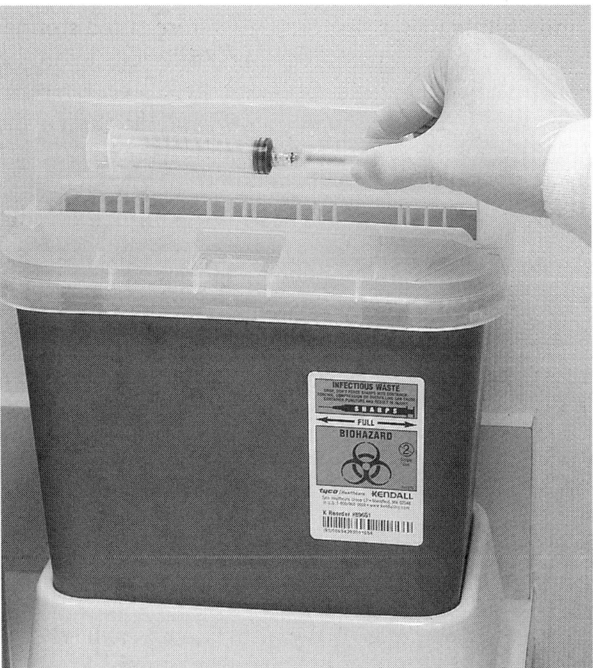

Figure 7–3 Syringe assembly disposal.

technical tip Do not hold evacuated collection tubes in your hand when filling them from a syringe. Place the tubes in the correct order of fill in a rack to prevent possible accidental needlesticks.

technical tip Forcing blood into the evacuated collection tube by pushing the syringe plunger can hemolyze the blood and create blood splatter when removing the needle from the stopper. The extra pressure may force the tube stopper to pop off and splatter blood.

underfilling of the first tube; therefore, a red stopper tube or discard tube should be collected before an anticoagulated tube to maintain the correct blood to anticoagulant ratio. To prevent hemolysis when using a small (23- or 25-gauge) needle, pediatric-size evacuated tubes should be used. When using, be sure to attach the adapter and not just push the tubes onto the back of the rubber sheathed needle. This will avoid an accidental needlestick exposure from the stopper-puncturing needle. Tubes are positioned downward to fill from the bottom up and in the same order of draw as in routine venipuncture. If blood has been collected into a syringe, the winged infusion set is removed from the syringe, a new 21-gauge needle attached, and the tubes are filled in the same manner as described earlier. Again, a safer alternative is to attach the BD blood transfer device to the syringe on removal of the winged infusion set (Fig. 7–2).

When disposing of the winged infusion set, use extreme care, because many accidental sticks result from unexpected movement of the tubing. Placing the needle into a sharps container before removing the syringe and then allowing the tubing to fall into the container when the syringe is removed can prevent accidents. Always hold a butterfly apparatus by the wings, not by the tubing. Using an apparatus with automatic resheathing capability or activating a device on the needle set that advances a safety blunt before removing the needle from the vein is recommended to prevent accidental needle punctures. Do not push the apparatus manually into a full sharps container.

The venipuncture procedure using a winged infusion set is shown in Figure 7–4.

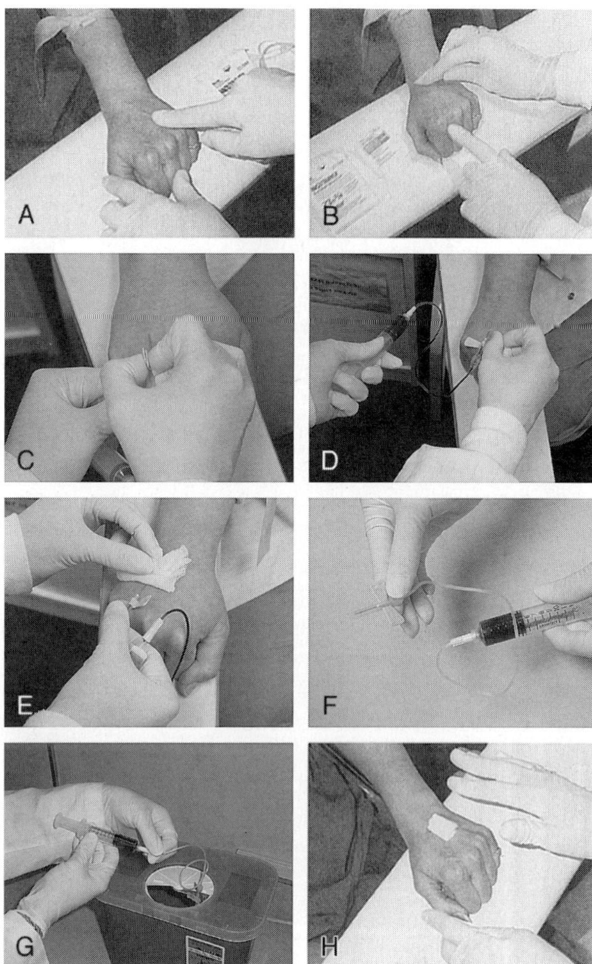

Figure 7–4 Venipuncture using a butterfly. *(A)* Hand vein palpation. *(B)* Cleansing the puncture site. *(C)* Inserting the needle. *(D)* Collecting blood in a syringe. *(E)* Removing the needle. *(F)* Activating the needle safety guard. *(G)* Disposing of the butterfly apparatus. *(H)* Patient's hand with pressure bandage.

Using Central Venous Access Devices

Blood specimens may be obtained from devices called ***central venous access devices*** (**CVADs**). However, this procedure must be performed by specially trained personnel, usually a member of the nursing staff, and physician authorization is required. Specific procedures must be followed for flushing the **catheters** with saline, and possibly heparin, when blood collection is completed (see Appendix II). Sterile technique procedures must be strictly adhered to when entering IV lines, because they provide a direct path for infectious organisms to enter the patient's bloodstream.

A CVAD is a device that has a catheter with a tip lying in the superior vena cava. It can be used for administration of fluids, drugs, blood products, and nutritional solutions, and to obtain blood specimens. Four major categories of CVADs used include the following:

1 Nontunneled
2 Tunneled
3 Implanted Portacaths
4 Peripherally inserted central catheters (**PICCs**)

The nontunneled CVAD is used for short-term dwell times and is percutaneously inserted into the jugular, subclavian, or femoral vein and threaded to the superior vena cava by a physician during surgery or in a hospital room with local anesthetic. It can be a single-, double-, or triple-lumen catheter. When using multilumen catheters, the proximal lumen is the preferred lumen from which to obtain a blood specimen. The lumens not being used should be clamped when drawing blood, to avoid contamination of the blood sample. A dressing covers the insertion site, and flushes are necessary to maintain patency of the CVAD.

The tunneled CVAD is considered more permanent and is used for long-term dwell times, such as administration of chemotherapy. The Hickman and Groshong catheters are examples of this single- or double-lumen type of catheter. A surgeon performs a cut-down of the vein with local or IV sedation and tunnels the catheter in subcutaneous tissue under the skin to the exit site, with the catheter tip in the superior vena cava. Dressing changes and flushing with heparin or saline are required maintenance for this type of catheter.

The implanted Portacath is a small chamber attached to a catheter that is also considered more permanent. It is used for long-term access to the central venous system for a patient requiring frequent IVs or receiving chemotherapy. Using local or IV sedation, a surgeon implants the Portacath in subcutaneous tissue under the skin with the catheter tip placed in the superior vena cava. The self-sealing septum of the device withstands 1000 to 2000 needle punctures; however, only noncoring needles can be used. The advantages of this CVAD are that there is no visible catheter tubing and no site care is needed when it is not being used. It is flushed monthly with heparin or saline.

The PICC is placed in the basilic or cephalic vein in the antecubital area of the arm, with the tip threaded to the superior vena cava. PICCs can be placed by IV team nurses or physicians and can be used for weeks to months. The advantage of a PICC is that it has few risks and causes minimal discomfort to the patient. A disadvantage of blood collection from a PICC is that the catheter walls are easily collapsed.

When intravenous fluids are being administered through the CVAD, the flow should be stopped for 5 minutes before collecting the sample. Syringes larger than 20 mL should not be used because the high negative pressure produced may collapse the catheter wall. At all times, the first 5 mL of blood must be discarded and a new syringe must be used to collect the sample. Drawing coagulation tests from a venous catheter is not recommended, but if this is necessary, they should be collected after 20 mL (or five to six times the volume of the catheter) of blood has been discarded or used for other tests.

The order of tube fill may vary slightly to accommodate the amount of blood that must be drawn before a coagulation test. As with other procedures, blood cultures are always collected first. Blood cultures are drawn from CVADs primarily to detect infection of the catheter tip and should be compared with results from blood cultures drawn from a peripheral vein. If these are ordered, the draw will satisfy the additional discard needed for coagulation tests. Therefore, the order of fill is as follows:

1. First syringe—5 mL discard
2. Second syringe—blood cultures
3. Third syringe—anticoagulated tubes (light blue, lavender, green, and gray)
4. Clotted tubes (red and serum separator tube [SST])

If blood cultures are not ordered, the coagulation tests (light blue stopper tube) can be collected with a new syringe after the other specimens have been collected using the order shown earlier. Phlebotomists are frequently responsible for assisting the nurse who is collecting blood from the CVAD and should understand these specimen collection requirements. The source of the specimen should be noted on the requisition form. Under no circumstances should a person without specialized training collect specimens from a CVAD.

technical tip When blood is collected from a CVAD, blood should not be left in the syringe while extensive flushing of the CVAD is performed. Anticoagulation of the specimen also is important.

Failure to Obtain Blood

Not all venipunctures result in the immediate appearance of blood; however, in many instances, this is only a temporary setback that can be corrected by slight movement of the needle. It is important for

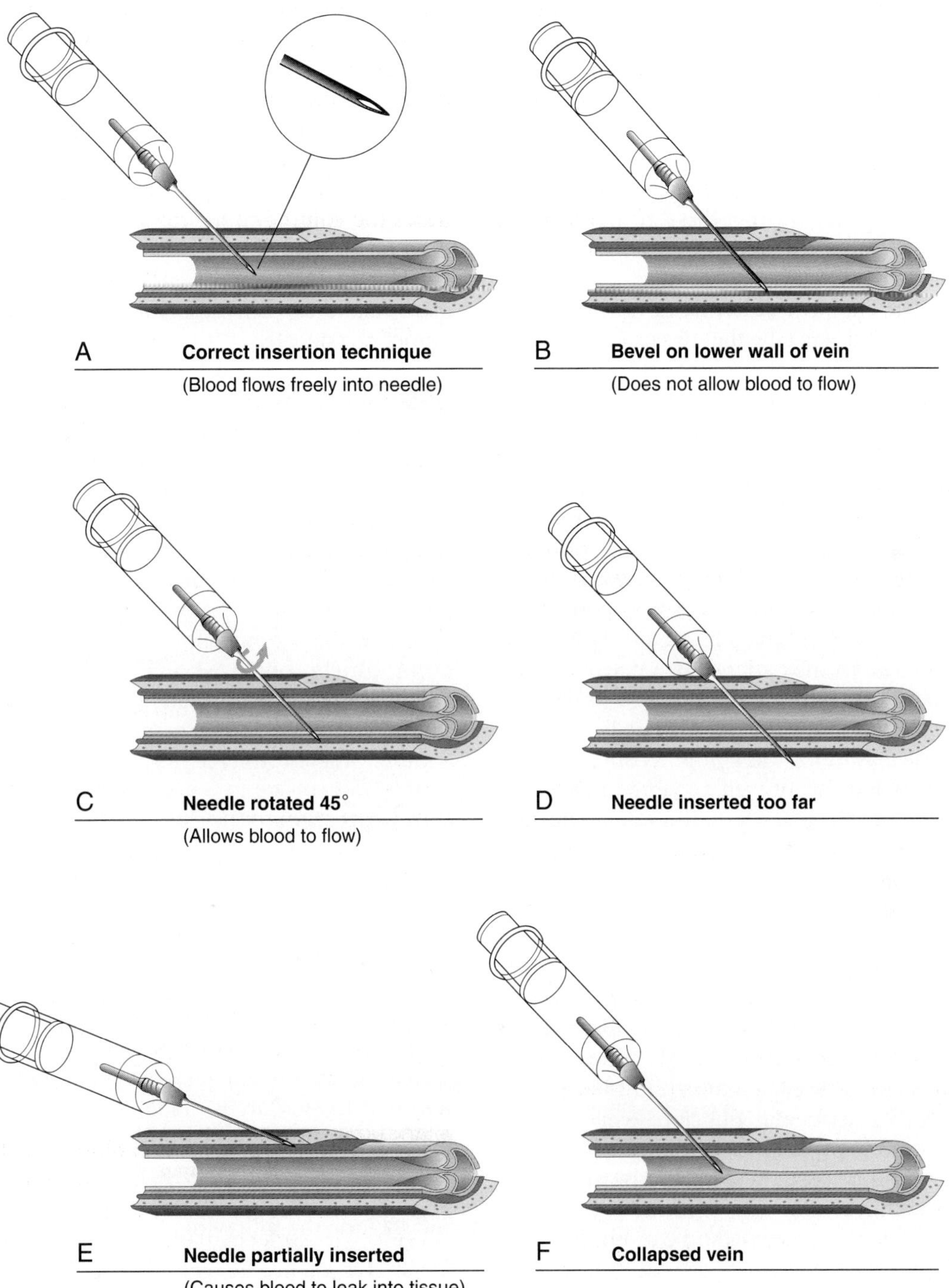

Figure 7–5 Possible reasons for failure to obtain blood.

beginning phlebotomists to know these techniques, because they have a tendency to immediately remove the needle when blood does not appear. The patient must then be repunctured when it may not have been necessary. Figure 7–5 illustrates possible causes of failure to obtain blood.

As shown in Figure 7–5*B* and *C*, the bevel of the needle may be resting against the wall of the vein, and rotating the needle a quarter of a turn will allow blood to flow freely.

Slowly advancing a needle that is not fully in a vein or pulling back a needle that has passed through a vein also may correct the problem (Fig. 7–5*D* and *E*). When the angle of needle insertion is too steep (greater than 30 degrees), the needle may penetrate through the vein into the tissue. Gently pulling the needle back may produce blood flow. If the needle angle is too shallow (less than 15 degrees), the needle may only partially enter the lumen of the vein, causing blood to leak into the tissues. Slowly advancing the needle into the vein may correct the problem. Failure to hold the adapter steady by bracing the hand against the patient's arm may cause the needle to be pushed through the vein or pulled out of the vein when tubes are being changed.

A frequent reason for the failure to obtain blood occurs when a vein is not well anchored before the puncture. The needle may slip to the side of the vein without actual penetration ("rolling vein"). Gentle touching of the area around the needle with the cleansed gloved finger may determine the positions of the vein and the needle, and allow the needle to be slightly redirected. To avoid having to repuncture the patient, withdraw the needle until the bevel is just under the skin, reanchor the vein, and redirect the needle into the vein. If the needle appears to be in the vein, a faulty evacuated tube (either by manufacturer error or accidental puncture when assembling the equipment) may be the problem, and a new tube should be used. Remember always to have extra tubes within reach.

Using too large an evacuated tube or pulling back on the plunger of a syringe too quickly creates suction pressure that can cause a vein to collapse and stop blood flow (Fig 7–5*F*). Using a smaller evacuated tube may remedy the situation. If it does not, another puncture must be performed, possibly using a syringe or butterfly.

Movement of the needle should not include vigorous probing because this is not only painful to the patient but also enlarges the puncture site so that blood can leak into the tissues and form a hematoma. The most critical permanent injury in the venipuncture procedure that can be caused by vigorous probing is damage to the median antebrachial cutaneous nerve. Errors in technique that can cause injury include selecting high-risk venipuncture sites, employing an excessive angle of needle insertion, and excessive manipulation of the needle. NCCLS (Standard H3-A4) limits the needle manipulation to only a forward or backward relocation of the needle.

technical tip Specimens collected following vigorous probing are frequently hemolyzed and must be recollected.

When blood is not obtained from the initial venipuncture, the phlebotomist should select another site, either in the other arm or below the previous site, and repeat the procedure using a new needle. If the second puncture is not successful, the same phlebotomist should not make another attempt. Following hospital policy, the phlebotomist should notify the nursing station and request that another phlebotomist perform the venipuncture.

Hemolyzed Specimens

Hemolysis may be detected by the presence of pink or red plasma or serum. Rupture of the red blood cell membrane releases cellular contents into the serum or plasma and produces interference with many test results so that the specimen may need to be redrawn. Hemolysis that is not visibly noticeable may be present and will affect test results of analytes such as potassium and lactic acid that are particularly sensitive to hemolysis. Table 7–3 summarizes the major tests affected by hemolysis.

Errors in performance of the venipuncture account for the majority of hemolyzed specimens and include the following:

1 Using a needle with too small a diameter (above 23 gauge)
2 Using a small needle with a large evacuated tube
3 Using an improperly attached needle on a syringe so that frothing occurs as the blood enters the syringe
4 Pulling the plunger of a syringe back too fast

TABLE 7-3
Laboratory Tests Affected by Hemolysis

Seriously Affected	Noticeably Affected	Slightly Affected
Potassium (K)	Serum iron (Fe)	Phosphorus (P)
Lactic dehydrogenase (LD)	Alanine aminotransferase (ALT)	Total protein (TP)
Aspartate aminotransferase (AST)	Thyroxine (T_4)	Albumin
Complete blood count (CBC)		Magnesium (Mg)
		Calcium (Ca)
		Acid phosphatase

5 Drawing blood from a site containing a hematoma
6 Vigorously mixing tubes
7 Forcing blood from a syringe into an evacuated tube
8 Failing to allow the blood to run down the side of an evacuated tube when using a syringe to fill it
9 Collecting specimens from IV lines when not recommended by the manufacturer
10 Applying the tourniquet too close to the puncture site or for too long

technical tip Hemolysis that is not evident to the naked eye can elevate critical potassium values.

Removal of the Needle

Improper technique when removing the needle is a frequent (although not the only) cause of a hematoma appearing on the patient's arm. The skin discoloration and swelling that accompanies a hematoma is often a cause of anxiety and discomfort to the patient. Errors in technique that cause blood to leak or be forced into the surrounding tissue and produce hematomas include:

1 Failure to remove the tourniquet before removing the needle
2 Applying inadequate pressure to the site after removal of the needle
3 Bending the arm while applying pressure
4 Excessive probing to obtain blood
5 Failure to insert the needle far enough into the vein
6 Inserting the needle through the vein

Under normal conditions, the elasticity of the vein walls prevents the leakage of blood around the needle during venipuncture. A decrease in the elasticity of the vein walls in older patients causes them to be more prone to developing hematomas. Using small-bore needles and firmly anchoring the veins before needle insertion may prevent a hematoma in older patients. If a hematoma begins to form while blood is being collected, immediately remove the tourniquet and needle and apply pressure to the site. An alternate site should be chosen for the repeat venipuncture. The goal of successful blood collection is not only to obtain the sample, but also to preserve the site for future venipunctures. It is critical to prevent hematoma formation.

Disposal of the Needle

There should be no deviations from the methods for needle disposal discussed in Chapter 5.

technical tip When removing the butterfly needle from the vein, always hold the base of the needle or the wings until it has been placed in the biohazard sharp container. The needle safety mechanism should be activated immediately.

Labeling the Tubes

Information contained on the labels of tubes from unidentified patients must follow the protocol used by the institution to provide a temporary but clear designation of the patient. When available, stickers from the patient's ID band should be attached to all specimens for the blood bank.

If preprinted labels are being used, it is important to double check the name on the label while attaching it to the tube.

Bandaging the Patient's Arm

Patients receiving anticoagulant medications or large amounts of aspirin or herbs, or patients with coagulation disorders, may continue to bleed after pressure has been applied for 5 minutes. The phlebotomist should continue to apply pressure until the bleeding has stopped. The nurse should be notified in cases of excessive bleeding. A CoBan pressure dressing can be used.

In the case of an accidental arterial puncture, which can usually be detected by the appearance of unusually red blood that spurts into the tube, the phlebotomist, not the patient, should apply pressure to the site for 10 minutes. The fact that the specimen is arterial blood should be recorded on the requisition form.

Some patients are allergic to adhesive bandages, and it may be necessary to wrap gauze around the arm before applying the adhesive tape or paper tape. Omitting the bandage in these patients and those with hairy arms is another option, particularly if the patient requests it. Bandages are not recommended for children younger than 2 years old, because children may put bandages in their mouths.

Leaving the Patient

Patients often request that the phlebotomist change the position of their bed or provide them with a drink of water. Because this may not be in the best interest of the patient, the phlebotomist should tell the patient that she or he will inform the nurse of the request. Leave the room in the condition in which you found it (bed and bed rails in the same position).

Completing the Venipuncture Procedure

Specimens brought to the laboratory may be rejected if conditions are present that would compromise the validity of the test results. Major reasons for specimen rejection are the following:

1 Unlabeled or mislabeled specimens
2 Inadequate volume
3 Collection in the wrong tube
4 Hemolysis
5 Lipemia
6 Clotted blood in an anticoagulant tube
7 Improper handling during transport, such as not chilling the specimen
8 Specimens without a requisition form
9 Contaminated specimen containers

Phlebotomists should make sure that none of these conditions exist in the specimens they deliver to the laboratory.

Bibliography

Boyles, S: Many Herbal Remedies May Interact with Popular Blood Thinner, http://my/webmd.com/content/article/1728.59275

Henry, JB, and Kurec, AS: The clinical laboratory: organization, purposes, and practices. In Henry, JB (ed): Clinical Diagnosis and Management by Laboratory Methods. WB Saunders, Philadelphia, 1996.

National Committee for Clinical Laboratory Standards Approved Standard H3-A4: Procedures for Collection of Diagnostic Blood Specimens by Venipuncture. NCCLS, Wayne, PA, 1998.

National Committee for Clinical Laboratory Standards Approved Guideline H18-A2: Procedures for the Handling and Processing of Blood Specimens. NCCLS, Wayne, PA, 1999.

National Committee for Clinical Laboratory Standards Approved Standard H21-A3: Collection, Transport, and Preparation of Blood for Coagulation Testing and Performance of General Coagulation Assays. NCCLS, Wayne, PA, 1999.

Read, DC, Viera, H, and Arkin, C: Effect of drawing blood specimens proximal to an in-place but discontinued intravenous solution. Am J Clin Pathol 90:702–706, 1988.

Study Questions

1. What two additional things should a phlebotomist do when encountering a patient who is sleeping?

   a. ______________________________

   b. ______________________________

2. Under what circumstance would a phlebotomist interrupt a physician-patient visit?

   ____

3. A phlebotomist encounters an inpatient without an ID band. When can the blood be drawn?

   ____

4. Why do phlebotomists perform their routine blood collections early in the morning?

   ____

5. Match the following patient variables with the possible effect on test results.

Effect		Variable
a. ________	Increased Hgb	1. Prolonged fasting
b. ________	Decreased glucose	2. Stress
c. ________	Increased adrenal hormones	3. Erect posture
d. ________	Increased sex hormones	4. Long-term exercise
e. ________	Increased albumin	5. Tobacco
f. ________	Increased aldolase	

6. Will a patient who has just awakened have a higher or lower WBC count than he or she would have after going to physical therapy. Why?

   ____

   ____

7. Which cellular element in the blood is affected when a patient is taking aspirin?

   ____

8. If a phlebotomist notices a preanalytical variable that might affect a patient's test results, what should the phlebotomist do?

____

9. When should the needle be removed if the patient develops syncope?

____

10. True or false. A patient can refuse to have blood drawn.

____

11. When a blood pressure cuff is used as a tourniquet, how will inflation of the cuff to a pressure above the patient's systolic pressure affect blood flow?

____

12. What two errors in test results can be caused by prolonged tourniquet application?

    a. ____

    b. ____

13. If a vein is not easily located in the patient's dominant arm, what is the first thing the phlebotomist should do?

____

14. Why are veins in the legs and feet avoided as venipuncture sites, if at all possible?

____

____

15. Indicate if each of the following are acceptable or unacceptable venipuncture sites by placing an "A" or a "U" in front of the statement. Explain all "U" answers, using the words contamination, infection, hemolysis, or decreased blood flow in the appropriate space.

    If "U"

    a. __________ Antecubital area above an IV drip that has been discontinued for 5 minutes __________________________

    b. __________ The wrist below an antecubital hematoma __________________

    c. __________ Antecubital area containing a tattoo __________________

    d. __________ Vein surrounded by a hematoma __________________

    e. __________ Wrist below an IV drip that has been discontinued for 5 minutes

    ____

f. __________ Wrist containing scar tissue ______________________________

g. __________ Arm with a fistula ______________________________

h. __________ Right arm of a patient with a right mastectomy ______________

i. __________ Veins on the back of the hand ______________________________

j. __________ Vein that feels hard ______________________________

16. Why is specialized training required for personnel collecting samples from CVADs?

____

____

17. What additional precaution must be taken when coagulation tests are drawn from CVADs?

____

18. True or False. The phlebotomist can draw from the T-connection of a dialysis patient's cannula. ______________________________

19. List three site cleansing solutions other than isopropyl alcohol and state a reason for their use.

Solution	**Reason**
a. ______________	______________
b. ______________	______________
c. ______________	______________

20. State two problems that may occur if the plunger of the syringe is pulled back too fast.

a. ____

b. ____

21. How do the wings on a butterfly aid the phlebotomist?

____

____

22. How could a phlebotomist who has correctly activated the needle safety device on a butterfly still receive an accidental needlestick?

____

23. List three reasons why blood may not be obtained even though the needle is in the vein.

    a. ______

    b. ______

    c. ______

24. What causes a vein to collapse?

    ______

25. State two tests that could be affected by nonvisible hemolysis.

    a. ______

    b. ______

26. List three causes of hematoma formation associated with needle removal.

    a. ______

    b. ______

    c. ______

27. List three causes of hematoma formation associated with needle insertion.

    a. ______

    b. ______

    c. ______

28. State two reasons why a phlebotomist may need to apply additional pressure to the puncture site after withdrawing the needle.

    a. ______

    b. ______

29. What should a phlebotomist do if a patient requests a glass of water?

    ______

30. List six possible causes of specimen rejection and state a *specific example of each.*

    a. ______

    ______

    b. ______

    ______

    c. ______

    ______

d. ____

____

e. ____

____

f. ____

____

Clinical Situations

1. A patient enters the outpatient drawing station, properly identifies herself, and states that she had a mastectomy 3 months ago. She holds her left arm out for the phlebotomist.

   a. What should the phlebotomist ask the patient?

   ____

   b. If blood is drawn from the wrong arm, state two possible dangers to the patient.

   ____

   ____

   c. If blood is drawn from the wrong arm, state two possible effects on laboratory tests.

   ____

   ____

   d. What body system has been affected by the mastectomy?

   ____

2. A patient has an IV drip running in the left forearm. From the following sites, indicate your first choice with a "1," your second choice with a "2," and an unacceptable site with an "X."

   a. ____________ The left wrist

   b. ____________ The left antecubital area

   c. ____________ The right antecubital area

3. While a CBC is being collected, the patient develops syncope and the phlebotomist immediately removes the needle and lowers the patient's head. When the patient has recovered, the phlebotomist labels the lavender stopper tube, which fortunately contains enough blood, and delivers it to the hematology section. Many results on this specimen are markedly lower than those on the patient's previous CBC.

   a. How could the quality of the specimen have caused this discrepancy?

   ____

b. How could the venipuncture complication have contributed to this error?

____

c. Could the phlebotomist have done anything differently? Explain your answer.

____

4. A nurse from the cardiac care unit reports that she is observing hematomas on the patients whenever phlebotomist X is assigned to the floor.

   a. Considering the medications commonly taken by cardiac patients, what is the most probable error being made by phlebotomist X?

   ____

   b. What should phlebotomist X be doing for these patients?

   ____

   c. Could the same problem occur with patients taking over-the-counter drugs? Explain your answer.

   ____

5. A patient with noticeable edema comes to the outpatient drawing area with a request for a cardiac risk profile. The patient has recently been hospitalized.

   a. What would be the best position of the phlebotomist to place the patient in before collecting the specimen?

   ____

   b. What two tests would be most affected by this patient's condition?

   ____

   ____

   c. What is the significance of the edema in this situation?

   ____

   d. Should the phlebotomist check to be sure this patient is fasting? Why or why not?

   ____

6. The phlebotomist has a requisition to collect a FANA, an RA, and a PT. No blood is obtained from the left antecubital area. The phlebotomist then moves to the right antecubital area and obtains a full red stopper tube, but cannot fill the light blue stopper tube.

   a. What should the phlebotomist do next?

   ____

   b. State two things the phlebotomist should do before deciding that the needle must be removed without filling the second tube.

   ____

   ____

7. The phlebotomist is assisting the nurse to collect a prothrombin time, CBC, and liver profile from an IV line.

   a. How many and what size syringes are needed?

   ____

   b. What will the phlebotomist do with blood collected in each syringe? (List the syringes in order of collection.)

   ____

   c. What should the phlebotomist write on the requisition form?

   ____

   d. What must the nurse do to the IV before collecting the specimen?

   ____

NAME ______________________________

Evaluation of Venipuncture Technique Using a Syringe

RATING SYSTEM 2 = SATISFACTORILY PERFORMED 1 = NEEDS IMPROVEMENT 0 = INCORRECT/DID NOT PERFORM

_________ 1. Examines requisition form

_________ 2. Greets patient, states procedure to be done

_________ 3. Identifies patient verbally

_________ 4. Examines patient's ID band

_________ 5. Compares requisition form with ID band

_________ 6. Washes hands and puts on gloves

_________ 7. Selects tubes and equipment for procedure

_________ 8. Positions patient's arm

_________ 9. Applies tourniquet

_________ 10. Identifies vein by palpation

_________ 11. Releases tourniquet

_________ 12. Cleanses site and allows it to air dry

_________ 13. Assembles and conveniently places equipment

_________ 14. Reapplies tourniquet

_________ 15. Does not touch puncture site with unclean finger

_________ 16. Checks plunger movement

_________ 17. Anchors vein below puncture site

_________ 18. Smoothly enters vein at appropriate angle with bevel up

_________ 19. Does not move needle when plunger is retracted

_________ 20. Collects appropriate amount of blood

_________ 21. Releases tourniquet

__________ 22. Covers puncture site with gauze

__________ 23. Removes needle smoothly and applies pressure

__________ 24. Uses correct and safe technique to fill tubes

__________ 25. Fills tubes in correct order

__________ 26. Mixes anticoagulated tubes promptly

__________ 27. Disposes of needle and syringe in sharps container

__________ 28. Labels tubes

__________ 29. Examines puncture site

__________ 30. Applies bandage

__________ 31. Disposes of used supplies

__________ 32. Removes gloves and washes hands

__________ 33. Thanks patient

__________ 34. Converses appropriately with patient during procedure

TOTAL POINTS __________

MAXIMUM POINTS - 68

Comments:

NAME ____________________

Evaluation of Venipuncture Technique Using a Butterfly

RATING SYSTEM 2 = SATISFACTORILY PERFORMED 1 = NEEDS IMPROVEMENT 0 = INCORRECT/DID NOT PERFORM

_______ 1. Examines requisition form

_______ 2. Greets patient, states procedure to be done

_______ 3. Identifies patient verbally

_______ 4. Examines patient's ID band

_______ 5. Compares requisition form with ID band

_______ 6. Washes hands and puts on gloves

_______ 7. Selects tubes and equipment for procedure

_______ 8. Positions patient's hand

_______ 9. Applies tourniquet

_______ 10. Identifies vein by palpation

_______ 11. Releases tourniquet

_______ 12. Cleanses site and allows it to air dry

_______ 13. Assembles and conveniently places equipment

_______ 14. Reapplies tourniquet

_______ 15. Does not touch puncture site with unclean finger

_______ 16. Anchors vein below puncture site

_______ 17. Holds needle appropriately

_______ 18. Enters vein smoothly at appropriate angle with bevel up

_______ 19. Maintains needle securely in vein

_______ 20. Smoothly operates syringe or evacuated tube adapter

_______ 21. Fills tubes in the correct order

_______ 22. Mixes anticoagulated tubes promptly

__________ 23. Collects appropriate amount of blood

__________ 24. Releases tourniquet

__________ 25. Covers puncture site with gauze

__________ 26. Removes needle smoothly and applies pressure

__________ 27. Disposes of apparatus in sharps container

__________ 28. Labels tubes

__________ 29. Examines puncture site

__________ 30. Applies bandage

__________ 31. Disposes of used supplies

__________ 32. Removes gloves and washes hands

__________ 33. Thanks patient

__________ 34. Converses appropriately with patient during procedure

TOTAL POINTS __________

MAXIMUM POINTS = 68

Comments:

Chapter 8

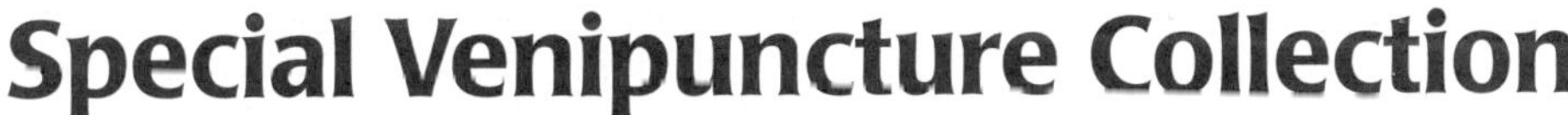

Special Venipuncture Collection

Chapter Outline

Collection Priorities
- Routine Specimens
- ASAP Specimens
- Stat Specimens

Fasting Specimens

Timed Specimens
- Two-Hour Postprandial Glucose
- Glucose Tolerance Test
- Diurnal Variation
- Therapeutic Drug Monitoring

Blood Cultures

Special Specimen Handling Procedures
- Cold Agglutinins
- Chilled Specimens
- Specimens Sensitive to Light
- Legal (Forensic) Specimens

Special Patient Populations
- Geriatric Population
- Pediatric Population

Learning Objectives

Upon completion of this chapter, the reader will be able to:

1 Define the various test collection priorities.

2 State two reasons why fasting specimens are requested, and name three tests affected by not fasting.

3 List four reasons for requesting timed specimens.

4 Explain the procedure for a 2-hour postprandial glucose test.

5 Correctly schedule specimen collections for a glucose tolerance test.

6 Using an example, discuss diurnal variation of blood constituents.

7 State two reasons for therapeutic drug monitoring.

8 Differentiate between a trough and a peak level.

9 Discuss three timing sequences for the collection of blood cultures, reasons for selecting a particular timing sequence, and the number of specimens collected.

10 Describe the aseptic techniques required when collecting blood cultures.

11 Describe the procedure for collecting specimens for cold agglutinins.

12 List seven tests that must be chilled immediately after collection.

13 List five tests that are affected by exposure to light.

14 Define chain of custody.

15 List three tests frequently requested for forensic studies.

16 Describe the physical and emotional changes in special patient populations and their effects on blood collection.

Key Terms

Aseptic
Chain of custody
Diurnal variation
Fasting
Forensic
Geriatric
Peak level
Postprandial
Septicemia
Trough level

Certain laboratory tests require the phlebotomist to use techniques that are not part of the routine venipuncture procedure. These special techniques may involve patient preparation, timing of specimen collection, venipuncture techniques, and specimen handling. Phlebotomists must know when these techniques are required, how to perform them, and how specimen integrity is affected when they are not properly performed.

Collection Priorities

Each test order is designated as routine, timed, **ASAP**, or stat. Collections lists and turnaround times (**TATs**) for test results are based on these designations and will vary for different institutions. The phlebotomist must prioritize his or her workload accordingly to accommodate the various test priorities.

Routine Specimens

Routine specimens are tests that are ordered by the healthcare provider to diagnose and monitor a patient's condition. Routine specimens are usually collected early in the morning, but can be collected throughout the day during scheduled "sweeps" (collection times) on the floors or from outpatients.

ASAP Specimens

ASAP means "as soon as possible." The response time for the collection of this test specimen is determined by each hospital or clinic and may vary by laboratory tests.

Stat Specimens

Stat means the specimen is to be collected and analyzed immediately. Stat tests have the highest priority and are usually ordered from the emergency room or for a critically ill patient whose treatment will be determined by the laboratory result. The specimen must be delivered to the laboratory promptly and the laboratory personnel notified.

Fasting Specimens

Certain laboratory tests must be collected from a patient who has been ***fasting***. Fasting differs from a basal state condition in that the patient must only have refrained from eating and drinking (except water) for 12 hours, whereas in the basal state, the patient must also have refrained from exercise. Drinking water is encouraged to avoid dehydration in the patient, which can affect laboratory results. A patient who is NPO is not allowed to have food or water because of possible complications with anesthesia during surgery or certain medical conditions.

Test results most critically affected in a nonfasting patient are those of glucose, cholesterol, and triglyceride tests. Prolonged fasting increases bilirubin and triglyceride values and markedly decreases glucose levels. When a fasting specimen is requested, it is the responsibility of the phlebotomist to determine whether the patient has been fasting for the required length of time. If the patient has not, this must be reported to a supervisor or the nurse and noted on the requisition form.

For glucose tolerance tests, the fasting patient should be instructed to abstain from food and drinks including coffee, except water, for 12 hours but not more than 16 hours before and during the test. Smoking and sugarless gum should be avoided during the test because they stimulate digestion and may cause inaccurate test results.

Timed Specimens

Requisitions are frequently received requesting that blood be drawn at a specific time. Reasons for timed specimens include the following:

1 Measurement of the body's ability to metabolize a particular substance
2 Monitoring changes in a patient's condition (such as a steady decrease in hemoglobin)
3 Determining blood levels of medications
4 Measuring substances that exhibit ***diurnal variation*** (normal changes in blood levels at different times of the day)
5 Measurement of cardiac markers following acute myocardial infarction

Phlebotomists should arrange their schedules to be available at the specified time, and should record the actual time of collection on the requisition and specimen tube. Specimens collected too early or too late may be falsely elevated or decreased. Misinterpretation of test results can cause improper treatment for the patient.

The most frequently encountered timed specimens are discussed in this chapter. Other diagnostic procedures may also require timed specimens, and any request for a timed specimen should be strictly followed.

Two-Hour ***Postprandial*** Glucose

Comparison of a patient's fasting glucose level with the glucose level 2 hours after eating a meal or ingesting a measured amount of glucose is used to evaluate diabetes mellitus. Ideally, the glucose level should return to the fasting level within 2 hours.

The phlebotomist must be able to explain the procedure to the patient, stressing the importance of eating a full meal and returning to the laboratory in time to have the blood drawn exactly 2 hours after the meal is completed.

Glucose Tolerance Test

The glucose tolerance test (GTT) is a procedure performed for the diagnosis of diabetes mellitus (hyperglycemia) and for evaluating persons with symptoms associated with low blood glucose (hypoglycemia). Phlebotomists are often responsible for the administration of this procedure, which includes patient instruction, administering the glucose solution, scheduling of samples, and the collection and organization of samples that consist of timed blood and possibly urine collections. If urine specimens are included in the procedure, patients are asked to collect them when the blood is drawn and they are labeled in the same manner as the blood samples. The procedure is scheduled for 3 hours to diagnose diabetes mellitus and may continue 5 or 6 hours to evaluate hypoglycemia.

GTT procedures should be scheduled to begin between 0700 and 0900 because glucose levels exhibit a diurnal variation. The phlebotomist draws a fasting glucose. The fasting blood specimen is tested before continuing the procedure to determine whether the patient can safely be given a large amount of glucose. The phlebotomist then asks the patient to drink a standardized amount of flavored glucose solution based on body weight within a period of 5 minutes. Timing for the remaining GTT specimens begins when the patient finishes drinking the glucose. Sample schedules are shown in Table 8–1. Notice that all timing is based on completion of the glucose drink.

Outpatients are given a copy of the schedule and instructed to continue fasting, to drink water to facilitate urine collection, and to return to the drawing station at the scheduled times. Patients are instructed to remain in the outpatient area and to continue to abstain from coffee, alcohol, food, smoking, or chewing gum throughout the entire procedure. Timing of inpatient collections is the responsibility of the phlebotomist.

Corresponding labels containing routinely required information and specimen order in the test sequence, such as $^1/_2$-hour (nonroutine), 1-hour, 2-hour, and so on, are placed on the blood and urine specimens. Blood specimens that will not be tested until the end of the sequence should be collected in gray stopper tubes. Timing of specimen collection is critical, because test results are related to the scheduled times; any discrepancies should be noted on the requisition. Consistency of venipuncture or dermal puncture must also be maintained, because glucose values differ between the two types of blood. The type of evacuated tube used must also be consistent.

Some patients may not be able to tolerate the glucose solution, and if vomiting occurs, the time of the vomiting must be reported to a supervisor and the healthcare provider contacted for a decision concerning whether to continue the test. Vomiting early in the procedure is considered to be the most critical, and in most situations, the tolerance test is discontinued when vomiting occurs in the first hour. During scheduled sample collections, phlebotomists should also observe patients for any changes in their

TABLE 8–1
Sample Glucose Tolerance Test Schedules

Test Procedure	3-Hour Test	6-Hour Test
Fasting blood and urine	0700	0700
Patient finishes glucose	0800	0800
$^1/_2$-Hour specimen (nonroutine)	0830	0830
1-Hour specimen	0900	0900
2-Hour specimen	1000	1000
3-Hour specimen	1100	1100
4-Hour specimen		1200
5-Hour specimen		1300
6-Hour specimen		1400

condition, such as dizziness, which might indicate a reaction to the glucose and should report any changes to a supervisor.

technical tip When collecting GTT specimens, closely observe the patient for symptoms of hyperglycemia or hypoglycemia.

Diurnal Variation

Substances and cell counts primarily affected by diurnal variation are corticosteroids, hormones, serum iron, glucose, white blood cell counts, and eosinophil counts. Phlebotomists are often requested to draw specimens for these tests at specific times, usually corresponding to the peak diurnal level. Certain variations can be substantial. Plasma cortisol levels drawn between 0800 and 1000 will be twice as high as levels drawn at 1600. Consequently, requests for plasma cortisol levels frequently specify that the test be drawn between 0800 and 1000, or at 1600. If the specimen cannot be collected at the specified time, the physician should be notified and the test rescheduled for the next day.

technical tip Patients must understand the importance of adhering to the scheduled blood collection times for accurate results.

Therapeutic Drug Monitoring

The fact that medications affect all patients differently frequently results in the need to change dosages or medications. Some medications can reach toxic levels in patients who do not metabolize or excrete them within an expected time frame. Likewise, there are patients who metabolize and excrete medications at an increased rate. To ensure patient safety and medication effectiveness, the blood levels of many therapeutic drugs are monitored.

Examples of frequently monitored therapeutic drugs are digoxin, phenobarbital, lithium, gentamicin, tobramycin, vancomycin, amikacin, and theophylline. Random specimens are occasionally requested; however, the most beneficial levels are those drawn before the next dosage is given (***trough level***) and shortly after the medication is given (***peak level***). Trough levels are collected 30 minutes before the drug is to be given and represent the lowest level in the blood. Ideally, trough levels should be tested before administering the next dose to ensure that the level is low enough for the patient to receive more medication safely. The time for collecting peak levels varies with the medication and the method of administration (intravenous, intramuscular, or oral). Information from drug manufacturers provides the recommended times for collection of peak levels. To ensure correct documentation of the peak and trough levels, requisitions and specimen tube labels should include the time and method of administration of the last dosage given, as well as the time that the specimen is drawn. Therapeutic drug monitoring collections are often coordinated with the pharmacy.

technical tip Depending on the half-life of the medication, the timing of peak levels in therapeutic drug monitoring can be critical.

Blood Cultures

One of the most difficult phlebotomy procedures is collection of blood cultures. This is because of the strict ***aseptic*** technique required and the need to collect multiple specimens in special containers. Blood cultures are requested on patients when symptoms of fever and chills indicate a possible infection of the blood by pathogenic microorganisms (***septicemia***). The patient's initial diagnosis is often fever of unknown origin (FUO).

Blood cultures are usually ordered stat or as timed collections. Isolation of microorganisms from the blood is often difficult due to the small number of organisms needed to cause symptoms. Specimens are usually collected in sets of two or three drawn either 30 to 60 minutes apart or just before the patient's temperature reaches its highest point (spike). The concentration of microorganisms fluctuates and is often highest just before the patient's temperature spikes. This explains why collections may be ordered at specific intervals or ordered stat if a pattern has been observed in the patient's temperature chart. If antibiotics are to be started immediately, the sets are drawn at the same time from different sites. Specimens collected from multiple sites at the same time serve as a control for possible contamination and must be labeled as to the collection site, such as right arm antecubital vein, and their number in the series (#1, #2, or #3). A known skin

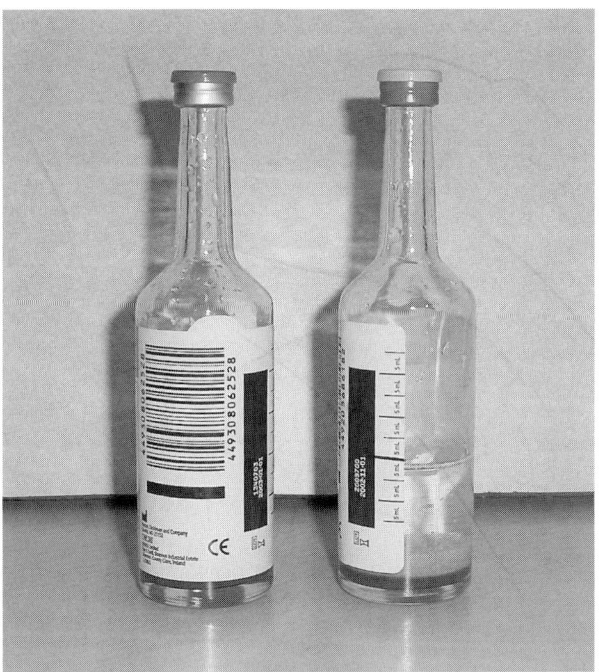
Figure 8–1 Adult blood culture collection bottles.

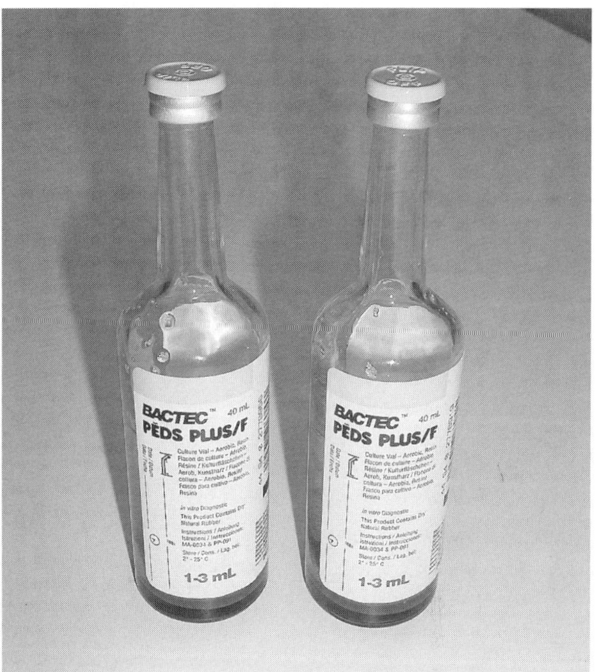

Figure 8–2 Pediatric blood culture collection bottles.

contaminant must be cultured from at least two of the sites for it to be considered a possible pathogen.

Figures 8–1 and 8–2 show examples of adult and pediatric blood culture collection systems. Blood also can be drawn into sterile, yellow stopper evacuated tubes and transferred to culture media in the laboratory.

A winged infusion set with a Luer adapter can be used with the Septi-Chek Blood Collection Adapter (Becton, Dickinson, Franklin Lakes, NJ) to transfer blood directly from the patient to bottles containing culture media. The Luer adapter on the butterfly apparatus attaches to the transfer device that contains a stopper-puncturing needle. Blood flows from the vein through the butterfly tubing, Luer adapter, and stopper-puncturing needle into the culture bottle.

Blood can be collected in a syringe and aseptically transferred to blood culture bottles at the bedside. Studies have shown that the earlier practice of putting a new needle on the syringe before inoculating the blood culture bottle is not necessary to avoid contamination. In fact, this practice increased the risk of an accidental needlestick.

An anticoagulant must be present in the tube or blood culture bottle to prevent microorganisms from being trapped within a clot, where they might be undetected; therefore, blood culture bottles must be mixed after the blood is added. The anticoagulant sodium polyanetholesulfonate is used for blood cultures because it does not inhibit bacterial growth and may, in fact, enhance it by inhibiting the action of phagocytes, complement, and some antibiotics. Other anticoagulants should not be used. Some blood culture collection systems have antimicrobial removal devices (ARDs) containing resin that inactivates antibiotics.

The venipuncture technique for collecting blood cultures follows the routine procedures, except for the increased aseptic preparation of the puncture site. Cleansing of the site begins with vigorous scrubbing of the site for 1 minute using isopropyl alcohol. This is followed by scrubbing the site with 2% iodine tincture or povidone-iodine for another minute and finishing by moving the iodine swab or applicator from the center of the puncture site to the outside area using concentric circles. Allow the iodine to dry on the site for at least 1 minute. Blood culture prep kits (Cepti-Seal Blood Culture Prep Kit II, Medi-Flex, Overland Park, KS) are available that contain a 70% isopropyl alcohol sponge and a 2% iodine tincture applicator (Fig. 8–3). The 2% iodine tincture

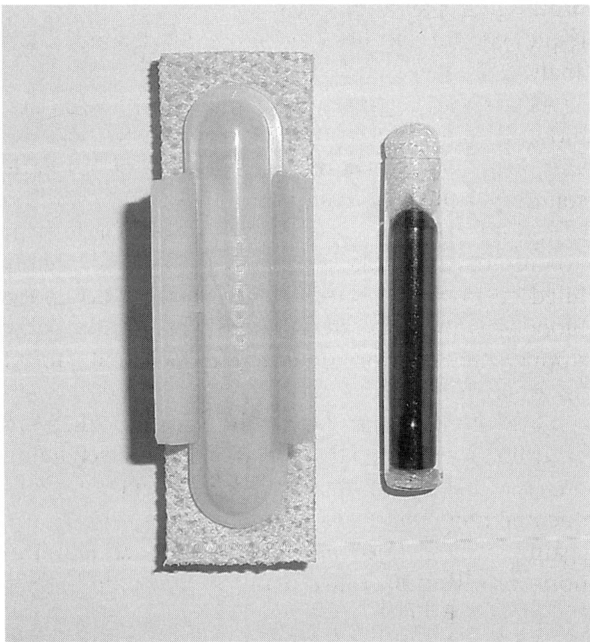

Figure 8–3 Cepti-Seal Blood Culture Prep Kit II.

contains 47% ethyl alcohol. Therefore, it dries more rapidly than the 2- to 3-minute drying time recommended after using the povidone-iodine solution. The iodine must be allowed to dry for 1 minute. The rapid drying time of the 2% iodine tincture has been reported to be more successful at reducing the rate of skin contamination. To prevent irritation of the patient's arm, the iodine is removed with alcohol when the procedure is complete.

technical tip The National Committee on Clinical Laboratory Standards (NCCLS) recommends removing the dried alcohol or iodine from the blood culture bottle stopper with clean gauze prior to inoculation.

Phlebotomists should take every precaution not to retouch the puncture site after it has been cleaned. If the vein must be repalpated, the gloved finger must be cleaned in the same manner as the puncture site.

The tops of the blood culture bottles also must be cleaned before inoculating them with blood. The rubber stoppers can be cleaned using alcohol only or with iodine that is allowed to dry and then wiped off with alcohol. The iodine should not remain on the stoppers because it can enter the culture during specimen inoculation and may cause deterioration of some stoppers during incubation.

Two specimens are routinely collected for each blood culture set, one to be incubated aerobically and the other anaerobically. When a syringe is used, the anaerobic bottle should be inoculated first to prevent possible exposure to air. When the specimen is collected using a winged infusion set, the aerobic bottle is inoculated first so that the air in the tubing does not enter the anaerobic bottle. Pediatric blood culture volume requirements are based on the child's weight and pediatric bottles are inoculated. Draw 1 mL of blood for every 5 kg (approximately 10 pounds) of patient weight. The specimen of a child heavier than 45 kg is treated as that of an adult. Draw 1 mL of blood on babies weighing less than 5 kg, and place all the blood in one pediatric bottle.

Because the number of organisms present in the blood is often small, the amount of blood inoculated into each container is critical. There should be at least a 1:10 ratio of blood to media. Phlebotomists should follow the instructions for the system being used. Overfilling of bottles should be avoided because this may cause false-positive results with automated systems.

Special Specimen Handling Procedures

Cold Agglutinins

Cold agglutinins are autoantibodies produced by persons infected with *Mycoplasma pneumoniae* (atypical pneumonia) or with autoimmune hemolytic anemias. The autoantibodies react with red blood cells at temperatures below body temperature.

Because the cold agglutinins in the serum attach to red blood cells when the blood cools to below body temperature, the specimen must be kept warm until the serum can be separated from the cells. Specimens are collected in tubes that have been warmed in an incubator at 37°C for 30 minutes and that contain no additives or gels that could interfere with the test. The phlebotomist can carry the warmed tube to the patient's room in a warm container or possibly a tightly closed fist, collect the specimen as quickly as possible, return the specimen to the laboratory in the same manner, and place it back in the incubator. Failure to keep a specimen warm before serum separation will produce falsely decreased test results.

Chilled Specimens

Specimens for arterial blood gases (ABGs), ammonia, lactic acid, pyruvate, gastrin, glucagons, **adrenocorticotropic hormone (ACTH)**, parathyroid hormone, and some coagulation studies may require chilling after collection to prevent deterioration. The National Committee for Laboratory Standards (NCCLS) recommends not to ice ABGs unless collecting them in conjunction with lactic acid (see Chapter 11). For adequate chilling, the specimen must be placed in crushed ice or a mixture of ice and water at the bedside. Placing a specimen in or on ice cubes is not acceptable because uniform chilling will not occur and may cause part of the specimen to freeze, resulting in hemolysis. It is important that these specimens be immediately delivered to the laboratory for processing.

Specimens Sensitive to Light

Exposure to light decreases the concentration of bilirubin, beta-carotene, vitamins A and B_{12}, folate, and porphyrins. Wrapping the tubes in aluminum foil can protect specimens.

technical tip Bilirubin is rapidly destroyed in specimens exposed to light.

Legal (*Forensic*) Specimens

When drawing specimens for test results that may be used as evidence in legal proceedings, phlebotomists must use extreme care to follow the stated policies exactly. Documentation of specimen handling, called the ***chain of custody***, is essential. It begins with patient identification and continues until testing is completed and results reported. Special forms are provided for this documentation, and special containers and seals may be required (Fig. 8–4). For each person handling the specimen, documentation must include the date, the time, and the identification of the handler. Patient identification and specimen collection should be done in the presence of a witness, frequently a law enforcement officer. Identification may include fingerprinting or heel printing in paternity cases. Tests most frequently requested are alcohol and drug levels and DNA analysis.

As stated in the previous chapter, when collecting blood alcohol levels, the site should be cleansed with soap and water or a nonalcoholic antiseptic solution such as benzalkonium chloride (Zephiran Chloride). To prevent the escape of the volatile alcohol into the atmosphere, tubes should be completely filled and not uncapped for longer than necessary. Blood alcohol levels are frequently collected in gray stopper tubes; however, laboratory protocol should be strictly followed.

Phlebotomists may be involved in the collection of urine specimens that are part of a screening process for the use of illegal drugs. Following and documenting the chain of custody procedures are again essential. Specimen substitution, contamination, or dilution must also be prevented. (See Chapter 12.)

technical tip Technical errors and failure to follow chain-of-custody protocol are primary targets of the defense in legal proceedings.

Special Patient Populations

Phlebotomists encounter patients of all ages, which will require different technical and communication skills appropriate for each age group. The Joint Commission on Accreditation of Healthcare Organizations recommends that phlebotomists be proficient with all age groups and that age-specific competencies be demonstrated and evaluated. Sometimes modifications to blood collection techniques and equipment are necessary to successfully accommodate the challenges of blood collection for the pediatric and ***geriatric*** population. Phlebotomists must develop and increase their knowledge and skills in working with all age groups of patients while performing blood collection procedures. An example of a phlebotomy department checklist for age-specific competency is shown in Figure 8–5.

Geriatric Population

Blood collection in the older patient population presents a unique challenge for the phlebotomist.

Saint Joseph Hospital Toxicology Laboratory
601 N. 30th Street
Omaha, NE 68131-2197
(402) 449-4940

Drug Testing Custody & Control Form
NON-DOT/NON-HHS (NON-NIDA)

SPECIMEN ID NO. LABORATORY ACCESSION NO.

▶ STEP 1: TO BE COMPLETED BY COLLECTOR OR EMPLOYER REPRESENTATIVE

A. Name, Address and I.D. No.

B. MRO Name and Address

C. Tests to be Performed: ☐ DS1 ☐ DS2 ☐ NON-NIDA5 ☐ URINE ALCOHOL ☐ BLOOD ALCOHOL

D. Reason for Test: ☐ pre-employment ☐ current employment ☐ periodic ☐ reasonable susp/cause ☐ post accident ☐ other ______ specify

E. Donor I.D. ______

▶ STEP 2: TO BE COMPLETED BY COLLECTOR - Specimen temperature must be read within 4 minutes of collection.

Specimen temperature within range: ☐ Yes, 90.5° - 99.8°F/32.5° - 37.7°C ☐ No, Record specimen temperature here ______

▶ STEP 3: TO BE COMPLETED BY COLLECTOR AND DONOR - Collector affixes bottle seal(s) to bottle(s). Collector dates seal(s). Donor initials seal(s).

▶ STEP 4: TO BE COMPLETED BY DONOR - Go to copy 2 (pink page); STEP 4.

▶ STEP 5: TO BE COMPLETED BY COLLECTOR

COLLECTION SITE LOCATION:

______ Collection Facility ( ) ______ Collector's Business Phone No.

______ Address ______ City ______ State ______ Zip

REMARKS: ______

I certify that the specimen identified on this form is the specimen presented to me by the donor providing the certification on Copy 2 of this form, that it bears the same specimen identification number as that set forth above, and that it has been collected, labeled and sealed.

______ (PRINT) Collector's Name (First, MI, Last) X ______ Signature of Collector / / Date (Mo./Day/Yr.) ______ AM PM Time

▶ STEP 6: TO BE INITIATED BY THE COLLECTOR AND COMPLETED AS NECESSARY THEREAFTER

DATE MO. DAY YR.	SPECIMEN RELEASED BY	SPECIMEN RECEIVED BY	PURPOSE OF CHANGE
/ /	DONOR - NO SIGNATURE	Signature Name	PROVIDE SPECIMEN FOR TESTING
/ /	Signature Name	Signature **Courier** Name	TRANSPORT TO LABORATORY
/ /	Signature **Courier** Name	Signature Name	

– INTENTIONALLY LEFT BLANK –

______ Date (Mo. Day. Yr.)
______ Donor's Initials

PLACE OVER CAP

SPECIMEN ID NO.

______ Date (Mo. Day. Yr.)
______ Donor's Initials

PLACE OVER CAP

SPECIMEN ID NO.

TRANSPORT BOX CUSTODY SEAL

COLLECTOR'S INITIALS ______ DATE ______

COPY 1 - ORIGINAL - MUST ACCOMPANY SPECIMEN TO LABORATORY

Figure 8–4 Sample chain-of-custody form. (Courtesy of Creighton University Medical Center, Omaha, NE.)

EMPLOYEE: Write examples of care you have provided specific to your job, department, and patient population. Please give one example for each category for all of the age groups you have identified.

1. Provides care to **infant and toddler patients** through utilization of the following:
   a. Communication: Recognize and respond to communication cues.
   b. Health: Assists in creating an environment so infants are able to get ample sleep.
   c. Safety: Limits number of strangers.

2. Provides care to **young children** through utilization of the following:
   a. Communication: Explains procedure and equipment.
   b. Health: Provide rest periods.
   c. Safety: Provide safety habits.

3. Provides care to **older children** through utilization of the following:
   a. Communication: Involves patient whenever possible to help them feel useful.
   b. Health: Promote good nutrition and hygiene.
   c. Safety: Promote safety habits.

4. Provides care to **adolescent patients** through utilization of the following:
   a. Communication: Explain procedure and equipment supplementing explanations with reasons.
   b. Health: Encourage discussions and listen to issues on sexual responsibility and substance abuse without being judgmental.
   c. Safety: Prevent sports accidents.

5. Provides care to **young adults** through utilization of the following:
   a. Communication: Provide privacy.
   b. Health: Encourage decision-making regarding personal healthcare.
   c. Safety: Assist in adjustment to physical/psychosocial changes related to illness

6. Provides care to **middle adults** through utilization of the following:
   a. Communication: Realizes need for self-reflection.
   b. Health: Encourage discussion and actively listen to issues regarding active retirement without being judgmental.
   c. Safety: Encourage preventative practice in relation to injuries.

7. Provides care to **older patients** through utilization of the following:
   a. Communication: Recognize need for some control due to multiple losses.
   b. Health: Plan for a balance between activity and rest during the day.
   c. Safety: Focuses object directly in line of vision if patient experiences decreased visual acuity.

8. Provides care to **adults ages 80 and older** through utilization of the following:
   a. Communication: Encourage discussion and listen to end-of-life concerns without being judgmental.
   b. Health: Plan for a balance between activity and rest during the day.
   c. Safety: Orient patient well to surroundings, remind patient to use call button, if assistance is needed.

______________________________	______________________________
Employee's Signature	Date
______________________________	______________________________
Supervisor's Signature	**Date**

Figure 8–5 Department-specific checklist for age-specific competency. (Adapted from Nebraska Methodist Hospital, courtesy of Diane Wolff, MLT [ASCP] Phlebotomy Team Leader, Omaha, NE.)

Physical and emotional factors related to the aging process can cause difficulty with the blood collection procedure and specimen integrity. The goal is to perform an atraumatic venipuncture without bruising or excessive bleeding and provide a quality specimen for analysis.

Normal aging often results in gradual hearing loss and failing eyesight. The other senses of taste, smell, and feeling are also affected. The phlebotomist may have to speak louder or repeat instructions. The patient may have to be guided to the blood drawing chair and have help being seated. Muscle weakness may cause the patient to drop things or be unable to make a fist before venipuncture or to hold the gauze after the venipuncture. Memory loss may cause the older patient to not remember medications he or she may have taken that can affect laboratory test results. A patient's inability to remember when he or she has last eaten can affect a test requiring fasting. Malnutrition or dehydration because of not eating or drinking adequately can make locating veins for venipuncture difficult because of decreased plasma volume and can affect laboratory test results. Certain disease states found predominantly in the older patient contribute to the challenge of venipuncture. A patient with Alzheimer's disease may be confused or combative, which can cause problems with identification and performing the procedure. Assistance from a family member or the patient's caretaker is necessary. Stroke patients may have paralysis requiring assistance in positioning and holding the arm. Patients in a coma should be treated as if they can hear what is being said. Again, assistance will be required when holding the arm. Arthritic patients may be in pain and may require assistance gently positioning and holding the arm. Older patients may have tremors, as evidenced in Parkinson's disease, and cannot hold the arm still for the venipuncture procedure. Patients are often embarrassed by these conditions, which may cause anxiety or fear of blood collection.

As a part of the normal aging process, physiologic changes occur that affect venipuncture. Normally the epidermis layer of skin regularly sheds dead cells and replaces them with new cells. In the older patient, there can be a delay in epidermal cell replacement, increasing the chance of infection. If the patient already has a weakened immune system, the patient may not heal as quickly or have the ability to fight bacteria that can be introduced during venipuncture. Extra care must be taken when preparing the site for venipuncture. Always wash hands before applying gloves and use gloves when palpating for the vein.

Because of the difficulty in locating and anchoring veins and the presence of hematomas from previous venipunctures in the elderly patient, the antecubital fossa may not be the best site selection. The veins in the hand or forearm may be a better choice. It may require taking a little extra time and using the techniques previously described for making veins more prominent. An exception to these techniques is tapping the vein, which can cause bruising in an older patient. Applying heat compresses and stimulating the area with alcohol can make the vein more prominent. With aging, the epithelium and subcutaneous tissues and muscle mass become thinner, causing veins to be less stable and harder to anchor. The phlebotomist must firmly anchor the vein below the site so that the vein does not move when punctured. The angle of the needle may need to be decreased for venipuncture. Older patients often feel cold because of the decreased fatty tissue layer, and warming of the site may be required. Aging veins have decreased collagen and elasticity, making them less firm and more difficult to puncture and therefore more prone to hematoma formation. Arteries and veins often become sclerotic in the older patient, making them poor sites for venipuncture because of the compromised blood flow. Blood pressure cuffs can be used for the thin patient with small, hard-to-find veins. Elderly patients are prone to bruising when applying the tourniquet or adhesive bandages. Therefore, it is preferable to use a self-adhering pressure-dressing bandage (e.g., CoBan) because adhesive bandages on the fragile skin of older patients can actually take off a layer of skin when they are removed and leave a raw wound susceptible to infection. A better alternative is for the phlebotomist to hold pressure on the site for 3 to 5 minutes or until the bleeding has stopped. The extra time and consideration given to the patient is well spent.

technical tip Direct light on the venipuncture sight may help locate hard-to-find veins in the older patient. Using a dilute iodine cleansing may color the site to help locate the vein. Confirm that the patient is not allergic to iodine by asking if he or she is allergic to shellfish.

Equipment Selection

Because of the small, fragile veins frequently seen in the older patient, the evacuated tube system is usually not the best choice of equipment. A better choice is a butterfly with a 23- to 25-gauge needle attached to a syringe that will allow the phlebotomist to control the suction pressure on the vein. A small-gauge needle with a syringe is also an option. If an evacuated tube system is used, the smallest possible tubes should be filled. Because of the tendency to develop anemia by older patients, the volume of blood collected also should be kept to the minimum acceptable amount.

Additional Considerations

When identifying older patients without identification bands be sure to have them state their names. An elderly patient who is confused or who has difficulty hearing is very likely to answer "yes" to any question.

As previously stated, emotional stress can alter blood composition and laboratory testing. In addition to the physical changes of aging, the older patient often faces the loss of career, spouse, family members, and friends. These life changes can bring about depression, sadness, and anger. The fear of pain or the expense associated with venipuncture may make the patient anxious or even tearful. All of these physical and emotional factors can alter test results, and the phlebotomist must be sensitive to them. In preparing the patient for venipuncture, it is important to take more time than usual to assist and reassure the patient. Treat patients with respect and dignity, giving them a sense of control. When identifying patients, address them by their rightful title and not by their first name. Always be considerate and thank the patient.

Dermal puncture, when possible, should be performed on the older patient as a way of avoiding complications such as hematomas, bruising, collapsed veins, and anemia. The advances in point-of-caretesting (see Chapter 13) have made it possible to perform many types of tests on a small amount of blood that can be obtained by a dermal puncture.

Pediatric Population

Ideally, children younger than 2 years of age should have blood collected by a dermal puncture procedure (see Chapter 9) . However, special tests for coagulation, erythrocyte sedimentation rates, special diagnostic studies, or blood cultures require more blood than can be collected from a finger or heel stick and must be collected by venipuncture. Pediatric blood collection involves preparing both the child and parent, using certain restraining procedures, and special equipment. Pediatric phlebotomy presents emotional as well technical difficulties and should be performed by only experienced phlebotomists. Often, there is only one chance to attempt a venipuncture on a child. The phlebotomist must develop interpersonal skills to successfully gain both the young patients' and parents' trust and cooperation as well as be skilled with the special types of equipment used for pediatric venipuncture. It is important to keep the patient as calm as possible during the procedure because as previously discussed, emotional stress and crying can affect blood analytes and cause erroneous test results.

Techniques for dealing with children vary depending on the child's age. It is best to establish guidelines and to be honest with both the patient and parent. Newborns and infants are totally dependent on their parents. The phlebotomist should introduce himself or herself to the parents and explain the procedure. If possible, have the parent hold the child. The parents must identify the child if it is an outpatient setting. Hospitalized patients will have an identification band.

Toddlers have limited language skills and fear of strangers. It is important to talk to the child calmly and maintain eye contact. Demonstrate the procedure using toys. Allow children to have their comfort toys or blanket and develop strategies to distract or entertain them. Again, it is helpful to have the parents assist with holding and comforting the child. Reward the child with praise and stickers. Thank the child and parent for their cooperation.

Older children are more willing to participate. Explain the procedure and demonstrate the equipment. Demonstrate and allow the child to touch the tourniquet or other clean equipment. Answer their questions honestly. Never tell a child it will not hurt. Explain that "it will hurt a little bit, but if you hold very still, it will be over quickly." Enlist the child's help in holding the gauze.

Teenagers are more independent and often embarrassed to show their emotions. Use adult language with teenagers for identification and explanation of the procedure. Ask them if they have fainted or had any reaction to a previous venipuncture procedure. Encourage them to ask questions about the procedure. They may or may not want their parents present.

Never draw blood from a small child without some type of assistance. Physical restraint may be required to immobilize the young child and steady the arm for the venipuncture procedure. This can be accomplished by having someone hold the child or by using a papoose board. Either a vertical or horizontal restraint will work. In the vertical position, the parent holds the child in an upright position on the lap. The parent places an arm around the toddler to hold the arm not being used. The other arm holds the child's venipuncture arm firmly from behind, at the bend of the elbow, in a downward position.

In the horizontal restraint, the child lies down, with the parent on one side of the bed and the phlebotomist on the opposite side. The parent leans over the child holding the near arm and body securely while reaching over the body to hold the opposite venipuncture arm for the phlebotomist.

Older children can usually sit in a drawing chair by themselves. An infant cradle pad (see Chapter 5) facilitates blood collection for infants.

In some instances, a child may become extremely combative. The procedure should be discontinued to avoid the risk of injury to the patient or phlebotomist and the healthcare provider notified.

Equipment Selection

The minimum amount of blood required for laboratory testing should be collected from infants and small children because drawing excessive amounts of blood can cause anemia. The amount of blood collected within a 24-hour period must be monitored owing to the small blood volume in newborns and small children. When using an evacuated tube system, select the smallest evacuated pediatric tubes available to collect the least amount of blood and to avoid causing the vein to collapse. Evacuated tubes as small as 1.8 mL are available. A 23- to 25-gauge winged infusion set needle with a syringe is recommended because of the small, fragile veins. Using an evacuated tube system on older children is acceptable. Pediatric-sized tourniquets are also available. Assemble equipment out of view of the child and cover threatening looking equipment when approaching the pediatric patient.

A local topical anesthetic, eutectic mixture of local anesthetics (**EMLA**), is ideal for use on an apprehensive child before venipuncture. This emulsion of lidocaine and prilocaine is applied directly to intact skin and covered with an occlusive dressing. EMLA penetrates to a depth of 5 mm through the epidermal and dermal layer of the skin. It takes 60 minutes to reach its optimum effect and lasts for 2 or 3 hours. Because of the length of time necessary to anesthetize the area, it is necessary that accurate vein selection is made or more than one site treated. EMLA should not be used on infants younger than 1

Dorsal Hand Vein Technique

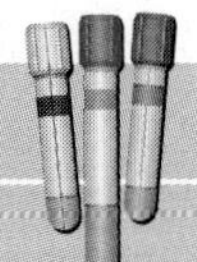

- Obtain and examine the requisition form
- Greet the parent
- Put on gloves
- Identify the infant/child
- Immobilize the infant/child
- Select the vein by encircling the wrist and gently bending it downward. Bending the wrist too much may cause the vein to flatten out and be hard to see or may cause the vein to collapse.
- Do not use a tourniquet
- Cleanse the site with alcohol and allow it to air dry
- Select a 23- to 25-gauge hypodermic needle with a clear hub and appropriate Microtainers
- Encircle the vein with the thumb underneath and the index and middle finger on top of the wrist and apply pressure with the index finger
- Insert the needle with the bevel up into the vein at a 15-degree angle to the skin. Stop advancing the needle as soon as blood appears in the hub.
- Fill Microtainers directly from the blood that drips from the hub of the needle
- Release the finger pressure intermittently to allow the blood to continue to flow
- After collection of specimens, place sterile gauze over the needle
- Remove the needle and apply pressure for 2 to 3 minutes or until the bleeding stops
- Do not apply a bandage
- Label the tubes
- Perform appropriate specimen handling
- Dispose of used supplies in biohazard containers
- Remove gloves and wash hands
- Enter blood collection volume in the nursery log book
- Deliver specimens promptly to the laboratory

month of age or if the child is allergic to local anesthetics. One side effect of this emulsion may be pallor at the site or a slight redness because of the adhesive covering.

Site Selection

The veins located in the antecubital fossa are the best choice for children older than 2 years of age. Do not use deep veins. Site selection and technique is similar to that used for adults (see Chapter 6).

Dorsal hand venipuncture can be used for children younger than 2 years of age. This technique can be used to collect specimens from a superficial hand vein directly into appropriate microspecimen containers. The advantage of this technique is that more blood can be collected from the vein as compared with a heel stick and there is less chance of hemolyzing the specimen or contaminating the specimen with tissue fluid. Use of this technique requires additional training and is an institutional decision, because saving all veins for intravenous therapy may be preferred. Use extreme care when disposing of the contaminated needle.

Bibliography

Henry, JB, and Kurec, AS: The clinical laboratory: organization, purpose, and practice. In Henry, JB (ed): Clinical Diagnosis and Management by Laboratory Methods. WB Saunders, Philadelphia, 1999.

Lotspeich, CA: Specimen collection and processing. In Bishop, ML (ed): Clinical Chemistry: Principles, Procedures and Correlations. JB Lippincott, Philadelphia, 1985.

National Committee for Clinical Laboratory Standards Approved Standard H3-A4: Procedures for Collection of Diagnostic Blood Specimens by Venipuncture. NCCLS, Wayne, PA, 1998.

National Committee for Clinical Laboratory Standards Approved Guideline H18-A2: Procedures for the Handling and Processing of Blood Specimens. NCCLS, Wayne, PA, 1999.

National Committee for Clinical Laboratory Standards Approved Standard H21-A3: Collection, Transport and Preparation of Blood for Coagulation Testing and Performance of General Coagulation Assays. NCCLS, Wayne, PA, 1999.

http://www.jcaho.org. search,HR.5 Copyright 2002 Joint Commission on Accreditation of Healthcare Organizations, One Renaissance Boulevard, Oakbrook Terrace, IL 60181, Site accessed June, 2002

Study Questions

1. Name three categories of test status and prioritize the order (1, 2, 3) in which they would be collected from different patients.

   a. ______

   b. ______

   c. ______

2. What is the difference between patients who have been fasting, NPO, and in a basal state?

   ______

   ______

   ______

3. What three tests are most affected by a nonfasting patient?

   a. ______

   b. ______

   c. ______

4. At 0730, the phlebotomist receives requests for a cortisol level on Unit 4B, a fasting blood sugar (FBS) on Unit 4A, and a stat crossmatch in the ER. In which order should the phlebotomist collect these specimens? Justify your answer.

   ______

   ______

   ______

5. Why should the fasting glucose specimen be tested before administering the glucose in a GTT?

   ______

6. Design a schedule for a 3-hour GTT assuming the patient has a fasting specimen drawn at 0715, the specimen is tested, and the patient completes drinking the glucose at 0745.

   ______

   ______

   ______

   ______

7. True or False. A phlebotomist who does not obtain the 2-hour sample in a GTT after the first venipuncture should immediately perform a capillary puncture. ______

8. When should trough and peak levels be drawn for therapeutic drug monitoring?

____

____

9. Which therapeutic drug monitoring level is used to determine whether the medication should be administered? _______________

10. Give two reasons why blood cultures are frequently ordered stat.

    a. _______________

    b. _______________

11. The condition represented by a positive blood culture is called _______________.

12. Describe the venipuncture site preparation when collecting a blood culture.

____

____

____

13. The major source of false-positive blood cultures is _______________.

14. True or False. A specimen for cold agglutinins will have a falsely decreased value if it is chilled immediately after collection. Explain your answer.

____

15. How will wrapping the collection tube in aluminum foil affect the results of a bilirubin test?

____

16. How will the results of a serum gastrin test be affected if the specimen is held tightly in the phlebotomist's fist when being delivered to the laboratory?

____

17. How is documentation of patient identification, specimen collection, and specimen handling performed when forensic studies are requested?

____

18. What precautions must be taken when applying tourniquets and adhesive bandages in the geriatric patient?

____

19. State the preferable venipuncture equipment used for both pediatric and geriatric patients.

____

20. Name four complications in performing venipuncture on the geriatric patient.

a. ______

b. ______

c. ______

d. ______

21. Name three differences between geriatric and pediatric venipuncture.

a. ______

b. ______

c. ______

22. How can a phlebotomist immobilize a child for venipuncture?

______

23. What is the preferred venipuncture technique for children younger than 2 years of age?

______

24. What can be used to alleviate venipuncture pain in the pediatric patient?

______

Clinical Situations

1. An outpatient comes to the laboratory at 13:00 with a requisition for a cardiac risk profile.

   A. Before collecting the specimen, what should the phlebotomist ask the patient?

   ______

   B. What specific tests requested on this patient are of concern to the phlebotomist?

   ______

   C. State the instructions that should have been given when the patient received the requisition.

   ______

2. An outpatient is scheduled for a 6-hour glucose tolerance test. After completion of the 2-hour blood collection, the patient decides to walk around the block to the hardware store while waiting for the 3-hour blood collection. The patient was brought back to the hospital by ambulance.

   A. Why did the hardware store clerk call an ambulance?

   ______

B. What instructions should have been given to the patient?

____

3. Two sets of blood cultures each consisting of an aerobic and an anaerobic bottle are drawn from a patient 1 hour apart. The first set is drawn using a syringe and the second set using a butterfly.

   A. Is this a common ordering pattern for blood cultures? Why or why not?

   ____

   B. What error in technique could cause a positive anaerobic culture from the first set and a negative anaerobic culture in the second set?

   ____

   C. What is the significance of a known skin contaminant growing in the aerobic bottle from the first set and not in the aerobic bottle from the second set?

   ____

   D. Would failure to mix the bottles after the blood is added most probably cause a false-positive or false-negative culture?

   ____

4. A phlebotomist collects a stat ammonia level and is then paged to collect a cold agglutinin on the next floor and a complete blood count (CBC) in the critical care unit (CCU). The phlebotomist sends the ammonia level to the laboratory in the pneumatic tube system; collects the cold agglutinin; goes to the CCU and draws the CBC; and delivers both specimens to the appropriate laboratory sections. How will the quality of these test results be affected and why?

   ____

   ____

   ____

5. While collecting blood from an elderly patient using an evacuated tube, the phlebotomist notices that the puncture site is beginning to swell.

   A. Why is this happening?

   ____

   B. What should the phlebotomist do?

   ____

   C. How could the specimen be collected?

   ____

6. State whether each of the following scenarios is acceptable or unacceptable and explain your answers.

   A. A physician requests two sets of blood cultures to be collected at the same time from two different arms.

   ____

   B. A trough level is requested 30 minutes after medication is given to the patient.

   ____

   C. Cortisol levels on a patient are ordered to be drawn at 0900 and 1600.

   ____

   D. A phlebotomist collects every other specimen for a GTT by dermal puncture when the test is being performed on an elderly patient.

   ____

7. As an attorney for a defendant with a blood alcohol level above the legal limit, you are questioning the phlebotomist.

   A. State three questions you would ask the phlebotomist to try to discredit the laboratory result.

   ____

   ____

   ____

   B. How should a competent phlebotomist answer these questions?

   ____

   ____

   ____

NAME ____________________

Evaluation of Blood Culture Collection Technique

RATING SYSTEM 2 = SATISFACTORILY PERFORMED 1 = NEEDS IMPROVEMENT 0 = INCORRECT/DID NOT PERFORM

_______ 1. Examines requisition and identifies patient

_______ 2. Correctly assembles equipment

_______ 3. Washes hands

_______ 4. Puts on gloves

_______ 5. Applies tourniquet

_______ 6. Selects puncture site

_______ 7. Releases tourniquet

_______ 8. Scrubs site with alcohol for 1 minute

_______ 9. Cleanses site with iodine

_______ 10. Completes iodine cleaning using concentric circles

_______ 11. Allows iodine to dry

_______ 12. Cleanses tops of blood culture containers

_______ 13. Cleanses palpating finger if necessary

_______ 14. Reapplies tourniquet

_______ 15. Performs venipuncture

_______ 16. Inoculates anaerobic container first from syringe or second from butterfly

_______ 17. Dispenses correct amount of blood into containers

_______ 18. Mixes containers

_______ 19. Disposes of used equipment and supplies

_______ 20. Removes iodine from patient's arm

_______ 21. Bandages patient's arm

_______ 22. Correctly labels blood culture containers

_______ 23. Overall aseptic technique

TOTAL POINTS

MAXIMUM POINTS = 46

Comments:

Chapter 9

Dermal Puncture

Chapter Outline

Composition of Capillary Blood

Dermal Puncture Equipment

- Dermal Puncture Devices
- Microspecimen Containers
- Additional Dermal Puncture Supplies

Dermal Puncture Procedure

- Phlebotomist Preparation
- Patient Identification and Preparation
- Site Selection
- Cleansing the Site
- Performing the Puncture
- Specimen Collection
- Order of Draw
- Bandaging the Patient
- Labeling the Specimen
- Completion of the Procedure
- Summary of Dermal Puncture Technique

Learning Objectives

Upon completion of this chapter, the reader will be able to:

1 State the complications associated with puncture of the deep veins in infants.

2 List six reasons for performing dermal punctures on adults.

3 Describe the composition of capillary blood and name four test results that may differ between capillary and venous blood.

4 Discuss the types of skin puncture devices available.

5 Describe the various types of microcollection containers, reasons for their use, method of collection, and advantages and disadvantages.

6 Discuss the purpose and methodology for warming the puncture site.

7 Identify the acceptable sites for performing heel and finger punctures and the conditions when each is performed.

8 List four unacceptable areas for heel puncture.

9 State the complications produced by the presence of alcohol at the puncture site.

10 State the correct positioning of the lancet for dermal puncture.

11 Name the major cause of microspecimen contamination.

12 State the order of collection for dermal puncture specimens.

13 Describe the correct labeling of microspecimens.

14 Correctly perform dermal punctures on the heel and the finger.

Key Terms

Calcaneus
Dermal
Ecchymoses
Microsample
Palmar
Plantar

Although venipuncture is the most frequently performed phlebotomy procedure, it is not appropriate in all circumstances. Current laboratory instrumentation and point-of-care testing make it possible to perform a majority of laboratory tests on ***microsamples*** of blood obtained by ***dermal*** puncture on both pediatric and adult patients.

In most institutions, dermal puncture is the method of choice for collecting blood from infants and children younger than 2 years of age. Locating **superficial** veins that are large enough to accept even a small-gauge needle is difficult in these patients, and available veins may need to be reserved for intravenous therapy. Use of deep veins, such as the femoral vein, can be dangerous and may cause complications including cardiac arrest, venous thrombosis, hemorrhage, damage to surrounding tissue and organs, infection, reflex arteriospasm (which can possibly result in gangrene), and injury caused by restraining the child. Drawing excessive amounts of blood from premature and small infants can rapidly cause anemia, because a 2-pound infant may have a total blood volume of only 150 mL.

Dermal puncture may be required in many adult patients, including:

1 Burned or scarred patients
2 Patients receiving chemotherapy who require frequent tests and whose veins must be reserved for therapy
3 Patients with thrombotic tendencies
4 Geriatric or other patients with very fragile veins
5 Patients with inaccessible veins
6 Patients requiring home glucose monitoring and point-of-care tests (see Chapter 13)

It may not be possible to obtain a satisfactory specimen by dermal puncture from patients who are severely dehydrated or who have poor peripheral circulation. Certain tests may not be collected by dermal puncture because of the larger amount of blood required; these include some coagulation studies, erythrocyte sedimentation rates, and blood cultures.

Correct collection techniques are critical because of the smaller amount of blood that is collected and the higher possibility of specimen contamination, microclots, and hemolysis. Hemolysis is more frequently seen in specimens collected by dermal puncture than it is in those collected by venipuncture. Excessive squeezing of the puncture site to obtain enough blood is often the cause of hemolysis. Newborns in general have increased numbers of red blood cells (RBCs) and increased RBC fragility, which raises the possibility that hemolysis may occur even in properly collected samples. The presence of hemolysis may not be detected in specimens containing bilirubin, but it interferes not only with the tests routinely affected by hemolysis but also with the frequently requested **neonatal** bilirubin determination.

Composition of Capillary Blood

Blood collected by dermal puncture comes from the capillaries, arterioles, and venules. Therefore it is a mixture of arterial and venous blood and may contain small amounts of tissue fluid. Because of arterial pressure, the composition of this blood more closely resembles arterial rather than venous blood. Warming the site before specimen collection increases blood flow as much as sevenfold, thereby producing a specimen that is very close to the composition of arterial blood.

With the exception of arterial blood gases, very few chemical differences exist between arterial and venous blood. The concentration of glucose is higher in blood obtained by dermal puncture, and the concentrations of potassium, total protein, and calcium are lower. Therefore, when dermal punctures are performed, this factor should be noted on the requisition form. Alternating between dermal puncture and venipuncture should not be done when results are to be compared.

technical tip By documenting that the specimen was collected by dermal puncture, the healthcare provider can consider the collection technique when interpreting results.

Dermal Puncture Equipment

In addition to the previously discussed venipuncture equipment, a phlebotomy collection tray or drawing station should contain skin puncture devices, microsample collection containers, glass slides, and possibly a heel warmer for use in performing dermal punctures.(Fig. 9–1).

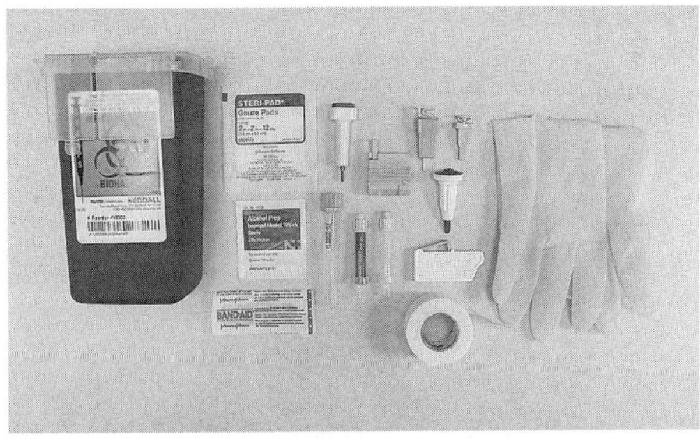

Figure 9–1 Dermal puncture equipment.

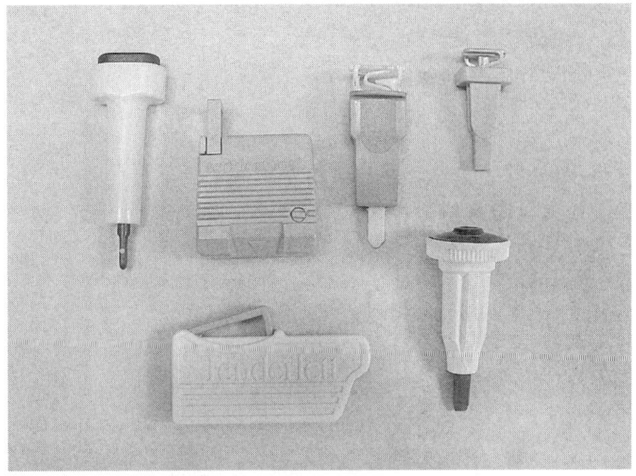

Figure 9–2 Dermal puncture devices. (Courtesy of Becton, Dickinson and Company © 2002 BD.)

Dermal Puncture Devices

As shown in Figure 9–2, a variety of skin puncture devices are commercially available, ranging from simple manual and automatic lancets, with and without retractable blades, to laser lancets. Most are safety devices that retract and lock after use to prevent reuse and accidental puncture. Many studies have been performed comparing the various devices with respect to efficiency of collection, specimen hemolysis, and the formation of *ecchymoses* (bruising) at the collection site. No single method appears to be superior.

To prevent contact with bone, the depth of the puncture is critical. The National Committee for Clinical Laboratory Standards (NCCLS) recommends that the incision depth should not exceed 2.0 mm in a device used to perform heel sticks. There is concern that even this may be too deep in certain infants, particularly premature infants. The length of manual lancets, the spring release mechanism, and the use of platforms in automatic devices control the puncture depth. Punctures should never be performed using an uncontrolled surgical blade. Manufacturers provide separate devices designed for heel sticks on premature infants, newborns, and babies; fingersticks on toddlers and older children; and fingersticks on adults. The depth of the puncture can range from 0.85 mm in the Tender-foot/Premi (Technidyne Corp., Edison, NJ, or BD Quikheel Lancet, Franklin Lakes, NJ) to 3.0 mm with the orange platform Autolet for adults (Ulster Scientific, New Paltz, NY).

To produce adequate blood flow, the depth of the puncture is actually much less important than the width of the incision. This is because the major vascular area of the skin is located at the dermal-subcutaneous junction, which in a newborn is only 0.35 to 1.6 mm below the skin and can range to 3.0 mm in a large adult (Fig. 9–3). Designated puncture devices can easily reach it. Therefore, the number of severed capillaries depends on the incision width. Incision widths vary from needle stabs to 2.5 mm. Sufficient blood flow should be obtained from incision widths no larger than 2.5 mm. Longer incisions should be avoided because they will produce unnecessary damage to the heel or finger.

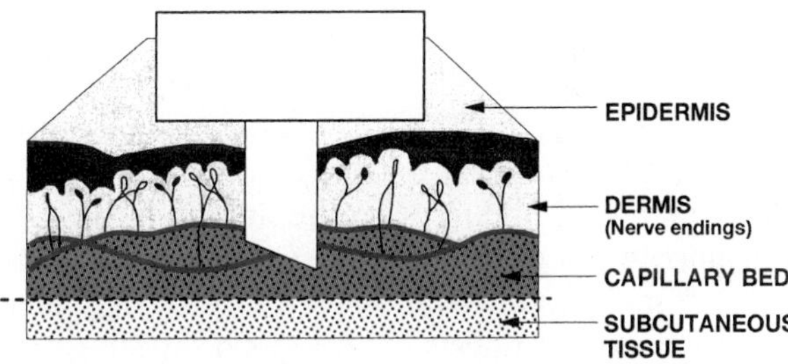

Figure 9–3 Vascular area of the skin, at the juncture between the dermis and the subcutaneous tissue. (Adapted from product literature, Becton, Dickinson and Company © 2002 BD.)

As illustrated in the following examples, lancets are available in varying depths and widths. BD Vacutainer Safety Flow Lancets (Becton, Dickinson, Franklin Lakes, NJ) are available in depths ranging from 2.2 mm to 1.4 mm and widths of 1.0 mm and 0.5 mm. The BD Genie Lancet (Becton, Dickinson, Franklin Lakes, NJ) is a safety puncture device in

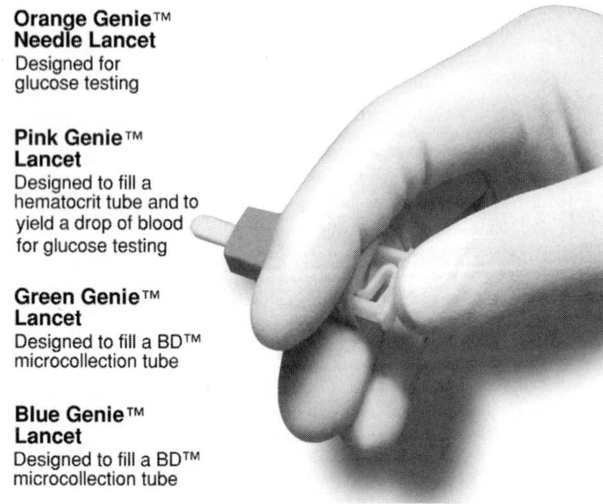

Orange Genie™
Needle Lancet
Designed for
glucose testing
Pink Genie™
Lancet
Designed to fill a
hematocrit tube and to
yield a drop of blood
for glucose testing
Green Genie™
Lancet
Designed to fill a BD™
microcollection tube
Blue Genie™
Lancet
Designed to fill a BD™
microcollection tube

Figure 9–4 Genie™ safety lancets. (Courtesy of Becton, Dickinson and Company © 2002 BD.)

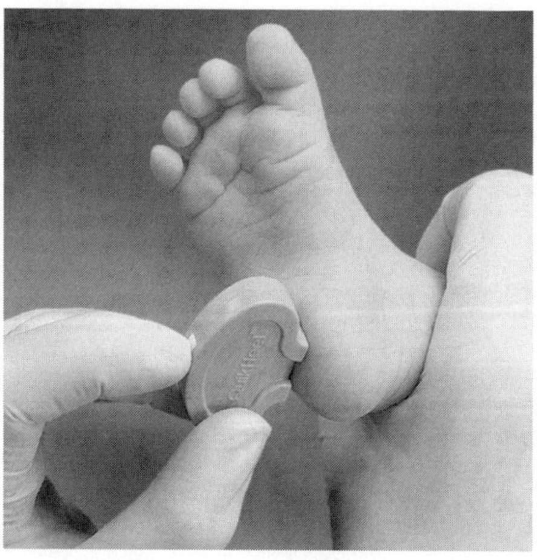

Figure 9–5 QuikHeel™ lancet. (Courtesy of Becton, Dickinson and Company © 2002 BD.)

varying depths (Fig. 9–4). The lavender Genie needle lancet (1.25 mm x 28-G needle) provides a single drop of blood and is used for infant heel sticks for glucose testing. The orange Genie needle lancet (2.25 mm x 23-G needle) is used to provide a drop of blood from a fingerstick for glucose testing. The pink Genie lancet blade (1.0 mm depth, 1.5 mm width) is used for low blood flow, the green Genie lancet blade (1.5 mm depth, 1.5 mm width) for medium blood flow, and the blue Genie lancet blade (2.0 mm depth, 1.5 mm width) for medium to high blood flow. A color-coded heel stick device designed specifically for premature infants, newborns, and babies is the BD Quikheel Lancet with a permanent retractable blade to minimize possible injury and prevent reuse. The pink lancet has a depth of 0.85 mm and a width of 1.75 mm for premature infants, and the green lancet has a depth of 1.0 mm and a width of 2.50 mm (Fig. 9–5).

International Technidyne Corporation (Edison, NJ) provides a range of color-coded, fully automated, single-use, retractable, disposable devices in varying depths. Tenderfoot and Tenderlett devices are designed for heel and finger punctures, respectively. Models are available ranging from the Tenderfoot for preemies to the Tenderlett for toddlers, juniors, and adults.

The Autolet system (Ulster Scientific, Inc., New Paltz, NY) uses disposable platforms to control the depth of the spring-activated puncture devices. The color-coded platforms are available in three depths ranging from 1.8 mm to 3.0 mm deep.

Laser lancets (Lasette® Plus, Cell Robotics International, Inc., Albuquerque, NM) are available for clinical and home use, and are approved by the Food and Drug Administration **(FDA)** for adults and children older than 5 years of age. The lightweight, portable, battery-operated device eliminates the risks of accidental punctures and the need for sharps containers. The laser light penetrates the skin 1 to 2 mm, producing a small hole by vaporizing water in the skin. This creates a smaller wound, reduces the pain and soreness associated with capillary puncture, and allows up to 100 μL of blood to be collected (Fig. 9–6).

technical tip Select the puncture device that will safely provide the appropriate volume of blood to perform the required tests.

Microspecimen Containers

Figure 9–7 illustrates some of the major specimen containers available for collection of microsamples, including capillary tubes, micropipets, microcollection tubes, and micropipets with dilution systems. Some containers are designated for a specific test, and others serve multiple purposes. The type of container chosen is usually related to laboratory preference, because advantages and disadvantages can be associated with each system.

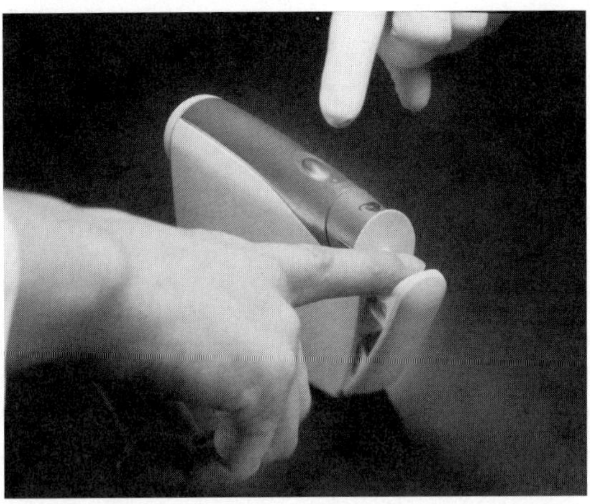

Figure 9–6 Laser lancet, the Lasette® Plus. (Courtesy of Cell Robotics, Inc., Albuquerque, NM.)

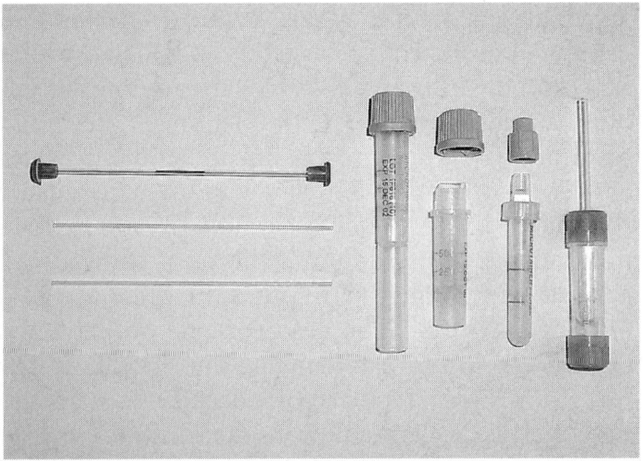

Figure 9–7 Microspecimen containers (note extender).

Capillary Tubes

Capillary tubes, which are frequently referred to as microhematocrit tubes, are small tubes used to collect approximately 50 to 75 μL of blood for the primary purpose of performing a microhematocrit test. The tubes are designed to fit into a hematocrit centrifuge and its corresponding hematocrit reader. Tubes are available plain or coated with ammonium heparin, and they are color-coded, with a red band for heparinized tubes and a blue band for plain tubes. Heparinized tubes should be used for hematocrits collected by dermal puncture, and plain tubes are used when the test is being performed on previously anticoagulated blood. When sufficient blood has been collected, the end of the capillary tube that has not been used to collect the specimen is closed with clay sealant or a plastic plug. Phlebotomists should use extreme care to prevent breakage when collecting specimens and sealing the tubes. As discussed in Chapter 3, a government alert issued in 1999 recommends that all glass capillary tubes be replaced with plastic tubes and tubes be sealed by methods other than clay plugs.

technical tip Use of plastic capillary tubes is strongly recommended.

Micropipets

Larger capillary tubes, called Caraway or Natelson pipets, are used when tests requiring more blood than a microhematocrit are requested. The pipets have a tapered end for specimen collection and fill by capillary action. Pipet lengths vary from 75 mm for Caraway pipets to 150 mm for Natelson pipets. The capacity varies from 330 to 470 μL in Caraway pipets to 220 to 420 μL in Natelson pipets. Pipets are available plain or with ammonium heparin and are color-coded respectively with blue or red bands. After collection of the sample, the nontapered ends are sealed with specifically matched soft plastic caps. Tubes designed for arterial blood gas analysis are also available.

For collection of serum or plasma, the tubes are centrifuged by carefully balancing them in cushioned centrifuge carriers. Inserting a syringe needle into the tapered end and slowly drawing the specimen away from the red cells can remove serum or plasma.

Microcollection Tubes

Plastic collection tubes such as the Microtainer (Becton, Dickinson, Franklin Lakes, NJ) provide a larger collection volume and present no danger from broken glass. A variety of anticoagulants and additives, including separator gel, are available, and the tubes are color coded in the same way as evacuated tubes. Some tubes are supplied with a capillary scoop collector top that is replaced by a color-coded plastic sealer top after the specimen is collected. Microtainer tubes are designed to hold approximately 600 μL of blood. BD Microtainer tubes with BD Microgard closures are designed to reduce the risk of blood splatter and blood leakage. The Microgard closure is removed by twisting and lifting.

Tubes have a wider diameter, textured interior, and integrated blood collection scoop to enhance blood flow into the tube and eliminate the need to assemble the equipment. After completion of the blood collection, the cap is placed on the container, and anticoagulated tubes are gently inverted to ensure complete mixing. Tubes have markings to indicate minimum and maximum collection amounts to prevent underfilling or overfilling that could cause erroneous results. Tube extenders are available for this system to facilitate labeling and handling (see Fig. 9–7). Other capillary blood collection devices have plastic capillary tubes inserted into the collection container (SAFE-T-FILL capillary blood collection system, RAM Scientific Co., Needham, MA). After blood has been collected, the capillary tube is removed and the appropriate color-coded cap closes the tube.

Mixing of anticoagulated specimens is enhanced by the presence of small plastic beads in some collection tube systems. Separation of serum or plasma is achieved by centrifugation in specifically designed centrifuges.

technical tip Mint green PST Microtainer tubes, gold SST Microtainer tubes, and amber Microtainer tubes are available for light-sensitive analyte testing.

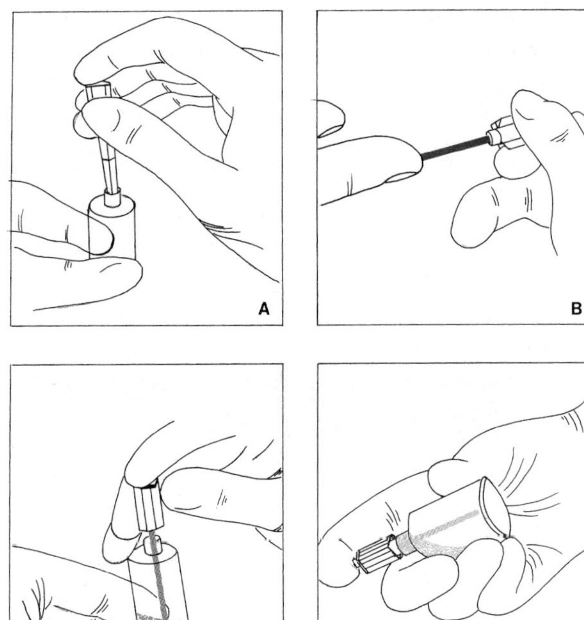

Figure 9–8 Unopette procedure. (*A*) Puncturing reservoir diaphragm. (*B*) Filling capillary pipet. (*C*) Transferring specimen to reservoir. (*D*) Mixing the reservoir. (From Wedding, ME, and Toenjes, SA: Medical Laboratory Procedures, ed. 2. FA Davis, Philadelphia, 1997, p 235, with permission.)

Micropipet and Dilution System

The Unopette™ System (Becton, Dickinson, Franklin Lakes, NJ) is designed for tests that can be performed on diluted whole blood, primarily hematology tests. The system consists of a sealed plastic reservoir containing a measured amount of diluent, a calibrated capillary pipet, and a plastic pipet shield. The amount and type of diluent and the size of the capillary pipet correspond to the specific test to be run. Pipets are designed to collect only the amount of blood for which they are calibrated.

The procedure for use of the Unopette System is shown in Figure 9–8*A* through *D* and includes:

1. Puncturing the diaphragm of the reservoir with the point of the pipet shield
2. Filling the capillary pipet and wiping excess blood from the outside
3. Slightly squeezing the reservoir
4. Placing the index finger over the opening in the pipet holder and inserting the pipet into the reservoir
5. Releasing pressure on the reservoir and removing the finger from the holder opening to cause blood to be drawn into the diluent
6. Carefully rinsing the pipet by squeezing the reservoir without overflowing the pipet
7. Placing the index finger over the opening and inverting the reservoir to mix

Additional Dermal Puncture Supplies

Alcohol pads, sterile gauze, and sharps containers are required for the dermal puncture just as they are for the venipuncture. Blood smears used for the white blood cell differential and the examination of RBC morphology must be made during the dermal puncture procedure and require a supply of glass slides. Phlebotomists prepare these slides using the procedure discussed in Chapter 10.

As discussed previously, warming the puncture site increases blood flow to the area. This can be accomplished by using warm washcloths or towels, or a commercial heel warmer. A heel warmer is a packet containing sodium thiosulfate and glycerin that produces heat when the chemicals are mixed together by gentle squeezing of the packet. The packet should be wrapped in a towel and held away from the face during the initial activation.

Dermal Puncture Procedure

Many of the procedures associated with the venipuncture also apply to the dermal puncture. Therefore, major emphasis in this chapter is placed on the techniques and complications that are unique to the dermal puncture.

Phlebotomist Preparation

Before performing a dermal puncture, the phlebotomist must have a requisition form containing the same information required for the venipuncture. When a specimen is collected by dermal puncture, this must be noted on the requisition form because, as discussed previously, the concentration of some analytes differs between venous and capillary blood.

Because of the variety of puncture devices and collection containers available for dermal puncture, phlebotomists should carefully examine the information on the requisition form to ensure that they have the appropriate equipment to collect all required specimens as well as the skin puncture device that corresponds to the age of the patient.

Phlebotomists frequently perform dermal punctures in the nursery and must observe its specified isolation procedures, such as the wearing of gowns and gloves, extensive handwashing, and carrying only the necessary equipment to the patient area. Equipment should be kept out of reach of the patient at all times.

Patient Identification and Preparation

Patients for dermal puncture must be identified using the same procedures as those used for venipuncture (requisition form, verbal identification, and ID band). In the nursery, an identification band *must* be present on the infant and not just on the bassinet. Verbal identification of pediatric outpatients may have to be obtained from the parents.

Approaching pediatric patients can be difficult, and the phlebotomist must present a friendly, confident appearance while explaining the procedure to the child and the parents. Do not say the procedure will not hurt, and explain the necessity of remaining very still.

Parents should be given the choice of staying with the child or leaving the room. If they choose to stay, they may be asked to assist in holding and comforting the child. Very agitated children may need to have their legs and free hand restrained, as discussed in Chapter 8. This can be accomplished by a parent or coworker, or by confining the child in a blanket or commercially available papoose-style wrap. If a restraint is used, parental consent must be obtained and documented in the patient's medical record.

technical tip Consider giving the parents the option to stay with a child or leave the room.

For optimum blood flow, the finger or heel from which the sample is to be taken may be warmed. This is primarily required for patients with very cold or cyanotic fingers, for heel sticks to collect multiple samples, and for the collection of capillary blood gases. Warming dilates the blood vessels and increases arterial blood flow. Moistening a towel with warm water (42°C) or activating a commercial heel warmer and covering the site for 3 to 5 minutes effectively warms the site. Use caution in moistening the towel to ensure the water temperature is not greater than 42°C to avoid burning the patient. The site should not be warmed for longer than 10 minutes or test results may be altered.

Site Selection

As mentioned in the discussion of skin puncture devices, a primary danger in dermal puncture is accidental contact with the bone, followed by infection (**osteomyelitis**). This problem can be avoided by selection of puncture sites that provide sufficient distance between the skin and the bone. The primary dermal puncture sites are the heel and the distal segments of the third and fourth fingers. The plantar surface of the large toe is also acceptable. Performing dermal punctures on earlobes is usually not recommended. The choice of a puncture area is based on the age and size of the patient.

Areas selected for dermal puncture should not be callused, scarred, bruised, edematous, cold or cyanotic, or infected. Punctures should *never* be made through previous puncture sites because this practice can easily introduce microorganisms into the puncture and allow them to reach the bone.

Heel Puncture Sites

The heel is used for dermal punctures on infants younger than 1 year of age because it contains more tissue than the fingers and has not yet become callused from walking.

Acceptable areas for heel puncture are shown in Figure 9–9 and are described as the medial and lateral areas of the ***plantar*** (bottom) surface of the heel. These areas can be determined by drawing imaginary lines extending back from the middle of the large toe and from between the fourth and fifth toes. It is in these areas that the distance between the skin and the ***calcaneus*** (heel bone) is greatest. Notice the short distance between the back (posterior curvature) of the heel and the calcaneus (see Fig. 9–9). This is the reason why this area is never acceptable for heel puncture.

Punctures should not be performed in other areas of the foot, and particularly not in the arch, where they may cause damage to nerves and tendons. In larger infants, the plantar surface of the large toe may be used.

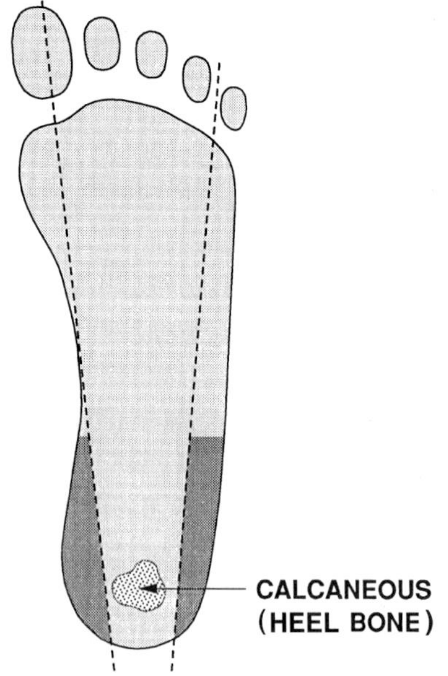

Figure 9–9 Acceptable heel puncture sites.

Finger Puncture Sites

Finger punctures are performed on adults and children over 1 year of age. Fingers of infants younger than 1 year of age may not contain enough tissue to prevent contact with the bone.

The fleshy areas located near the center of the third and fourth fingers on the ***palmar*** side of the nondominant hand are the sites of choice for finger puncture (Fig. 9–10). Because the tip and sides of the finger contain only about half the tissue mass of the central area, the possibility of bone injury is increased in these areas. Problems associated with use of the other fingers include possible calluses on the thumb, increased nerve endings in the index finger, and decreased tissue in the fifth finger. Patients who routinely perform home glucose monitoring may request a specific finger, and their wishes should be accommodated.

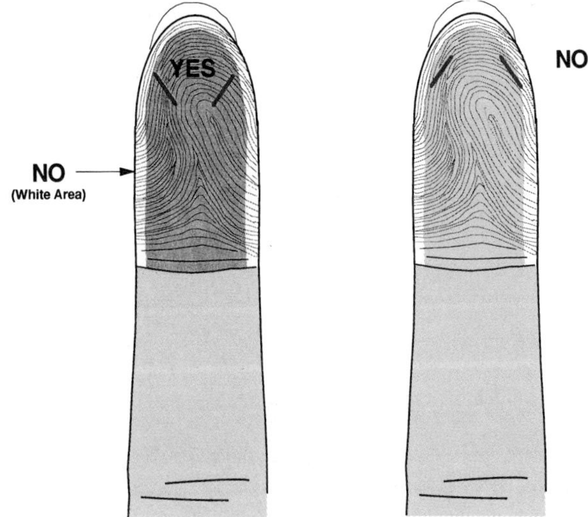

Figure 9–10 Acceptable finger puncture sites and correct puncture angle.

Summary of Dermal Puncture Site Selection

- Use the medial and lateral areas of the plantar surface of the heel.
- Use the central fleshy area of the third or fourth finger.
- Do not use the back of the heel.
- Do not use the arch of the foot.
- Do not puncture through old sites.
- Do not use areas with visible damage.

Cleansing the Site

The selected site is cleansed with 70% isopropyl alcohol, using a circular motion. The alcohol should be allowed to dry on the skin for maximum antiseptic action, and the residue may be removed with sterile gauze to prevent interference with certain tests. Failure to allow the alcohol to dry:

1. Causes a stinging sensation for the patient
2. Contaminates the specimen
3. Hemolyzes RBCs
4. Prevents formation of a rounded blood drop because blood will mix with the alcohol and run down the finger

Use of povidone-iodine is not recommended for dermal punctures because specimen contamination may elevate some test results, including bilirubin, phosphorus, uric acid, and potassium.

Performing the Puncture

While the puncture is performed, the heel or finger should be well supported and held firmly, without squeezing the puncture area. Massaging the area before the puncture may increase blood flow to the area. The heel is held between the thumb and index finger of the nondominant hand, with the index finger held over the heel and the thumb below the heel (Fig. 9–11). The finger is held between the thumb and index finger, with the palmar surface facing up and the finger pointing downward to increase blood flow.

Punctures performed with a manual lancet should be made with one continuous motion, and automatic devices should be placed firmly on the puncture site. Depress the lancet and hold for a moment, then release. Pressure must be maintained because

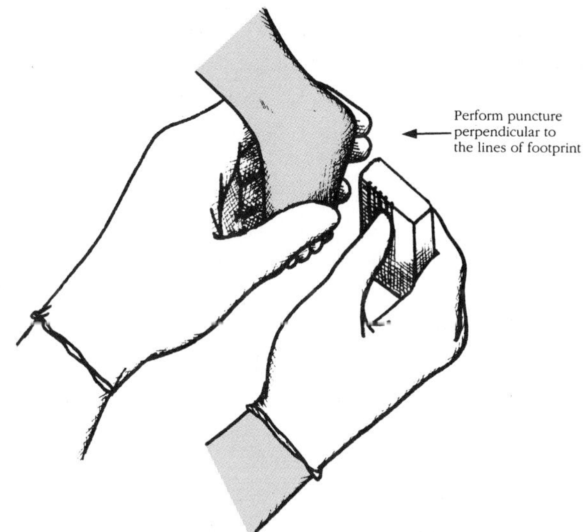
Perform puncture perpendicular to the lines of footprint

Figure 9–11 Correct position for heel puncture.

the elasticity of the skin naturally inhibits penetration of the blade. Removal of the lancet before the puncture is complete will yield a low blood flow. Be sure the device chosen for the puncture corresponds to the size of the patient. As shown in Figure 9–11, the blade of the lancet should be aligned to cut across (perpendicular to) the grooves of the fingerprint or heel print. This aids in the formation of a rounded drop because the blood will not have a tendency to run into the grooves.

technical tip Failure to place puncture devices firmly on the skin is the primary cause of insufficient blood flow. One firm puncture is less painful for the patient than two "mini" punctures.

After completing the puncture, the puncture device should be placed in an appropriate sharps container. A new puncture device must be used if an additional puncture is required.

Specimen Collection

Before beginning the blood collection, the first drop of blood must be wiped away with sterile gauze. This will prevent contamination of the specimen with residual alcohol and tissue fluid released during the puncture. When collecting microspecimens, even a minute amount of contamination can severely affect the sample quality. Therefore, blood should be freely flowing from the puncture site as a result of firm pressure and should not be obtained by milking of the surrounding tissue, which will release tissue fluid. Alternately applying pressure to the area and releasing it will produce the most satisfactory blood flow. Tightly squeezing the area with no relaxation cuts off blood flow to the puncture site.

technical tip Applying pressure about 1/2 inch away from the puncture site frequently produces better blood flow than pressure very close to the site.

Because collection containers fill by capillary action, the collection tip can be lightly touched to the drop of blood and the blood will be drawn into the container. Collection devices should not touch the puncture site and should not be scraped over the skin because this will produce specimen contamination and hemolysis. Fingers are positioned slightly downward with the palmar surface facing up during the collection procedure (Fig. 9–12).

technical tip While the sample is being collected, the patient's hand does not have to be completely turned over. Rotating the hand 90 degrees allows the phlebotomist to clearly see the blood drops without placing himself or herself in an awkward position and produces adequate blood flow.

To prevent the introduction of air bubbles, capillary tubes and micropipets are held horizontally while being filled. The presence of air bubbles limits the amount of blood that can be collected per tube and will interfere with blood gas determinations and tests performed with Unopettes. When the tubes are filled, they are sealed with sealant clay or designated plastic caps.

Microcollection tubes are slanted down during the collection, and blood is allowed to run through the capillary collection scoop and down the side of the tube. The tip of the collection container is placed beneath the puncture site and touches the underside of the drop. The first three drops of blood provide the channel to allow blood to freely flow into the container. Gently tapping the bottom of the tube may be necessary to force blood to the bottom. When a tube is filled, the color-coded top is attached. Tubes with anticoagulants should be inverted 8 to 20 times (lavender top tubes). If blood flow is slow, it may be necessary to mix the tube while the collection is in progress. It is important to work quickly, because blood that takes more than 2 minutes to collect may form microclots in an anticoagulated Microtainer.

technical tip Fast collection and mixing ensure more accurate test results.

technical tip Clotting is triggered immediately on skin puncture and represents the greatest obstacle in collecting quality specimens.

Order of Draw

The order of draw for collecting multiple specimens from a dermal puncture is important because of the tendency of platelets to accumulate at the site of a wound. Blood to be used for tests for the evaluation of platelets, such as the blood smear, platelet count, and CBC, must be collected first. The blood smear should be made first, followed by the Unopette System or the EDTA tube, other anticoagulated tubes, and then serum tubes.

Bandaging the Patient

When sufficient blood has been collected, pressure is applied to the puncture site with sterile gauze. The finger or heel is elevated and pressure is applied until the bleeding stops. Confirm that bleeding has stopped before removing the pressure.

Bandages are not used for children younger than 2 years because the children may remove the bandages, place them in their mouth, and possibly aspirate the bandages. Adhesive may also cause irritation to or tear sensitive skin, particularly the fragile skin of a newborn or older adult patient.

Labeling the Specimen

Microsamples must be labeled with the same information required for venipuncture specimens. Labels can be wrapped around microcollection tubes or groups of capillary pipets. For transport, capillary pipets are then placed in a large tube because the outside of the capillary pipets may be contaminated with blood. This procedure also helps to prevent breakage.

BD Microtainer tubes have extenders that can be attached to the container. This allows the computer label to be applied vertically (see Fig. 9–12).

Completion of the Procedure

The dermal puncture procedure is completed in the same manner as the venipuncture by disposing of all used materials in appropriate containers, removing gloves, washing hands, and thanking the patient and/or the parents for their cooperation. Figure 9–12 shows the procedures unique to the finger puncture.

All special handling procedures associated with venipuncture specimens also apply to microspecimens. Observe test collection priorities.

To prevent excessive removal of blood from small infants, many nurseries have a log sheet for documenting the amount of blood collected each time a procedure is requested. The phlebotomist should record the amount of blood collected on the log sheet before leaving the area.

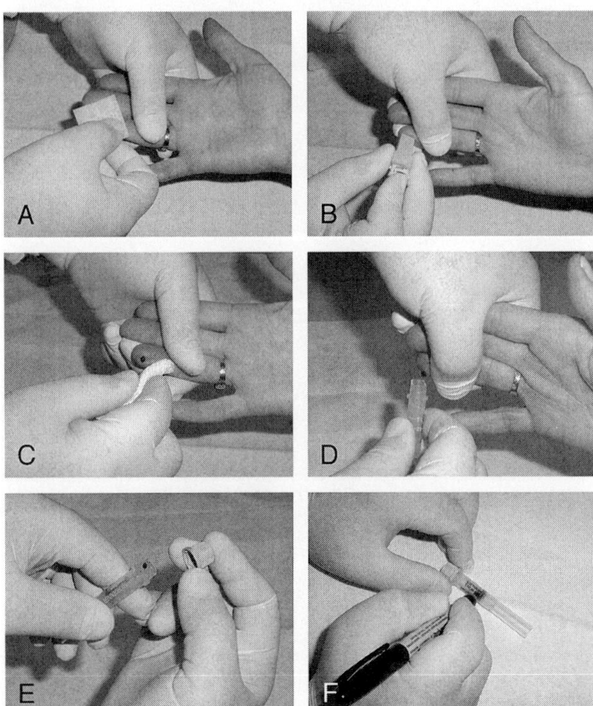

Figure 9–12 Finger puncture procedure. (*A*)Cleansing the finger site. (*B*) Puncturing the finger with an automatic safety lancet. (*C*,)Wiping away the first drop of blood. (*D*) Collecting blood in a Microtainer. (*E*) Capping the Microtainer for inversion. (*F*) Labeling the Microtainer (note extender).

As with venipuncture, it is recommended that only two punctures be attempted to collect blood. When a second puncture must be made to collect the sufficient amount of blood, the blood should not be added to the previously collected tube. This can cause erroneous results as a result of microclots and hemolysis. The puncture also must be performed at a different site using a new puncture device.

Summary of Dermal Puncture Technique

1. Obtain and examine the requisition form.
2. Organize equipment and supplies.
3. Greet the patient and/or the parents.
4. Identify the patient.
5. Position the patient and the parents.
6. Wash hands.
7. Put on gloves.
8. Select the puncture site.
9. Warm the puncture site if necessary.
10. Cleanse and dry the puncture site.
11. Prepare equipment.
12. Perform the puncture.
13. Wipe away the first drop of blood.
14. Make blood smears if requested.
15. Collect the hematology specimen and then other specimens.
16. Mix the specimens if necessary.
17. Apply pressure.
18. Dispose of the puncture device.
19. Label the specimens.
20. Perform appropriate specimen handling.
21. Examine the site for stoppage of bleeding.
22. Thank the patient and/or the parents.
23. Dispose of used supplies.
24. Remove and dispose of gloves.
25. Wash hands.
26. Complete any required paperwork.
27. Deliver specimens to the appropriate locations.

Bibliography

National Committee for Clinical Laboratory Standards Approved Standard H4-A4: Procedures for the Collection of Diagnostic Blood Specimens by Skin Puncture. NCCLS, Wayne, PA, 1999.

Study Questions

1. List six possible complications associated with femoral puncture in infants.
   a. ______
   b. ______
   c. ______
   d. ______
   e. ______
   f. ______

2. Daily collection of 3 mL of blood from a premature infant may produce ______.

3. Why are dermal punctures often performed on (a) patients receiving chemotherapy, (b) geriatric patients, and (c) diabetic patients?
   a. ______
   b. ______
   c. ______

4. State a major concern when collecting a specimen for potassium and bilirubin by dermal puncture.

   ______

5. Describe the composition of capillary blood.

   ______

6. Can dermal puncture and venipuncture collections be alternated on a patient receiving 4-hour hemoglobin and hematocrit (H & H) tests? Why?

   ______

7. The maximum length of a puncture device used on the heel is ______

8. True or False. Surgical blades should be used when collecting more than 100 μL of blood.

   ______

9. The location of the major vascular area of the skin is ______.

10. Which is more important for producing adequate blood flow, the width or depth of the puncture?

    ______

11. Collection of a microhematocrit by dermal puncture is performed using a tube that is color coded (red) (blue). Circle one.

12. What is the recommended safety precaution associated with capillary tubes?

____

13. True or False. Caraway and Natelson pipets can be used to collect serum or plasma specimens.

____

14. A lavender-top Microtainer contains _______________ and is used for tests performed in the _______________ section of the laboratory.

15. What types of tests can be performed using the Unopette System?

____

16. What is the approximate temperature used for heel warming?

____

17. List three precautions to be observed when collecting specimens in the nursery.

a. _______________

b. _______________

c. _______________

18. List six visible reasons for avoiding a particular area as a skin puncture site.

a. _______________

b. _______________

c. _______________

d. _______________

e. _______________

f. _______________

19. Name two possible causes of osteomyelitis associated with dermal puncture.

a. _______________

b. _______________

20. Name two areas of the foot where dermal puncture should not be performed.

a. _______________

b. _______________

21. State a reason for not selecting each of the following as a puncture site.

    a. Thumb

    b. Index finger

    c. Fifth finger

    d. Tip of the finger

22. State four reasons for removing alcohol from the site before performing the puncture.

    a.

    b.

    c.

    d.

23. How should a dermal puncture be performed to encourage the formation of a rounded drop?

24. List three sources of microspecimen contamination.

    a.

    b.

    c.

25. In what order should the following be collected: bilirubin, blood smear, and CBC?

26. State two reasons for not applying a bandage to the puncture site on a 1-year-old child.

    a.

    b.

27. State two reasons for placing filled capillary tubes in a large tube when transporting them.

    a.

    b.

28. What is the purpose of a collection volume log sheet in the nursery?

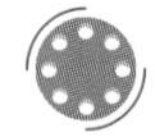

Clinical Situations

1. An adult patient receiving chemotherapy must have weekly platelet counts.
   a. What collection method would be least traumatic for the patient?
   ____
   b. State two types of specimen containers that could be used for this procedure.
   ____
   c. How could using a different collection method affect the patient's treatment?
   ____
2. The phlebotomy supervisor is informed that many of the specimens collected by the personnel on the pediatric unit are hemolyzed. The supervisor schedules a continuing education in-service for the unit.
   a. Why should preparation of the collection site be stressed?
   ____
   b. Why is it important for the personnel to obtain rounded drops of blood to prevent hemolysis?
   ____
   c. Should the inservice include the procedure to follow when a second puncture must be performed to obtain a full tube of blood? Why or why not?
   ____
   ____
3. A phlebotomist enters the nursery, performs the specified isolation procedures, checks the infant's name on the bassinet, selects an area of the plantar surface of the heel, cleanses the area with iodine, collects and labels the specimen, and bandages the heel. What is wrong with this scenario?
   ____
   ____
4. After failing to collect a sufficient amount of blood from two dermal punctures, the phlebotomist asks a coworker to complete the collection. What additional technique could the second phlebotomist perform to obtain sufficient blood flow?
   ____

5. A phlebotomist delivers a lavender-top Microtainer to hematology and two red-top Microtainers to the chemistry lab. The hematology supervisor is concerned because the platelet count is much lower than the previous day's count and all other CBC parameters match the previous values. Could the phlebotomy technique have caused this? Why or why not?

____

6. A phlebotomy student is having difficulty obtaining rounded drops of blood. Why should the instructor check the following parts of the student's technique?

   a. Site cleansing

   ____

   b. Alignment of the puncture device

   ____

   c. Puncture technique

   ____

   d. Application of pressure

   ____

7. While selecting a site for a heel puncture, the phlebotomist notices that a previous puncture has been performed on the back of the heel. What should the phlebotomist do?

____

8. Why are dermal puncture devices usually color coded?

____

NAME ______________________________

Evaluation of a Microtainer Collection by Heel Stick

RATING SYSTEM 2 = SATISFACTORILY PERFORMED 1 = NEEDS IMPROVEMENT 0 = INCORRECT/DID NOT PERFORM

_________ 1. Places collection tray in designated area

_________ 2. Checks requisition and selects necessary equipment

_________ 3. Washes hands, puts on gown and gloves

_________ 4. Assembles equipment and carries it to patient

_________ 5. Identifies patient using ID band

_________ 6. Warms heel

_________ 7. Selects appropriate puncture site

_________ 8. Cleanses puncture site with alcohol and allows it to air dry

_________ 9. Does not contaminate puncture device

_________ 10. Performs puncture smoothly

_________ 11. Wipes away first drop of blood

_________ 12. Collects rounded drops into Microtainer without scraping

_________ 13. Does not milk site

_________ 14. Collects adequate amount of blood

_________ 15. Mixes Microtainer eight to 20 times

_________ 16. Cleanses site and applies pressure until bleeding stops

_________ 17. Removes all collection equipment from area

_________ 18. Disposes of puncture device in sharps container

_________ 19. Disposes of used supplies

_________ 20. Labels tube

_________ 21. Removes and disposes of gloves and gown

_________ 22. Washes hands

_________ 23. Completes nursery log sheet

TOTAL POINTS _________

MAXIMUM POINTS = 46

Comments:

NAME ______________________________

Evaluation of Finger Stick on an Adult Patient

RATING SYSTEM 2 = SATISFACTORILY PERFORMED 1 = NEEDS IMPROVEMENT 0 = INCORRECT/DID NOT PERFORM

__________ 1. Greets patient and explains procedure

__________ 2. Examines requisition form

__________ 3. Asks patient to state full name

__________ 4. Compares requisition and patient's statement

__________ 5. Organizes and assembles equipment

__________ 6. Washes hands

__________ 7. Puts on gloves

__________ 8. Selects appropriate finger

__________ 9. Warms finger, if necessary

__________ 10. Gently massages finger

__________ 11. Cleanses site with alcohol and allows to air dry

__________ 12. Does not contaminate puncture device

__________ 13. Smoothly performs puncture across fingerprint

__________ 14. Wipes away first drop of blood

__________ 15. Collects two microhematocrit tubes without air bubbles

__________ 16. Seals tubes

__________ 17. Asks patient to apply pressure with gauze

__________ 18. Labels tubes

__________ 19. Examines site for stoppage of bleeding and applies bandage

__________ 20. Thanks patient

__________ 21. Disposes of puncture device in sharps container

__________ 22. Disposes of used supplies

__________ 23. Removes gloves

__________ 24. Washes hands

TOTAL POINTS

MAXIMUM POINTS = 48

Comments:

NAME ______________________________

Evaluation of Unopette Collection on a 2-Year-Old Child

RATING SYSTEM 2 = SATISFACTORILY PERFORMED 1 = NEEDS IMPROVEMENT 0 = INCORRECT/DID NOT PERFORM

__________ 1. Greets patient and parent

__________ 2. Examines requisition

__________ 3. Identifies patient using correct verbal ID procedure

__________ 4. Explains procedure to patient and parent

__________ 5. Determines if parent needs/wants to hold patient

__________ 6. Washes hands

__________ 7. Puts on gloves

__________ 8. Organizes equipment

__________ 9. Punctures reservoir diaphragm

__________ 10. Gently massages finger

__________ 11. Cleanses site with alcohol and allows to air dry

__________ 12. Does not contaminate puncture device

__________ 13. Smoothly performs puncture across fingerprint

__________ 14. Wipes away first drop of blood

__________ 15. Removes pipet shield

__________ 16. Completely fills pipet with no air bubbles

__________ 17. Wipes blood from outside of pipet without drawing blood out of the pipet

__________ 18. Places index finger over opening in overflow chamber

__________ 19. Squeezes reservoir

__________ 20. Places pipet firmly into reservoir

__________ 21. Removes index finger and releases reservoir

__________ 22. Rinses pipet by squeezing reservoir

_____________ 23. Does not force fluid out of overflow chamber

_____________ 24. Places shield on overflow chamber

_____________ 25. Mixes container

_____________ 26. Applies pressure to site until bleeding stops

_____________ 27. Applies bandage

_____________ 28. Labels Unopette

_____________ 29. Disposes of puncture device in sharps container

_____________ 30. Disposes of used supplies

_____________ 31. Thanks patient and parents

_____________ 32. Removes gloves and washes hands

TOTAL POINTS

MAXIMUM POINTS = 64

Comments:

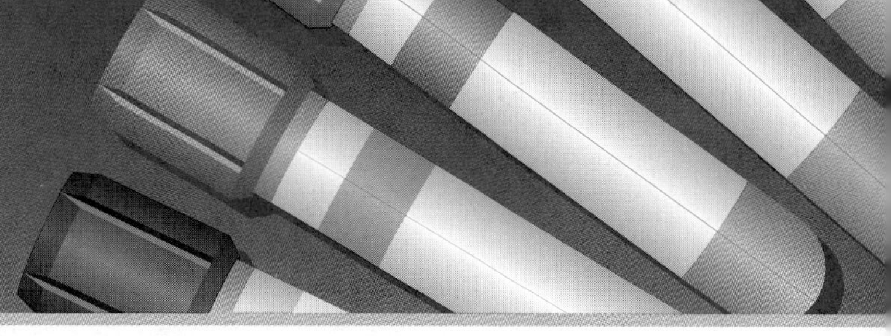

Chapter 10

Special Dermal Puncture

Chapter Outline

Learning Objectives

Upon completion of this chapter, the reader will be able to:

1. Discuss the necessary precautions for collecting high-quality specimens for neonatal bilirubin tests.
2. Briefly discuss why and how neonatal filter paper screening tests are collected.
3. Describe the appearance of an acceptable blood smear.
4. List six possible errors in technique that cause unacceptable blood smears.
5. Prepare an acceptable blood smear using the instructions provided.
6. State the purpose of the bleeding time and three reasons why it may be prolonged.
7. Discuss the standardization of the bleeding time and errors in technique that affect test results.
8. Correctly perform a bleeding time following the instructions provided in the text or by the manufacturer of the incision device.

Key Terms

Feathered edge	*Phenylalanine*	*Platelet plug*
Jaundiced	*Phenylketonuria*	*Volar*

Several of the special collection techniques discussed in Chapter 8 also apply to specimens collected by dermal puncture. These include:

1. Fasting specimens
2. Specimens for glucose tolerance tests
3. Timed specimens for postprandial glucose. (It is recommended that sodium fluoride be used when collecting neonatal glucose tests because the normally high red blood cell count increases glycolysis.)
4. Specimens for therapeutic drug monitoring
5. Specimens affected by diurnal variation
6. Specimens that must be warmed or chilled during transport
7. Forensic specimens

Procedures primarily associated with dermal punctures are as follows:

1. Collection of neonatal bilirubin
2. Collection of neonatal filter paper screening tests
3. Preparation of blood smears
4. Bleeding time (BT) test
5. Point-of-care testing (POCT) (see Chapter 13)

Collection of Neonatal Bilirubin

One of the most frequently performed tests on newborns measures bilirubin levels, and specimens for this determination are often collected at timed intervals over several days. Bilirubin is a very light-sensitive chemical and is rapidly destroyed when exposed to light.

Increased serum bilirubin in newborns may be caused by the presence of hemolytic disease of the newborn, or it may simply occur because the liver of newborns (particularly premature infants) is often not developed enough to process the bilirubin produced from the normal breakdown of red blood cells. Bilirubin test results are critical to infant survival and mental health because the blood-brain barrier is not fully developed in neonates, a condition that allows bilirubin to accumulate in the brain and cause permanent or lethal damage. Bilirubin levels reaching 18.0 mg/dL (hyperbilirubinemia) or rising at a rate of 0.5 mg/dL per hour indicate the need for an **exchange transfusion**.

Phlebotomy technique is critical to the determination of accurate bilirubin results, and specimens must be protected from excess light during and after the collection. Infants who appear ***jaundiced*** are frequently placed under an ultraviolet light (bililight) to lower the level of circulating bilirubin. This light must be turned off during specimen collection. Amber-colored microcollection tubes are available for collecting bilirubin, or if multiple capillary pipets are used, the filled tubes should be shielded from light. Hemolysis must be avoided; it will falsely lower bilirubin results in some procedures and must be corrected for in others. Also, specimens must be collected at the specified time so that the rate of bilirubin increase can be determined. Noninvasive transcutaneous bilirubin measurements in neonates are discussed in Chapter 13.

technical tip When collecting specimens for neonatal bilirubin tests, turn off the bililight during collection unless it is a newer model that is strapped directly to the infant.

Neonatal Screening

Screening of newborns for 50 inherited **metabolic** disorders can currently be performed from blood collected by heel stick and placed on specially designed filter paper. Most states have laws requiring the screening of newborns for the presence of the most prevalent disorders: ***phenylketonuria* (PKU)**, which is caused by the lack of the enzyme needed to metabolize ***phenylalanine***, and **hypothyroidism**. Both disorders produce severe mental retardation, but retardation can be avoided by changes in diet and the use of medication if these disorders are detected within the first few weeks after birth. Routine screening is not usually performed for other disorders, but screening may be requested when symptoms or family history indicates a need or when state law requires a more extensive battery of neonatal tests.

The filter paper blood screening test for PKU uses bacterial growth to determine the presence or absence of phenylalanine in the blood. The blood-impregnated filter paper disks are placed on culture media containing bacteria, and the media are then observed for bacterial growth, as shown in

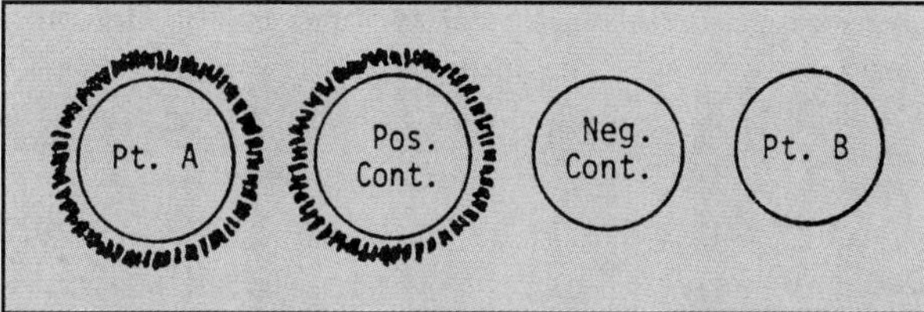

Figure 10–1 Sample bacterial inhibition test. (From Strasinger, SK, and Di Lorenzo, MS: Urinalysis and Body Fluids, ed. 4. FA Davis, Philadelphia, 2001, p. 137, with permission.)

Figure 10–1. Hypothyroidism is detected by performing immunochemical analysis of the dried blood.

It can be understood from this brief explanation of the bacterial testing procedure that correct collection of the blood specimen is critical for accurate test results. Special collection kits are used, consisting of a patient information form attached to specifically designed filter paper that has been preprinted with an appropriate number of $^1/_2$-inch-diameter circles (Fig. 10–2). The filter paper and the ink must be biologically inactive and approved by the Food and Drug Administration (FDA). The phlebotomist must be careful not to touch or contaminate the area inside the circles or to touch the dried blood spots.

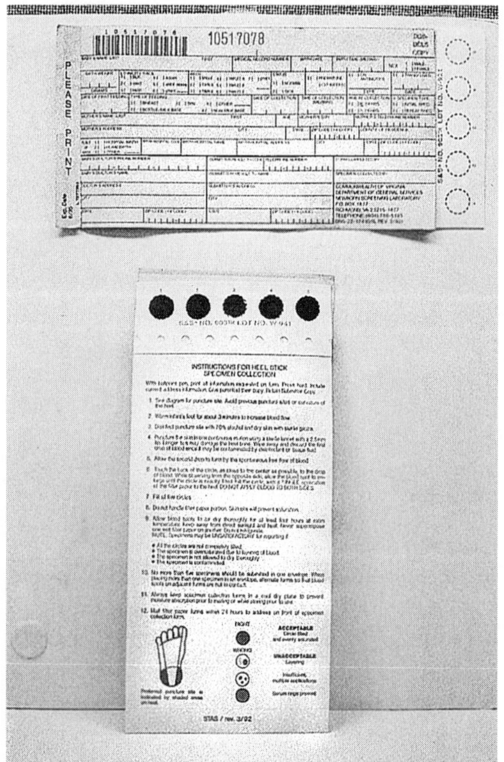

Figure 10–2 Collection kit for neonatal screening tests. (From Strasinger, SK, and Di Lorenzo, MS: Skills for the Patient Care Technician. FA Davis, Philadelphia, 1999, p. 225, with permission.)

The heel stick is performed in the routine manner, and the first drop of blood is wiped away. A large drop of blood is then applied directly into a filter paper circle. To obtain an even layer of blood, only one drop should be used to fill a circle. Blood is applied to only one side of the filter paper, and there must be enough to soak through the paper and be visible on the other side. As shown in Figure 10–3, if a circle is not evenly or completely filled, a new circle and a larger drop of blood should be used. The collected specimen must be allowed to air dry in a suspended horizontal position, at room temperature, and away from direct sunlight. To prevent cross-contamination, specimens should not be stacked during or after the drying process.

Collection of blood in heparinized capillary pipets followed by its immediate transfer to the filter paper circles is an acceptable but not recommended technique. Each circle requires 100 µL of blood, which must be added without scratching or denting the filter paper with the capillary tip.

technical tip Be sure that all required patient information is filled out on the neonatal screening test form.

Preparation of Blood Smears

Blood smears are needed for the microscopic examination of blood cells that is performed for the differential blood cell count, for special staining procedures, and for nonautomated reticulocyte

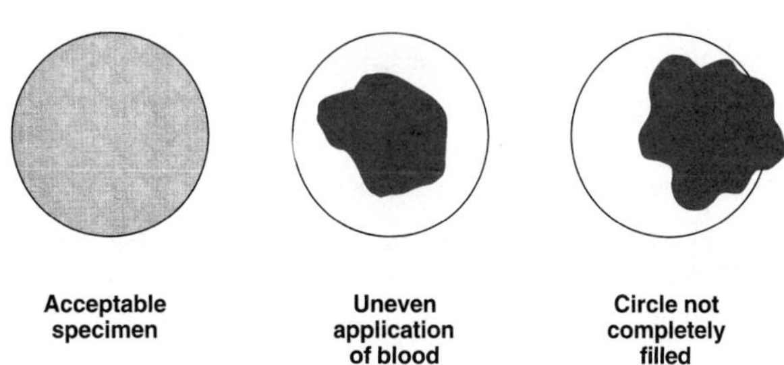

Figure 10–3 Correct and incorrect blood collection with filter paper.

technical tip Uneven or incomplete saturation of PKU filter paper circles because of layering from multidrop application or scratches from capillary pipets will yield an unacceptable specimen for testing.

counts. Phlebotomists may make smears when one of these tests is ordered and a dermal puncture is performed. When specimens are collected by venipuncture, the smear is usually made in the laboratory from the ethylenediaminetetraacetic acid (EDTA) tube. Blood smears should be made within 1 hour of collection to avoid cell distortion caused by the EDTA anticoagulant. Performing smears at the bedside after a venipuncture may sometimes be necessary to be sure there is no anticoagulant interference. This practice can be dangerous, however, because blood must be forced from the needle onto the slide and the needle cannot be disposed of until the smear has been made. In addition, blood smears must be considered infectious until they have been fixed with alcohol in the laboratory, and gloves must be worn when handling them. Carrying numerous smears in a crowded collection tray can cause contamination of equipment and ungloved hands.

Learning to prepare an acceptable blood smear requires considerable practice and can be a source of frustration for beginning phlebotomists. Once the technique is mastered, however, it is seldom that an acceptable smear is not achieved on the first attempt. The technique for preparing a blood smear is described here and illustrated in Figures 10–4 and 10–5.

1 Obtain three clean glass slides and perform the dermal puncture in the manner discussed in Chapter 9. Be sure to wipe away the first drop of blood.
2 Place the second drop of blood in the center of a glass slide approximately $^1/_2$ to 1 inch from the end or just below the frosted end by lightly touching the drop with the slide. The drop should be 1 to 2 mm in diameter.
3 Immediately place the slide in one of the positions shown in Figure 10–5. Choose the one that works best for you.
4 Place a second slide (spreader slide) with a clean, smooth edge in front of the drop at a 30- to 40-degree angle inclined over the blood.

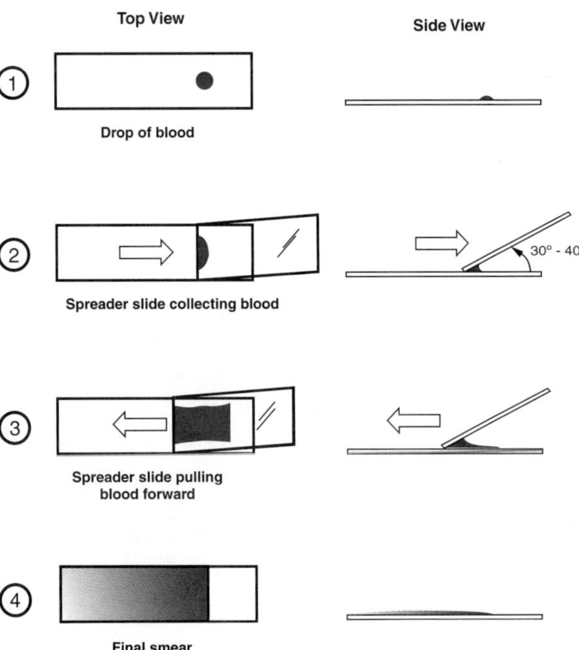

Figure 10–4 Preparation of a blood smear.

5 Draw the spreader slide back to the edge of the drop of blood, allowing the blood to spread across the end.
6 When blood is evenly distributed across the spreader slide, lightly push the spreader slide forward with a continuous movement all the way past the end of the smear slide. Be sure to maintain the 30- to 40-degree angle, and do not apply pressure to the spreader slide.
7 Place the slide in an area in which it can dry undisturbed and repeat the procedure for the second smear.
8 Smears collected on slides with frosted ends are labeled by writing the patient information on the frosted area with a pencil. Labels containing the appropriate information are attached to the thick end of smear slides that do not have frosted ends.

A properly prepared blood smear has a smooth film of blood that covers approximately one-half to two-thirds of the slide, does not contain ridges or holes, and has a lightly ***feathered edge*** without

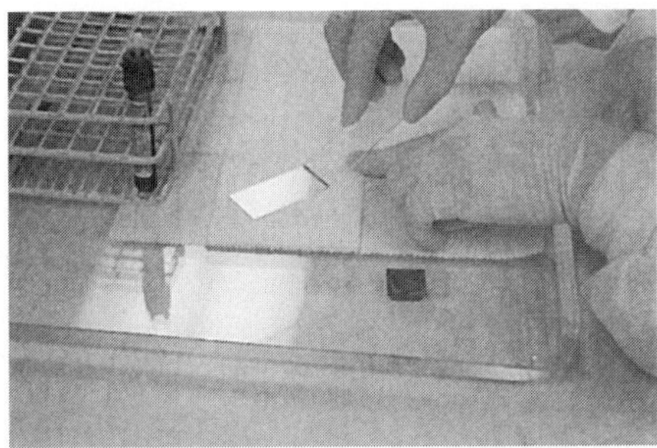

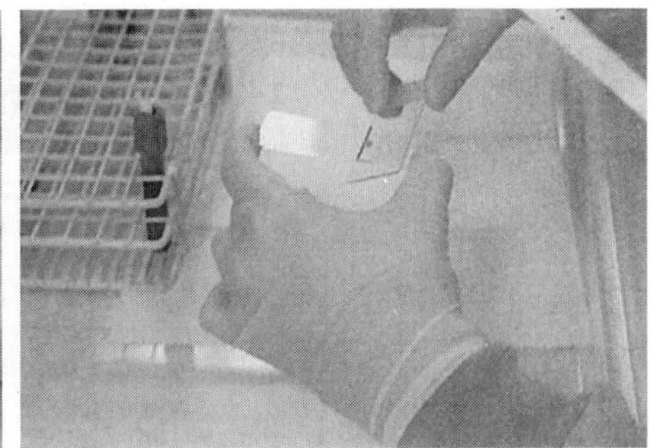

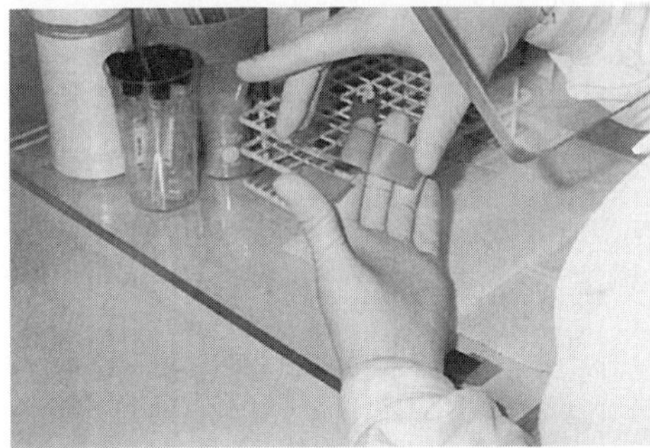

Figure 10–5 Examples of slide positioning for blood smear preparation.

streaks. The microscopic examination is performed in the area of the feathered edge because here the cells have been spread into a single layer. An uneven smear indicates that the cells are not evenly distributed; therefore test results will not be truly representative of the patient's blood. Errors in technique that result in an unacceptable specimen are summarized in Table 10–1.

Blood Smears for Malaria

The parasites (*Plasmodium* species) that cause malaria invade the red blood cells, and their presence is detected by microscopic examination of thick and thin blood smears. Patients with malaria exhibit periodic episodes of fever and chills related to the multiplication of the parasites within the red blood

TABLE 10–1
Effects of Technical Errors on Blood Smears

Discrepancy	Possible Causes
Uneven distribution of blood (ridges)	Increased pressure on the spreader slide Movement of the spreader slide not continuous Delay in making slide after drop is placed on slide
Holes in the smear	Dirty slide Contamination with glove powder
No feathered edge	Spreader slide not pushed the entire length of the smear slide
Streaks in the feathered edge	Chipped or dirty spreader slide Spreader slide not placed flush against the smear slide Pulling the spreader slide into the drop of blood so that the blood is pushed instead of pulled Drop of blood starts to dry out owing to delay in making smear
Smear too thick and short	Drop of blood is too big Angle of spreader slide is greater than 40 degrees
Smear too thin and long	Drop of blood is too small Angle of spreader slide is less than 30 degrees Spreader slide pushed too slowly

technical tip An EDTA anticoagulated blood specimen must be mixed at least 2 minutes before making blood smears to ensure a uniform specimen.

cells. Therefore specimen collection is frequently requested on an emergent or timed basis similar to that of blood cultures. Smears may be prepared from EDTA anticoagulated blood unless a dermal puncture must be performed.

Thin smears (two or three) are prepared in the manner previously described. Thick smears are made by placing a large drop of blood in the center of a glass slide and then using a wooden applicator stick to spread the blood into a circle about the size of a dime. The smear must be allowed to dry for at least 2 hours before staining. Thick smears concentrate the specimen for detection of the parasites, and thin smears are then examined for parasitic morphology and identification.

Bleeding Time

BT is performed to measure the time required for platelets to form a plug strong enough to stop bleeding from an incision. The length of the BT is increased when the platelet count is low, when platelet disorders affect the ability of the platelets to stick to each other to form a plug, and in persons taking aspirin and certain other medications and herbs. Test results can also be affected by the type and condition of the patient's skin, vascularity, and temperature and the phlebotomist's technique. Therefore the BT is considered a screening test, and abnormal results are followed by additional testing. BTs are frequently ordered as part of a presurgical workup.

Measurement of the BT was first introduced by Duke in 1910 and was performed by timing the length of bleeding from a lancet puncture of the earlobe. The Duke method is not as well standardized as current methods are; however, it may occasionally be requested in special situations.

Standardization of the BT began in 1941, when Ivy modified the Duke method by performing the incision on the ***volar*** surface of the forearm and inflating a blood pressure cuff to 40 mm Hg to control blood flow to the area. These modifications are still a part of the BT procedure. In 1969, Mielke introduced a plastic template, used with a surgical blade rather than a lancet, to control the length and depth of the incision. Automated disposable incision devices, such as the Simplate R and Simplate-II (Organon Teknika Corp, Durham, NC) and Surgicutt® (International Technidyne Corp., Edison, NJ), that produce standardized incisions of 1 mm in depth and 5 mm in length have now replaced the original template method (Fig. 10–6).

Steps in performing the BT using an automated device are:

1 Identify the patient following routine protocol.
2 Explain the procedure to the patient, including the possibility of leaving a small scar, and obtain information about any prescribed or over-the-counter medications, particularly aspirin, that may have been taken in the last 7 to 10 days. Many medications contain salicylate (aspirin); therefore the contents of any medication mentioned by the patient should be checked before performing the test, and if salicylate has been taken, the physician should be notified. Ethanol, dextran, streptokinase, streptodornase, and various herbs may also cause a prolonged BT.
3 Wash hands and put on gloves.
4 Place the patient's arm on a steady surface with the volar surface facing up.
5 Select an area, approximately 5 cm below the antecubital crease and in the middle of the arm, that is free of surface veins, scars, bruises, and edema.

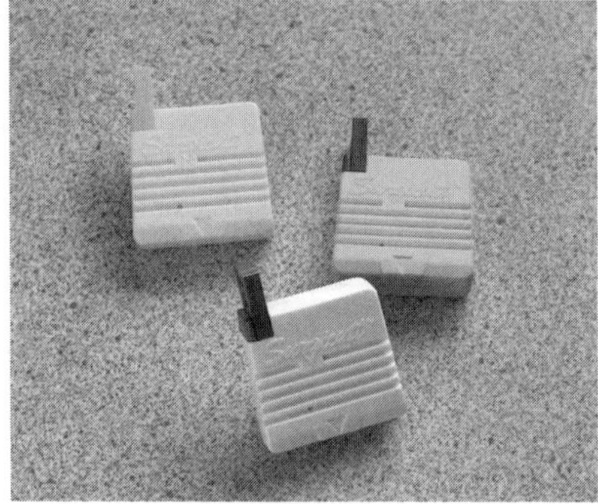

Figure 10–6 Surgicutt® incision devices. (Courtesy of International Technidyne Corporation, Edison, NJ.)

6 Cleanse the area with alcohol and allow it to dry.
7 Assemble required materials, filter paper, stopwatch, and bandages.
8 Place a blood pressure cuff on the upper arm.
9 Inflate the blood pressure cuff to 40 mm Hg. This pressure must be maintained throughout the procedure. The time between inflation of the blood pressure cuff and making the incision should be between 30 and 60 seconds.
10 Remove the incision device from its package and release the safety lock, being careful not to touch the blade area.
11 Place the incision device firmly, but without making an indentation, on the arm and position it so that the incision will be horizontal (parallel to the antecubital crease) (Fig. 10–7). In adults, horizontal incisions are slightly more sensitive to hemorrhagic disorders and are less likely to leave a scar, whereas in newborns, a vertical incision is preferable for the same reasons.
12 Depress the trigger, simultaneously start the stopwatch, and then remove the incision device.
13 After 30 seconds, remove the blood that has accumulated on the incision by gently "wicking" it onto a circle of Whatman No. 1 filter paper or Surgicutt® Bleeding Time Blotting Paper (International Technidyne Corp., Edison, NJ) (Fig. 10–8). Do not touch the incision because this disturbs formation of the ***platelet plug*** and prolongs the BT.
14 Continue to remove blood from the incision every 30 seconds in the manner described previously until the bleeding stops.
15 Record the time on the stopwatch to the nearest 30 seconds.
16 Deflate and remove the blood pressure cuff.
17 Clean the patient's arm and apply a butterfly bandage to hold the edges of the incision together tightly. Cover this bandage with a regular bandage. Instruct the patient to leave the bandages on for 24 hours.
18 Depending on the method and device used, normal BTs range from 2 to 10 minutes. The test can be discontinued after 15 minutes and reported as greater than 15 minutes to a supervisor. It is important to follow the manufacturer's procedure exactly for reproducible results.

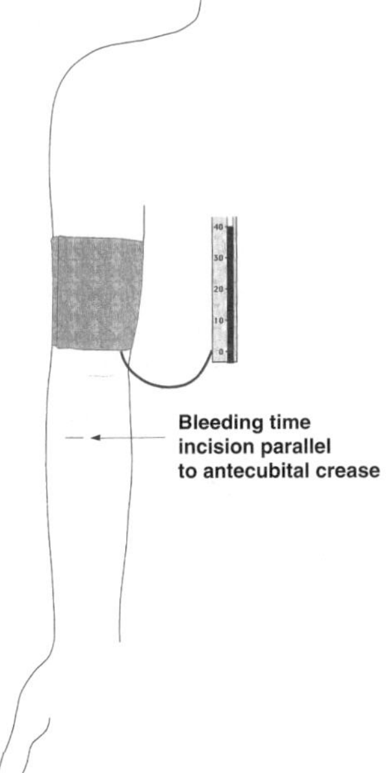

Figure 10–7 Template bleeding time procedure.

technical tip Consideration should be given to documenting that the patient understands the possibility of a scar.

technical tip Often patients do not consider aspirin and herbs medication and will not offer that specific information unless asked.

technical tip Never instruct a patient to stop taking prescribed medication. The healthcare provider must be notified and will make this decision before the bleeding time test is repeated.

Point-of-Care Testing

The development of portable handheld instruments capable of performing a variety of routine laboratory procedures has increased the efficiency of patient testing. Specimens can be collected by dermal puncture and tested by phlebotomists or other healthcare personnel in the patient area. Test results are available quickly and transportation of specimens to the laboratory is avoided. Dermal punctures are performed following the procedure detailed in Chapter 9, unless modifications are recommended by the instrument manufacturers. Phlebotomists performing POCT should follow all manufacturer recommendations. The most routinely performed POCTs are discussed in Chapter 13.

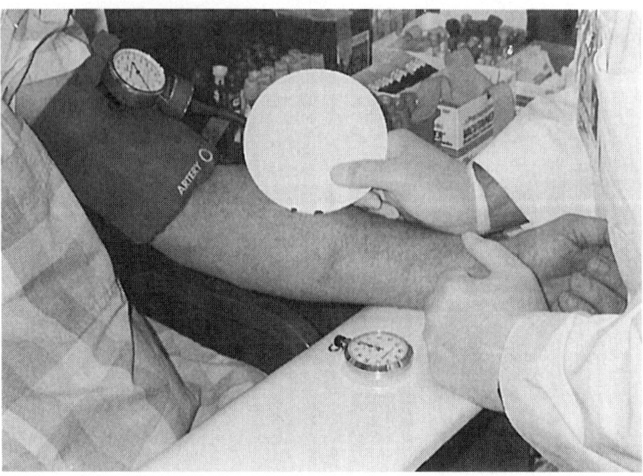

Figure 10–8 Wicking of blood during the bleeding time procedure.

Bibliography

Brown, BA: Hematology: Principles and Procedures, ed. 6. Lea & Febiger, Philadelphia, 1995.

Buchanan, GR, and Holtkamp, CA: A comparative study of variables affecting the bleeding time using two disposable devices. Am J Clin Pathol, 9(1), 1989.

Henry, JB: Clinical Diagnosis and Management by Laboratory Methods. WB Saunders, Philadelphia, 1999.

National Committee for Clinical Laboratory Standards Approved Standard LA4-A2: Blood Collection on Filter Paper for Neonatal Screening Programs. NCCLS, Villanova, PA, 1999.

Study Questions

1. List two reasons for elevated neonatal bilirubin.

   a. ______

   b. ______

2. Why is neonatal bilirubin frequently ordered as a timed test?

   ______

3. A neonatal bilirubin collected at 0600 is 10.0 mg/dL, the specimen collected at 1800 reads 12.0 mg/dL, and the specimen collected the next morning at 0600 has a value of 5.0 mg/dL.

   a. State an error in phlebotomy technique that could cause the last result.

   ______

   b. State a specimen characteristic that could cause the last result.

   ______

4. Name two disorders in which neonatal filter paper tests are frequently used for screening.

   a. ______

   b. ______

5. How should blood collected on a filter paper disk appear?

   ______

   ______

6. State a reason why collecting blood for filter paper testing with a capillary pipet or from a dorsal hand vein may not be recommended.

   ______

7. Name two tests that require a blood smear.

   a. ______

   b. ______

8. True or False. Unfixed blood smears are a biologic hazard. ______

9. The proper angle of the spreader slide when preparing a blood smear is

   ______

10. If the angle of the spreader slide is too large, the blood smear will be too ______ and ______ .

11. What is the purpose of the feathered edge on a blood smear?

____

12. A chipped spreader slide will cause

____

13. Why is a blood smear containing ridges or holes considered unacceptable?

____

14. What laboratory error could occur if only thin smears are prepared for a malaria test?

____

15. List three reasons for a BT to be prolonged.

    a. ____

    b. ____

    c. ____

16. State the basic principle of the BT.

____

____

17. True or False. To obtain an accurate BT result, the patient must be given aspirin before having the test performed. ____________

18. What is the purpose of "wicking?"

____

19. In adults, the BT incision is made (horizontal) (vertical) to the antecubital crease. (Circle one) Why?

____

20. The normal BT is approximately ______________ .

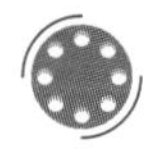

Clinical Situations

1. The phlebotomy supervisor is asked to present an inservice to the nurses who collect neonatal bilirubins on the night shift. Specimens are not hemolyzed; however, the test results are consistently lower than those of tests collected on the morning and evening shifts. What should the supervisor stress?

____

2. A phlebotomist collects three Caraway micropipets for a bilirubin, labels a large tube, places the sealed tubes into it, and leaves the tube on the counter in chemistry while everyone is at lunch. The chemistry supervisor rejects the specimen.

   a. Why is this specimen unacceptable?

   ____

   b. How could this have been avoided?

   ____

3. In what circumstance might a phlebotomist deliver a blood smear without a feathered edge to the hematology section?

   ____

4. BTs performed by a new employee are consistently prolonged.

   a. What part of the employee's technique should the supervisor observe most closely?

   ____

   b. Why?

   ____

5. A phlebotomist performs a BT on an outpatient using correct technique and the result is prolonged. The next day the physician sends the patient back to the laboratory for a repeat test. The phlebotomy supervisor prepares to perform the test, but after talking to the patient, she stops and calls the physician's office. The test is canceled. What had the first phlebotomist failed to do?

   ____

6. A phlebotomist with requisitions for two BTs is gone for 2 hours and returns with results of 40 minutes and 45 minutes. The phlebotomy supervisor tells the phlebotomist to reread the bleeding time procedure in the procedure manual. Why?

   ____

7. A phlebotomist with a requisition for a BT identifies the patient, checks on medications, selects and chooses an appropriate site, inflates the blood pressure cuff to halfway between the systolic and diastolic pressure, performs the puncture, wipes away the first drop of blood, starts the stopwatch, blots the area with gauze every 30 seconds until the bleeding stops, records the time, and completes the procedure. What is wrong with this scenario?

   ____

   ____

   ____

8. How could failure to wipe away the first drop of blood affect the results of a filter paper PKU?

____

9. A phlebotomist has requisitions for a blood smear and a BT.

   a. Can this be accomplished with one puncture?

   ____

   b. Why or why not?

   ____

NAME ____________________

Evaluation of Blood Smear Preparation

RATING SYSTEM 2 = SATISFACTORILY PERFORMED 1 = NEEDS IMPROVEMENT 0 = INCORRECT/DID NOT PERFORM

_______ 1. Obtains requisition form

_______ 2. Obtains three clean glass slides

_______ 3. Identifies patient

_______ 4. Puts on gloves

_______ 5. Selects and cleanses an appropriate site and allows it to air dry

_______ 6. Performs puncture

_______ 7. Wipes away first drop

_______ 8. Puts correct size drop on appropriate area of slide

_______ 9. Positions slide

_______ 10. Places spreader slide at correct angle

_______ 11. Pulls spreader slide back to blood drop

_______ 12. Allows blood to spread across spreader slide

_______ 13. Pushes spreader slide evenly forward

_______ 14. Places smear to dry

_______ 15. Collects second smear using correct technique

_______ 16. Labels smears

_______ 17. Smear has feathered edge with no streaks

_______ 18. Blood is evenly distributed

_______ 19. Smear does not have holes

_______ 20. Smear is not too long or too thick

_______ 21. Smear is not too short or too thin

_______ 22. Disposes of equipment and supplies

_______ 23. Removes gloves and washes hands

TOTAL POINTS _______

MAXIMUM POINTS = 46

Comments:

NAME ______________________________

Evaluation of Bleeding Time Technique

RATING SYSTEM 2 = SATISFACTORILY PERFORMED 1 = NEEDS IMPROVEMENT 0 = INCORRECT/DID NOT PERFORM

_______ 1. Obtains requisition form

_______ 2. Identifies patient

_______ 3. Explains procedure to patient

_______ 4. Asks patient about medications

_______ 5. Assembles equipment

_______ 6. Puts on gloves

_______ 7. Positions patient's arm

_______ 8. Selects appropriate site

_______ 9. Cleanses site and allows it to air dry

_______ 10. Puts blood pressure cuff on upper arm

_______ 11. Opens and does not contaminate puncture device

_______ 12. Inflates blood pressure cuff to 40 mm Hg

_______ 13. Correctly aligns puncture device on patient's arm

_______ 14. Simultaneously performs puncture and starts stopwatch

_______ 15. Quickly removes puncture device

_______ 16. Correctly wicks blood after 30 seconds

_______ 17. Continues wicking every 30 seconds

_______ 18. Recognizes endpoint and discontinues timing

_______ 19. Records stopwatch time

_______ 20. Deflates and removes blood pressure cuff

_______ 21. Cleans patient's arm

_______ 22. Applies butterfly bandage

__________ 23. Applies regular bandage

__________ 24. Instructs patient when to remove bandages

__________ 25. Disposes of equipment and supplies

__________ 26. Removes gloves and washes hands

TOTAL POINTS __________

MAXIMUM POINTS = 52

Comments:

NAME ________________________________

Evaluation of Neonatal Filter Paper Collection

RATING SYSTEM 2 = SATISFACTORILY PERFORMED 1 = NEEDS IMPROVEMENT 0 = INCORRECT/DID NOT PERFORM

______ 1. Obtains requisition

______ 2. Performs nursery isolation procedures

______ 3. Assembles equipment

______ 4. Identifies patient

______ 5. Puts on gloves

______ 6. Selects appropriate heel site

______ 7. Cleanses site and allows it to air dry

______ 8. Performs the puncture

______ 9. Wipes away first blood drop

______ 10. Evenly fills a circle

______ 11. Fills all required circles correctly

______ 12. Does not touch inside of circles or blood spots

______ 13. Places filter paper in appropriate transport position

______ 14. Applies pressure until bleeding stops

______ 15. Disposes of equipment and supplies

______ 16. Correctly completes all required paperwork

______ 17. Removes gown and gloves

______ 18. Washes hands

TOTAL POINTS ______

MAXIMUM POINTS = 36

Comments:

Chapter 11

Arterial Blood Collection

Chapter Outline

Arterial Blood Gases

Arterial Puncture Equipment

Arterial Puncture Procedure

- Phlebotomist Preparation
- Patient Preparation
- Site Selection
- Modified Allen Test
- Preparing the Site
- Performing the Puncture
- Completion of the Procedure
- Summary of Steps in the Arterial Puncture

Specimen Integrity

Arterial Puncture Complications

- Accidental Arterial Puncture

Capillary Blood Gases

Learning Objectives

Upon completion of this chapter, the reader will be able to:

1 Describe the recommended requirements for personnel performing arterial punctures.

2 Define arterial blood gases and describe their diagnostic function.

3 List the equipment and materials needed to perform arterial punctures and discuss preparation of materials.

4 Define "steady state" and list additional patient information that must be recorded when performing blood gas determinations.

5 State four factors that are considered when selecting a site for arterial puncture and name the preferred site.

6 Perform and state the purpose of the modified Allen test.

7 Describe the steps in the performance of an arterial puncture.

8 State five technical errors associated with arterial puncture and their effect on the specimen.

9 Discuss seven complications of arterial puncture, including their effect on the patient and the precautions taken to avoid them.

10 Describe the collection of capillary blood gases, including sources of technical error.

Key Terms

Arteriospasm
Collateral circulation
Local anesthetic
Luer tip
Partial pressure
Respiration rate
Steady state
Thrombolytic therapy
Thrombosis
Vasovagal reaction
Ventilation device

The composition of arterial blood is uniform throughout the body, whereas the composition of venous blood varies because it receives waste products from different parts of the body. However, the normal values for most laboratory tests are based on venous blood. This is because arterial blood collection is more uncomfortable and dangerous for the patient and is more difficult to perform. Arterial blood is primarily requested for the evaluation of blood gases (oxygen and carbon dioxide) and may be requested for the measurement of lactic acid and ammonia in certain metabolic conditions.

Performing arterial punctures is not a routine duty for phlebotomists. The National Committee for Clinical Laboratory Standards (NCCLS) recommends that all institutions require personnel performing arterial punctures to complete specialized training before performing the procedure. This training should include instruction on:

1. Complications associated with arterial punctures
2. Precautions taken to ensure a safe procedure
3. Specimen handling procedures to prevent alteration of test results
4. Correct puncture technique
5. Supervised puncture performance

Personnel trained to perform arterial punctures include physicians, nurses, medical technologists, respiratory therapists, and senior phlebotomists. In some institutions collecting and testing of arterial blood gases (ABGs) has become the responsibility of the respiratory therapy department. In institutions where the laboratory performs the testing, phlebotomists may be required to perform the puncture or to assist the person performing the puncture by preparing and delivering the specimen to the laboratory following special procedures.

To provide phlebotomists with a thorough understanding of arterial punctures, whether or not they are required to perform them, this chapter covers the equipment, patient preparation, puncture technique, specimen handling, and complications of the procedure. However, phlebotomists should *not* perform arterial punctures until they complete specialized training in their place of employment. Collection of capillary blood gases (**CBGs**), a procedure routinely performed by phlebotomists, is also covered.

Arterial Blood Gases

Testing of ABGs measures the ability of the lungs to exchange oxygen and carbon dioxide by determining the ***partial pressure*** of oxygen (Po_2) and carbon dioxide (Pco_2) present in the arterial blood, and the **pH** of the blood. Under normal conditions, arterial blood has a higher Po_2 than Pco_2 because oxygen enters the arterial blood flowing through the lungs and carbon dioxide released from the tissues accumulates in the venous blood. Conditions requiring the measurement of blood gases may be of respiratory or metabolic origin and include chronic obstructive pulmonary disease (**COPD**), cardiac and respiratory failures, severe shock, lung cancer, diabetic coma, open heart surgery, and respiratory distress syndrome (**RDS**) in premature infants. Patients requiring blood gas determinations are often critically ill.

Arterial Puncture Equipment

Arterial blood is collected and transported in specially prepared syringes. Specimens can be introduced directly into blood gas analyzers from the collection syringe as shown in Figure 11–1. This is necessary to protect the specimen from contact with room air. Syringes recommended by the NCCLS for arterial punctures are plastic with freely moving plungers and contain an appropriate anticoagulant. Based on the requirements of the testing instrument and the number of tests requested they may range in size from 1 to 5 mL. They should be no larger than the volume of specimen required. If the specimen cannot be analyzed within 30 minutes, a glass syringe should be used.

Based on the size and depth of the artery selected for puncture, acceptable needle sizes range from 20 to 25 gauge and are $^5/_8$ to $1^1/_2$ inches long. Smaller-gauge needles may not allow the plunger to move spontaneously from arterial pressure, and the collector must move the plunger slowly.

Heparin is the anticoagulant of choice for ABGs and must be present in the syringe when the specimen is collected. The type of heparin used must not interfere with any additional tests being performed on the sample. For example, sodium heparin would not be used if electrolytes were also requested. Plastic

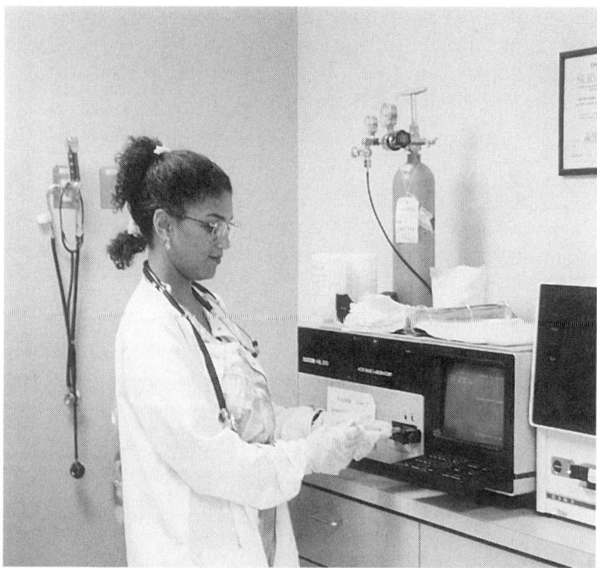

Figure 11–1 Technician performing arterial blood gas determination.

syringes containing the appropriate amount and type of dried heparin can be purchased. Liquid heparin can be used to prepare a glass syringe just before use. The plunger of a glass syringe must be lubricated before performing an arterial puncture to ensure smooth movement.

By expelling the heparin with the needle pointing downward, the space in the needle that would normally contain air contains heparin, so that air cannot be introduced into the specimen. It is important to expel the excess heparin from the syringe barrel because the presence of excess heparin will lower the pH value.

A tightly fitting cap must be available to place on the ***Luer tip*** of the collection syringe after the needle has been removed. It is also desirable to have a small rubber or plastic block to stick the needle into immediately after it is withdrawn from the patient. This procedure prevents air contamination while the patient is being cared for and until the phlebotomist is free to apply the Luer cap. Appropriate needle removal devices and puncture-resistant containers must be present. An arterial blood sampling kit with dry lithium heparin called PRO-VENT PLUS is available from Portex, Inc., Keene, NH. The kit includes a 3-mL plastic syringe with a 22-gauge × 1 inch needle with a Needle-Pro safety device attached and a Filter-Pro device that is applied to the hub of the syringe

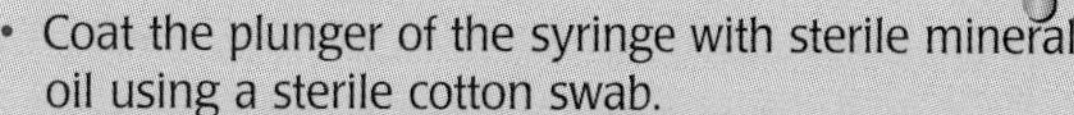

Heparin Preparation of a Lubricated and Heparinized Syringe

- Coat the plunger of the syringe with sterile mineral oil using a sterile cotton swab.
- Insert the plunger into the syringe with a circular motion to coat the inside of the syringe.
- Obtain a vial of heparin with a concentration of 1000 IU/mL.
- Attach a 20-gauge needle to the collection syringe.
- Cleanse the top of the heparin vial with alcohol.
- Draw 0.5 mL of heparin into the syringe.
- Pull the plunger back to expose the area of the syringe that will be in contact with the blood and rotate the syringe so that the entire surface has been heparinized.
- Remove the 20-gauge needle and replace it with the needle to be used for performing the puncture.
- Hold the syringe with the needle pointing up and expel the air; then point the needle down, expel the excess heparin, carefully remove the needle, and attach a new sterile needle. (When the heparin is expelled with the needle pointing downward, the space in the needle that would normally contain air contains heparin, so that air cannot be introduced into the specimen. It is important to expel the excess heparin from the syringe barrel because the presence of excess heparin will lower the pH value.)

for removing air bubbles from the sample and for specimen transport after needle removal (Fig. 11–2). Also available is the Point Lok device (Portex, Inc, Keene, NH), into which the needle can be inserted before removal (Fig. 11–3).

A container of crushed ice, or ice and water, is required for maintaining specimen integrity if the specimen cannot be tested within 30 minutes. The container must be large enough to cover the entire blood specimen with the ice and water. Materials used for specimen labeling must be waterproof if the specimen is placed in an ice bath.

Some institutions administer a ***local anesthetic*** before performing arterial punctures. This requires a 1-mL hypodermic syringe with a 25- or 26-gauge needle containing 0.5 mL of an anesthetic such as lidocaine.

Materials for care of the puncture site include povidone-iodine or chlorhexidine for cleansing the site, alcohol pads to remove the iodine after the

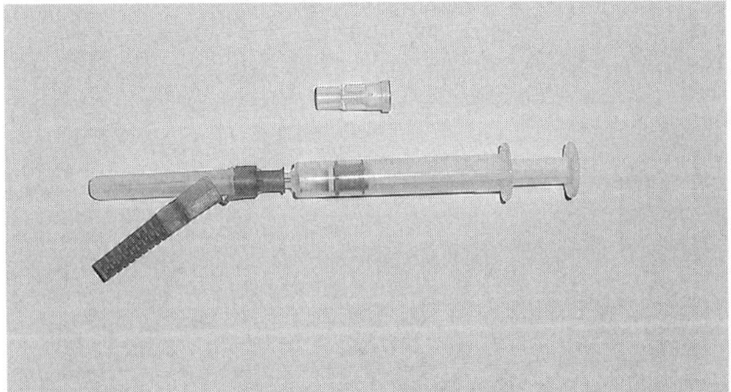

Figure 11–2 Portex, Inc. Pro-Vent Plus arterial blood sampling kit. (Courtesy of Portex, Inc., Keene, NH.)

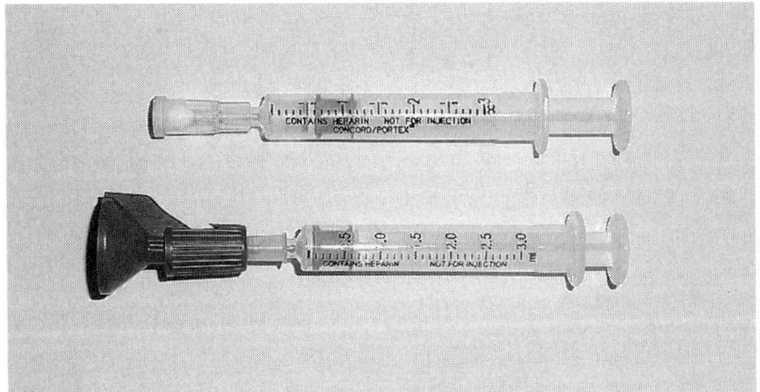

Figure 11–3 Portex, Inc. Point-Lok device and Filter-Pro. (Courtesy of Portex, Inc., Keene, NH.)

procedure is complete, gauze pads to apply pressure to the site, and bandages. Self-adhesive pressure dressing bandages such as CoBan are used for additional pressure.

Arterial Puncture Procedure

As discussed previously for the venipuncture and the dermal puncture, when an arterial puncture is performed, a requisition containing appropriate information is required, patients must be properly identified, and specimens must be labeled with required information.

Phlebotomist Preparation

After carefully examining the requisition form, the phlebotomist must collect all the required equipment, and if necessary, heparinize the collection syringe and prepare the syringe to administer the local anesthetic. All equipment must be conveniently accessible when the puncture is being performed.

Patient Preparation

Additional patient information concerning the conditions under which the specimen was obtained should be provided on either the requisition form or a designated ABG form. This information includes the following:

1 Time of collection
2 Patient's temperature
3 Patient's ***respiration rate***
4 Amount of oxygen the patient is receiving, specified either as room air or the concentration shown on the oxygen monitor, and the type of ***ventilation device*** in use
5 Patient activity, such as comatose, agitated, or anesthetized
6 Collection site (arterial puncture or cannula, capillary puncture)

The patient should have been receiving the specified amount of oxygen and have refrained from exercise for at least 20 to 30 minutes before obtaining the sample. This is referred to as a ***steady state***.

Patients are often apprehensive about arterial punctures, and considerable time and care must be taken to reassure them because an agitated patient will not be in a steady state. Telling the patient that a local anesthetic will be administered after the site has been selected may aid in relaxing an apprehensive patient. The patient should be in a relaxed state with normal breathing for at least 5 minutes.

technical tip Keeping the patient calm is extremely important for patient safety and specimen integrity. Specimen collection should not be performed hurriedly.

Site Selection

Arterial punctures can be hazardous, a situation that limits the number of acceptable sites. To be acceptable as a puncture site, an artery must be:

1 Large enough to accept at least a 25-gauge needle
2 Located near the skin surface so that deep puncture is not required
3 In an area where injury to surrounding tissues will not be critical

4 Located in an area where other arteries are present to supply blood (***collateral circulation***) in case the punctured artery is damaged

The radial artery, located on the thumb side of the wrist, and sometimes the brachial artery, located near the basilic vein in the antecubital area, are the only arterial sites used by phlebotomists. Physicians and specially trained personnel must collect specimens from sites such as the femoral artery, umbilical and scalp veins, and the foot artery (dorsalis pedis). These are also the only personnel authorized to insert and collect specimens from arterial cannulas. However, phlebotomists may be asked to assist in the collection of specimens from cannulas.

Although it is smaller than the brachial artery, the radial artery is the arterial puncture site of choice because:

1 The ulnar artery can provide collateral circulation to the hand.
2 It lies close to the surface of the wrist and is easily accessible.
3 It can be easily compressed against the wrist ligaments, so that pressure can be applied more effectively on the puncture site after removal of the needle and there is less chance of a hematoma.

In spite of its large size and the presence of adequate collateral circulation, the brachial artery is not routinely used; this is owing to its depth, its location near the basilic vein and median nerve, and the fact that it lies in soft tissue that does not provide adequate support for postpuncture pressure.

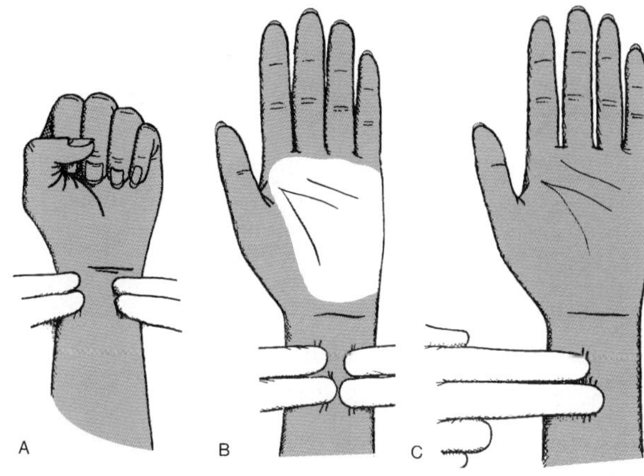

Figure 11–4 Modified Allen test procedure. (*A*) Apply pressure to the radial and ulnar arteries while the patient opens and closes the fist. (*B*) While applying pressure, look for blanching of the palm when fist is opened. (*C*) Release pressure only on the ulnar artery; if color returns to the palm, the test result is positive.

Modified Allen Test

Before performing a radial artery puncture, the modified Allen test can be performed to determine if the ulnar artery is capable of providing collateral circulation to the hand. Lack of available circulation could result in loss of the hand or its function, and another site should be chosen.

The modified Allen test (Fig. 11–4) is performed as follows:

1 Extend the patient's wrist over a rolled towel and ask the patient to form a tight fist.
2 Locate the pulses of the radial and ulnar arteries on the palmar surface of the wrist by palpating with the second and third fingers, not the thumb, which has a pulse.
3 Compress both arteries and, while they are occluded, have the patient open the fist and observe that the palm has become pale (blanched).
4 Release pressure on the *ulnar artery only* and watch to see that color returns to the palm. This should occur within 5 seconds if the ulnar artery is functioning.
5 If color does not appear (negative modified Allen test), the radial artery must not be used. If the modified Allen test is positive, proceed by palpating the radial artery to determine its depth, direction, and size.

Preparing the Site

The risk of infection is higher in arterial punctures than in venipunctures. Therefore the puncture site is cleansed with povidone-iodine or chlorhexidine and the area is allowed to air dry. The gloved palpating fingers are cleansed in the same manner.

A local anesthetic may be administered at this time. This is done by injecting a small amount of anesthetic just under the skin, or into the surrounding tissue if the artery is deep. Before injecting the anesthetic, gently pull back on the plunger and check for the appearance of blood, which would indicate that a blood vessel—rather than tissue—has been entered. Should this happen, a new anesthetic syringe must be prepared and a slightly different injection site must be chosen. Allow 2 minutes for the anesthetic to take effect, and if the patient is apprehensive, allow him or her to relax for 5 minutes.

Performing the Puncture

Just before performing the puncture, the artery is relocated with the cleansed finger of the nondominant hand. The finger is placed directly over the area where the needle should enter the artery—not where the needle enters the skin.

The heparinized syringe is held like a dart in the dominant hand and the needle is inserted about 5 to 10 mm below the palpating finger at a 30- to 45-degree angle with the bevel up (Fig. 11–5). The needle is slowly advanced into the artery until blood appears in the needle hub. At this time, arterial pressure should cause blood to pump into the syringe. The plunger may have to be very carefully pulled back when a plastic syringe and a small needle are used. If blood does not appear, the needle may be slightly redirected but must remain under the skin. Blood that does not pulse into the syringe and appears dark rather than bright red may be venous blood and should not be used.

When enough blood has been collected, remove the needle and apply firm pressure to the site with a gauze pad. The phlebotomist, not the patient, must apply firm pressure for a minimum of 3 to 5 minutes. Arterial punctures are often performed on patients receiving anticoagulant therapy (Coumadin or heparin) or ***thrombolytic therapy*** (tissue plasminogen activator [**tPA**], **streptokinase**, or **urokinase**). Application of pressure for longer than 5 minutes may be necessary for patients receiving this type of therapy.

With the hand holding the syringe, immediately expel any air that has entered the specimen and stick the end of the needle into the rubber or plastic block to prevent additional exposure to air. If using the Sims Portex ABG syringe, activate the needle protection shield or insert the needle into a Sims Portex Point Lock device. Rotate the syringe to mix the anticoagulant with the entire specimen. After 3 to 5 minutes, check the puncture site and, if bleeding has stopped, discontinue the pressure and remove the iodine with alcohol. If bleeding has not stopped, reapply pressure for an additional 2 minutes. Repeat this procedure until the bleeding has stopped. Notify patient care personnel if the bleeding does not stop.

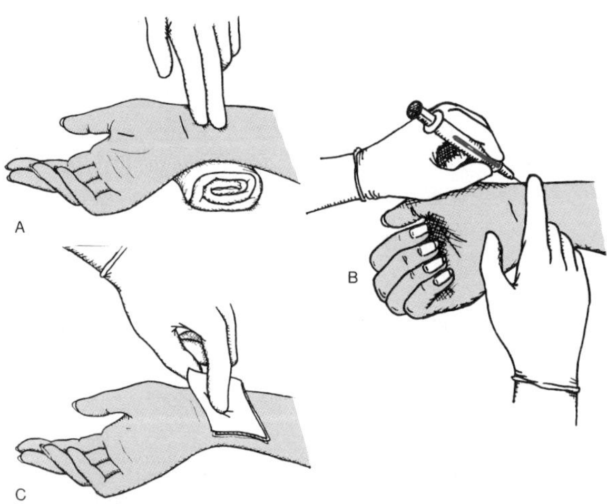

Figure 11–5 Arterial puncture procedure. (*A*) Palpate to locate the radial artery. (*B*) Holding the syringe like a dart, make the puncture at a 30- to 45-degree angle. (*C*) Apply firm pressure to the puncture site for 5 minutes.

Completion of the Procedure

When both hands are free, the needle is discarded in an appropriate container and the Luer cap (Filter-Pro device) is applied to the hub of the syringe. The specimen is labeled and, if necessary, placed in an ice-water bath.

After pressure has been removed for 2 minutes, the patient's arm is rechecked to be sure that a hematoma is not forming, in which case additional pressure is required.

The radial artery is checked for a pulse below the puncture site, and the nurse is notified if a pulse cannot be located.

A pressure bandage is applied if no complications are discovered.

In the same manner as discussed with previous phlebotomy procedures, before leaving the room, the phlebotomist disposes of used materials in appropriate containers, removes gloves, washes hands, and thanks the patient.

Summary of Steps in the Arterial Puncture

1. Obtain a requisition form.
2. Collect equipment.
3. Greet and identify the patient.
4. Explain the procedure and reassure the patient.
5. Obtain metabolic and oxygen therapy information and ensure a steady state.
6. Wash hands and put on gloves.
7. Organize equipment, heparinize the collection syringe, and prepare the anesthetic syringe if necessary.
8. Support and hyperextend the patient's wrist.
9. Perform the modified Allen test.
10. Locate and palpate the radial artery.
11. Cleanse the site and the palpating finger.
12. Administer the anesthetic, if necessary, and wait 2 minutes.
13. Place a cleansed, gloved finger over the arterial puncture site.
14. Insert needle, bevel up at a 30- to 45-degree angle, 10 to 15 mm below the palpating finger.
15. Allow syringe to fill.
16. Remove needle and apply pressure.
17. Expel any air bubbles from the syringe.
18. Stick needle into rubber or plastic block.
19. Roll syringe to mix.
20. Maintain pressure on puncture site for 3 to 5 minutes.
21. Examine puncture site and remove pressure if bleeding has stopped.
22. Remove needle from syringe using appropriate safety precautions and replace with Luer cap.
23. Dispose of needle.
24. Label specimen and place in an ice-water bath. if necessary.
25. Reexamine puncture site for hematoma formation.
26. Check for a radial pulse below the puncture site.
27. Apply a pressure bandage.
28. Dispose of used materials.
29. Remove gloves and wash hands.
30. Thank the patient.
31. Immediately deliver specimen to the laboratory.

Specimen Integrity

ABG test results can be noticeably affected by improper specimen collection and handling. Of primary importance is maintaining the specimen under strict anaerobic conditions. Specimen integrity also is compromised by improper amount of anticoagulant, failure to analyze the specimen in a timely manner, and collection of venous rather than arterial blood (Table 11–1).

Procedural errors that introduce air into the specimen include failure to firmly seat the plunger into the syringe, failure to immediately expel any bubbles from the syringe, and failure to seal the syringe or needle after collection. Excessive pulling of the syringe plunger resulting in increased suction may cause the aspiration of capillary blood into the specimen. The presence of excess heparin in the syringe falsely lowers the blood pH. When preparing heparinized syringes, all excess heparin must be expelled from the syringe. In contrast, an inadequate amount of heparin can allow the specimen to clot and prevent analysis. If this problem occurs, the specimen will not be a true representation of arterial blood.

TABLE 11–1
Effect of Technical Errors on ABG Results

Technical Error	Effect
Air bubbles present	Atmospheric oxygen enters the specimen, and carbon dioxide from the specimen enters the air bubbles
Too much heparin	pH is lowered
Too little heparin/inadequate mixing	Clots that interfere with the analyzer are present
Delayed analysis/improper cooling	Blood cells in the specimen continue their metabolism, utilizing oxygen and producing carbon dioxide and acids that lower the pH
Venous rather than arterial sample	Falsely decreased PO_2 and increased PCO_2

Current NCCLS recommendations state that specimens that will be analyzed within 30 minutes can be collected in plastic syringes and do not require the specimens to be placed in an ice bath. The exception to this is when lactates have been ordered with the ABG; lactates are iced immediately. Earlier recommendations to place all specimens immediately in ice to prevent use of oxygen by leukocytes and platelets present in the specimen have been amended to include only those specimens with elevated leukocyte or platelet counts. Specimens that cannot be analyzed within 30 minutes are still collected in glass syringes and placed in ice and water.

technical tip Every precaution should be taken to avoid the need to recollect an arterial specimen because of improper handling.

Arterial Puncture Complications

As mentioned previously, the arterial puncture is more dangerous for the patient than the venipuncture. Possible complications include hematoma formation, ***arteriospasm, vasovagal reaction, thrombosis***, hemorrhage, infection, and nerve damage (Table 11–2).

Hematomas are more common after arterial puncture because the increased pressure forces blood into the surrounding tissue. Failure of the phlebotomist to maintain pressure for at least 3 to 5 minutes and to check the site, use of arteries located in soft tissues where pressure is difficult to apply, and the decrease in elasticity in the arteries of older persons are frequent causes of hematomas.

An arteriospasm is a spontaneous, usually temporary constriction of an artery in response to a sensation such as pain. Closure of the artery prohibits collection of the specimen and prevents oxygen from reaching the tissues so that tissue destruction and possible gangrene may result. This is why the presence of collateral circulation is essential when performing arterial punctures.

Apprehensive patients may experience a vasovagal reaction resulting in a sudden loss of consciousness. Stimulation of the vagus nerve as a result of sudden stress or pain produces vascular dilation and a rapid drop in blood pressure (**hypotension**). Medical assistance should be summoned.

Formation of a clot (**thrombus**) on the inside wall of an artery or vein in response to a puncture hole can produce occlusion of the vessel, particularly if the thrombus continues to grow. This is most frequently caused by irritation from the continued presence of a cannula. Collateral circulation again becomes important.

Patients with coagulation disorders or receiving anticoagulant or thrombolytic therapy have an increased risk of bleeding after arterial puncture. Puncture of a large artery, such as the femoral artery, using a large-gauge needle can produce considerable hemorrhaging in these patients.

Failure to cleanse the arterial puncture site adequately, resulting in the introduction of microorganisms into the arterial circulation, is more likely to cause infection than if microorganisms are introduced into the venous circulation. In the arterial circulation, the organisms are easily carried into many areas of the body without coming in contact with the protective capabilities of the lymphatic system, which runs in close proximity to the venous circulation.

TABLE 11–2
Arterial Puncture Complications

Complication	Cause	Prevention
Hematoma	Arterial blood entering the tissue	Phlebotomist applies pressure until bleeding stops
Tissue destruction/gangrene	Arteriospasm	Evaluate collateral circulation
Vasovagal reaction	Apprehension/pain	Calming the patient, local anesthetic
Hemorrhage	Coagulation disorders and therapy	Increased pressure, smaller-gauge needles
Infection	Failure to adequately cleanse the site	Proper cleansing, sterile technique
Nerve damage	Deep punctures	Avoiding deep sites if possible, specialized training

The possibility of nerve damage is greater with arterial puncture because of the need to puncture more deeply into the tissue to reach the artery, thereby increasing the possibility of encountering a nerve. Remember, the brachial artery is located very near the median nerve.

Considering these possible complications, it is easy to understand why phlebotomists should perform arterial punctures only after receiving specialized training and when the requisition form indicates an arterial puncture. They should never perform an arterial puncture just because they have been unsuccessful with the venipuncture.

Accidental Arterial Puncture

Considering that the brachial artery is located near the basilic vein, it is possible for a phlebotomist to puncture this artery accidentally. Phlebotomists should be alert for the appearance of bright red blood that pulsates into the evacuated tube or syringe. If an arterial puncture is suspected, the phlebotomist must apply pressure in the manner previously described for arterial punctures. The specimen is submitted to the laboratory and the collection of arterial blood noted on the requisition form.

technical tip Never hesitate to report anything unusual observed while performing an arterial puncture.

Capillary Blood Gases

Performing deep arterial punctures in newborns and young children is usually not recommended; therefore, unless blood can be obtained from umbilical or scalp arteries, blood gases are performed on capillary blood. Blood is collected from the plantar area of the heel or big toe and the palmar area of the fingers, as described in Chapter 9. As discussed in Chapter 4, capillary blood is actually a mixture of venous and arterial blood, with a higher concentration of arterial blood. The concentration of arterial blood is also increased when the collection site is warmed. Therefore, when collecting capillary blood gases, it is essential to warm the collection site.

technical tip Do not forget to wipe away the first drop of blood before collecting a capillary specimen.

Specimens are collected in heparinized blood gas pipets designed to correspond with the volume and sampling requirements of the blood gas analyzer being used. Plugs or clay sealants are needed for both ends of the pipets, and a **magnetic "flea"** and circular magnet are used to mix the specimen.

After warming the site to 40°C to 42°C for 3 to 5 minutes to increase the flow of arterial blood, blood is collected using the technique discussed in Chapter 9. Pipets must be completely filled and must not contain air bubbles. When the pipet is full, one end is immediately sealed, the magnetic flea is inserted into the open end, the round magnet is slipped over the tube, and the other end is sealed. The blood is mixed by moving the magnet up and down the tube several times. The tubes are labeled, placed horizontally in an ice/water, and immediately transported to the laboratory water.

technical tip To avoid air bubbles, hold the tube in a horizontal position and be sure that blood flows easily from the puncture site.

Bibliography

National Committee for Clinical Laboratory Standards Approved Standard H11-A3: Procedures for the Collection of Arterial Blood Specimens. NCCLS, Wayne, PA, 1999.

Study Questions

1. List five components of an arterial puncture.
   a. ______
   b. ______
   c. ______
   d. ______
   e. ______

2. Name a hospital department other than the clinical laboratory that may be responsible for collecting and analyzing blood gases.

   ______

3. List and define the components of a blood gas analysis.

   ______

   ______

   ______

4. Why are specimens for ABGs not transferred into anticoagulant tubes after collection?

   ______

5. The primary anticoagulant used for ABGs is ______.

6. When preparing a syringe for collecting ABGs, why is the needle pointed downward when expelling the anticoagulant?

   ______

7. When are ABGs collected in glass syringes?

   ______

8 List five items of patient information required when collecting ABGs that are not required for routine venipuncture.
   a. ______
   b. ______
   c. ______
   d. ______
   e. ______

9. List three reasons why the radial artery is the artery of choice for arterial puncture.

   a. ______________________________

   b. ______________________________

   c. ______________________________

10. List three reasons why the brachial artery is not the artery of choice for arterial punctures.

   a. ______________________________

   b. ______________________________

   c. ______________________________

11. Place the following steps performed in the modified Allen test in the correct order, using the numbers 1 to 6:

   a. ________ Patient makes a fist.

   b. ________ Patient opens hand.

   c. ________ Ulnar artery is released.

   d. ________ Pressure is applied to radial and ulnar arteries.

   e. ________ Patient's palm is observed for blanching.

   f. ________ Patient's palm is observed for color.

12. True or False. When a negative modified Allen test is encountered, blood should be collected from the ulnar rather than the radial artery. ______________

13. What is the angle of needle insertion for arterial punctures, and why does it differ from the angle used for venipunctures?

   ____

14. Match the following complications of arterial puncture with the most possible cause or effect. Complications may be used more than once.

Cause/Effect	**Complication**
a. ________ Presence of an arterial cannula	1. Hematoma
b. ________ Pressure applied to the site for 2 minutes	2. Arteriospasm
c. ________ Patient receiving tPA	3. Thrombosis
d. ________ Gangrene of the fingers	4. Hemorrhage
e. ________ Use of the brachial artery	5. Vasovagal reaction
f. ________ Extremely apprehensive patient	

g. __________ Inability to obtain a radial pulse after the puncture

h. __________ Patient loses consciousness

15. Why must the site for collection of capillary blood gases be warmed before specimen collection?

____

Clinical Situations

1. When entering a patient's room to collect an ABG specimen, a phlebotomist learns that the patient has just returned from physical therapy and has been disconnected from a portable oxygen device and reconnected to the bedside oxygen system.
   a. When should the phlebotomist collect the specimen? Why?

   ____

   b. What additional information related to the patient's status should the phlebotomist obtain?

   ____

   ____

2. When performing an arterial puncture, the phlebotomist notices that the blood is not pulsating into the syringe.
   a. What other observation should the phlebotomist make?

   ____

   b. Should the phlebotomist be concerned? Why or why not?

   ____

   c. Which ABG test result could be falsely decreased? Increased?

   ____

3. A phlebotomist is performing an arterial puncture on a patient with an elevated white blood cell count.
   a. What type of syringe should be used? ____________________

   b. What two things must the phlebotomist do to prepare the syringe?

   ____

   ____

   c. How should the syringe be transported to the laboratory?

   ____

4. When performing a venipuncture in the antecubital area of an obese patient, the phlebotomist notices that blood is pulsating into the evacuated tube.

   a. What other observation should the phlebotomist make?

   ____

   b. What blood vessel may have been punctured?

   ____

   c. What additional precautions should the phlebotomist take to protect the patient?

   ____

   d. What is the most probable complication for this patient?

   ____

5. While sealing one end of a capillary blood gas tube, a phlebotomist accidentally allows some blood to flow out of the tube while adding the "magnetic flea."

   a. Will this be an acceptable specimen? Why or why not?

   ____

   b. What is the purpose of adding a "magnetic flea" to a capillary blood gas tube?

   ____

   c. If the "magnetic flea" is not added to the tube, how might this affect the analysis of the specimen?

   ____

NAME ________________________________

Evaluation of Modified Allen Test Performance

RATING SYSTEM 2 = SATISFACTORILY PERFORMED 1 = NEEDS IMPROVEMENT 0 = INCORRECT/DID NOT PERFORM

__________ 1. Explains procedure to patient

__________ 2. Extends patient's wrist

__________ 3. Asks patient to make a fist

__________ 4. Locates radial and ulnar arteries using appropriate fingers

__________ 5. Compresses both arteries

__________ 6. Asks patient to open the fist

__________ 7. Looks for blanching of patient's palm

__________ 8. Tells patient to leave hand open

__________ 9. Releases pressure on the ulnar artery only

__________ 10. Observes color of patient's palm

__________ 11. States if the test is positive or negative

__________ 12. Explains the significance of the test result

TOTAL POINTS

MAXIMUM POINTS = 24

Comments:

NAME ____________________

Evaluation of Arterial Puncture Technique

RATING SYSTEM 2 = SATISFACTORILY PERFORMED 1 = NEEDS IMPROVEMENT 0 = INCORRECT/DID NOT PERFORM

________ 1. Obtains requisition form

________ 2. Assembles equipment

________ 3. Identifies patient

________ 4. Explains procedure to the patient

________ 5. Determines that patient is in a steady state

________ 6. Obtains metabolic and oxygen therapy information

________ 7. Organizes equipment

________ 8. Washes hands and puts on gloves

________ 9. Prepares anesthetic syringe

________ 10. Supports and hyperextends the patient's wrist

________ 11. Performs and interprets the modified Allen test

________ 12. Locates and palpates the radial artery

________ 13. Cleanses the site with iodine; allows it to air dry

________ 14. Cleanses palpating finger

________ 15. Administers local anesthetic and waits 2 minutes

________ 16. Places palpating finger over puncture site

________ 17. Inserts needle, bevel up, at a 30- to 45-degree angle

________ 18. Inserts needle 10 to 15 mm below palpating finger

________ 19. Allows syringe to fill by arterial pressure

________ 20. Removes needle and applies pressure

________ 21. Consistently maintains pressure on site for 5 minutes

________ 22. Expels air bubbles from syringe

____________ 23. Sticks needle into rubber block

____________ 24. Rolls syringe to mix

____________ 25. Examines puncture site after 3 to 5 minutes

____________ 26. Replaces syringe needle with Luer cap

____________ 27. Disposes of needle

____________ 28. Labels specimen

____________ 29. Reexamines patient's arm

____________ 30. Checks for a radial pulse

____________ 31. Removes iodine and applies pressure bandage

____________ 32. Disposes of used supplies

____________ 33. Removes gloves and washes hands

____________ 34. Thanks patient

____________ 35. Immediately delivers specimen to the laboratory

TOTAL POINTS

MAXIMUM POINTS = 70

Comments:

NAME ______________________________

Evaluation of Capillary Blood Gas Collection

RATING SYSTEM 2 = SATISFACTORILY PERFORMED 1 = NEEDS IMPROVEMENT 0 = INCORRECT/DID NOT PERFORM

__________ 1. Obtains requisition

__________ 2. Performs nursery isolation procedures

__________ 3. Identifies patient

__________ 4. Begins 3- to 5-minute heel warming

__________ 5. Assembles equipment

__________ 6. Washes hands and puts on gloves

__________ 7. Selects appropriate heel site

__________ 8. Cleanses site, and allows it to air dry

__________ 9. Performs puncture

__________ 10. Wipes away first drop of blood

__________ 11. Fills capillary tube without bubbles

__________ 12. Seals one end of capillary tube

__________ 13. Adds magnetic "flea" and magnet

__________ 14. Seals second end of tube

__________ 15. Mixes specimen

__________ 16. Applies pressure to site until bleeding stops

__________ 17. Labels tube

__________ 18. Places tube in an ice-water bath.

__________ 19. Disposes of equipment and supplies

__________ 20. Removes gown and gloves

__________ 21. Washes hands

__________ 22. Immediately transports specimen to laboratory

TOTAL POINTS

MAXIMUM POINTS = 44

Comments:

Chapter 12

Additional Duties of the Phlebotomist

Chapter Outline

Patient Instruction
- Urine Specimen Collection
- Urine Drug Specimen Collection
- Fecal Specimen Collection
- Semen Specimen Collection

Collection of Throat Cultures

Collection of Sweat Electrolytes

Blood Donor Collection
- Donor Selection
- Donor Collection
- Additional Donor Collection

Receiving and Transporting Specimens

Specimen Processing, Accessioning, and Shipping
- Specimen Aliquoting
- Specimen Shipping
- Use of the Laboratory Computer

Learning Objectives

Upon completion of this chapter, the reader will be able to:

1. Provide patients with instructions and containers for the collection of random, first morning, midstream clean-catch, and 24-hour urine specimens.
2. Provide patients with instructions and containers for the collection of random and timed fecal specimens.
3. Provide patients with instructions and containers for the collection of semen specimens.
4. Correctly collect a throat culture.
5. Briefly describe the purpose of and the collection procedure for sweat electrolytes, including the precautions to protect specimen integrity.
6. Discuss the major components and concerns of the blood donor selection process.
7. Compare and contrast the blood donor collection process and the routine venipuncture.
8. Describe the distribution of tubes for cerebrospinal fluid (CSF) analysis.
9. Discuss the responsibilities of a phlebotomist when transporting or accepting specimens into the laboratory.
10. Describe the safety precautions associated with specimen processing.
11. State four rules for safe operation of a centrifuge.
12. State three routine phlebotomy duties that can involve a phlebotomist in the use of a laboratory information management system.

Key Terms

Aliquot
Apheresis
Autologous donation
Iontophoresis
Pilocarpine
Pneumatic tube system
Sweat electrolytes
Therapeutic phlebotomy

Although collection of quality blood specimens is the primary duty of phlebotomists, they are frequently assigned other responsibilities related to specimen collection and handling of nonblood specimens. These additional duties may include:

1. Providing instructions and materials to patients for the collection of urine, fecal, and semen specimens
2. Collecting throat cultures
3. Performing sweat electrolyte collections
4. Interviewing blood donors
5. Performing donor blood collections and therapeutic phlebotomies
6. Transporting and receiving nonblood specimens
7. Preparing specimens for delivery to laboratory sections or shipment to reference laboratories
8. Transporting specimens from off-site collection areas
9. Using the laboratory computer system to enter and retrieve patient and specimen information

The extent to which phlebotomists are assigned these duties varies greatly among laboratories, as do the protocols for performing them. This chapter is intended to provide phlebotomists with basic information associated with these additional functions.

Patient Instruction

The phlebotomy department is usually located in or near the laboratory patient and specimen reception area. Therefore, phlebotomists often provide instructions to patients and may receive calls from the healthcare provider's office personnel requesting instructions. Instructions may be given verbally, using guidelines stated in the laboratory procedure manual, or may be handed to the patient in written form. The phlebotomist should be prepared to answer questions regarding the instructions. Depending on the test requested, patients may be collecting the specimen while at the laboratory or collecting the specimen at home and returning it to the laboratory. The facilities for specimen collection should be at a location convenient to the laboratory.

Urine Specimen Collection

Frequently collected urine specimens include random, first morning, midstream clean-catch, and 24-hour (timed) specimens. Phlebotomists should explain to patients that the composition of urine changes quickly and specimens should be delivered promptly to the laboratory or refrigerated.

Random specimens are collected by patients while at the laboratory and are used primarily for routine urinalysis. Patients should be provided with a disposable urine container and directed to the bathroom facility.

A first morning specimen is the specimen of choice for urinalysis because it is more concentrated. It may be used to confirm results obtained from random specimens. Patients are provided with a container and instructed to collect the specimen immediately after arising and to return it to the laboratory within 2 hours or refrigerate the sample.

Midstream clean-catch specimens are used for urine cultures. Patients are provided with sterile containers and antiseptic materials for cleansing the genitalia. Mild antiseptic towelettes are recommended. Women should be instructed to spread the labia and cleanse from front to back. Men should cleanse the tip of the penis; the cleansing should include retraction of the foreskin if the man is uncircumcised. Patients are instructed to begin voiding into the toilet, then collect the specimen without touching the inside of the container, and finish voiding into the toilet. Midstream clean-catch specimens are collected at the laboratory and delivered immediately to the microbiology section.

technical tip Posting instructions for collection of midstream clean-catch specimens on bathroom walls is very helpful to patients.

A carefully timed (usually 24 hours) specimen is required for quantitative measurement of urine constituents. Patients are provided with large plastic containers that may contain a preservative. Phlebotomists should check the procedure manual or with a laboratory supervisor to be sure the appropriate preservative is supplied. Patients should be cautioned to avoid contact with the preservative in the container because some preservatives are caustic. For accurate results, it is critical that the patient

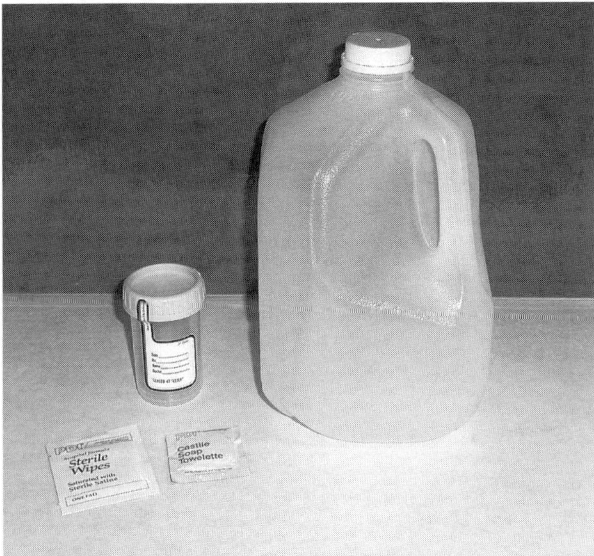

Figure 12–1 Containers for urine specimens.

understand that all urine produced during the collection period be placed in the container. Patients who indicate they have not been able to collect a complete sample should obtain a new specimen. To obtain an accurate timed specimen, it is necessary for the patient to begin and end the collection period with an empty bladder. Addition of urine produced before the start of the collection time or failure to include urine produced at the end of the collection period will affect the accuracy of the analysis. Examples of urine specimen containers and supplies are shown in Figure 12–1.

technical tip Failure to collect a complete timed specimen causes falsely decreased results.

Urine Drug Specimen Collection

Phlebotomists may be involved in the urine drug specimen collection from both outpatients and in-house healthcare workers. Specimen collection is the most vulnerable part of a drug-testing program. For urine specimens to withstand legal scrutiny, it is necessary to prove that no tampering (e.g., adulteration, substitution, or dilution) took place. Acceptable identification of the person requires picture identification, and as discussed in Chapter 8, the chain of custody (COC) must be carefully documented.

24-Hour (Timed) Specimen Collection Procedure

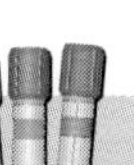

- Provide patient with written instructions and explain the collection procedure.
- Issue the proper collection container and preservative.
- Day 1—7 A.M. Patient voids and discards specimen. Patient collects all urine for the next 24 hours.
- Day 2—7 A.M. Patient voids and adds this urine to the previously collected urine.
- On arrival in the laboratory, the entire 24-hour specimen is thoroughly mixed, and the volume is accurately measured and recorded.
- An aliquot is saved for testing and additional or repeat testing. Discard remaining urine.

Urine specimen collection may be "witnessed" or "unwitnessed." The decision to obtain a witnessed collection is indicated when it is suspected that the donor may alter or substitute the specimen, or it is the policy of the client ordering the test. If a witnessed specimen collection is ordered, a same-gender collector will observe the collection of 30 to 45 mL of urine. Witnessed and unwitnessed collections should be immediately handed to the collector.

The urine temperature must be taken within 4 minutes from the time of collection to confirm the specimen has not been adulterated. The temperature should read within the range of 32.5°C to 37.7°C. If the specimen temperature is not within range, the specimen temperature should be recorded and the supervisor or employer contacted immediately. Urine temperatures outside of the recommended range may indicate specimen contamination. Recollection of a second specimen as soon as possible is necessary. The urine color is inspected to identify any signs of contaminants. A urine pH of greater than 9.0 suggests adulteration of the urine specimen and requires that the specimen be recollected if clinically necessary. A specific gravity of less than 1.005 could indicate dilution of the urine specimen and would require recollection of the specimen. The specimen is labeled, packaged, and transported following laboratory-specific instructions.

Fecal Specimen Collection

The laboratory provides patients with several types of containers for collection of fecal specimens

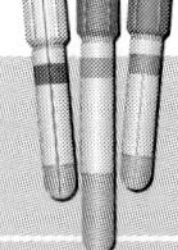

Urine Drug Specimen Collection Procedure

1. The collector washes hands and wears gloves.
2. The collector adds bluing agent (dye) to the toilet water reservoir to prevent an adulterated specimen.
3. The collector eliminates any source of water other than the toilet by taping the toilet lid and faucet handles.
4. The donor provides photo identification or positive identification from employer representative.
5. The collector completes step 1 of the COC form and has the donor sign the form.
6. The donor leaves his or her coat, briefcase, or purse outside the collection area to avoid the possibility of concealed substances contaminating the urine.
7. The donor washes his or her hands and receives a specimen cup.
8. The collector remains in the restroom but outside the stall, listening for unauthorized water use, unless a witnessed collection is requested.
9. The donor hands specimen cup to the collector.
10. The collector checks the urine for abnormal color and for the required amount (30 to 45 mL).
11. The collector checks that the temperature strip on the specimen cup reads between 32.5°C and 37.7°C. The collector records the in-range temperature on the COC form (COC step 2). If the specimen temperature is out of range or the specimen is suspected to have been diluted or adulterated, a new specimen must be collected and a supervisor notified.
12. The specimen must remain in the sight of the donor and collector at all times.
13. With the donor watching, the collector peels off the specimen identification strips from the COC form (COC step 3) and puts them on the capped bottle, covering both sides of the cap.
14. The donor initials the specimen bottle seals.
15. The date and time are written on the seals.
16. The donor completes step 4 on the COC form.
17. The collector completes step 5 on the COC form.
18. Each time the specimen is handled, transferred, or placed in storage, every individual must be identified and the date and purpose of the change recorded.
19. The collector follows laboratory-specific instructions for packaging the specimen bottles and laboratory copies of the COC form.
20. The collector distributes the COC copies to appropriate personnel.

(Fig. 12–2). Random specimens used for cultures, ova and parasites, microscopic examination for cells, fats and fibers, and detection of blood are collected in cardboard containers with wax-coated interiors or plastic containers with wide openings. Containers with preservatives may be required for certain microbiology tests, including ova and parasites. Phlebotomists should check the procedure manual before distributing containers for fecal specimens. Large paint can–style or plastic hat–style containers, as shown in Figure 12–2, are used for collection of 72-hour specimens for fecal fats. Kits containing reagent-impregnated filter paper are provided to screen for the presence of occult (hidden) blood (see Chapter 13)

technical tip Clean disposable plastic containers such as margarine tubs can be used to collect stool specimens.

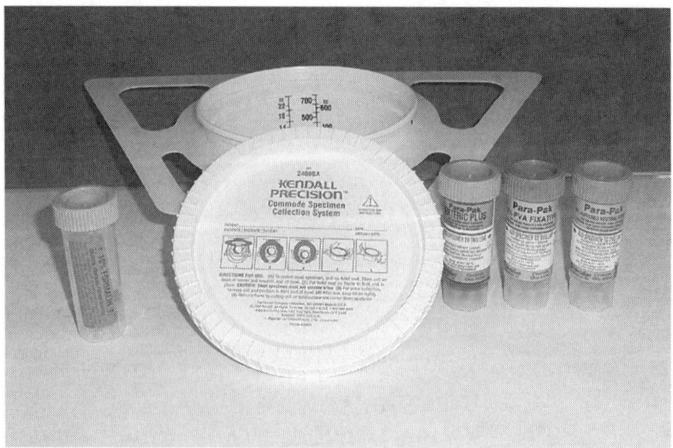

Figure 12–2 Containers for fecal specimens.

Patients should be instructed to return the specimen to the laboratory as soon as possible and to avoid contaminating the specimen with urine or toilet water. It may be necessary to collect the specimen in a large container such as a bedpan and then transfer it to the laboratory container. For purposes of safety, the outside of the container must not be contaminated.

Semen Specimen Collection

Patients presenting requisitions for semen analysis should be instructed to abstain from sexual activity for 3 days and not longer than 5 days before collecting the specimen. Ideally, the specimen should then be collected at the laboratory in a warm sterile container. Specimens for fertility studies must not be collected in a condom because condoms frequently contain spermicidal agents.

If the specimen is collected at home, it must be kept warm and delivered to the laboratory within 1 hour. When accepting a semen specimen, it is essential that the phlebotomist record the time of specimen collection, not specimen receipt, on the requisition form because certain parameters of the semen analysis are based on specimen life span.

Written instructions should be available for patients required to collect semen samples.

Collection of Throat Cultures

In some institutions, the duties of the phlebotomist may include collection of throat cultures from outpatients, often children. They are performed primarily for the detection of a streptococcal infection, "strep throat." Specimens may be collected for the purpose of performing a culture or a rapid immunologic Group A Strep test (see Chapter 13).

technical tip The purpose of the transport media in a culture swab kit is to keep the bacteria to be cultured alive during transport.

technical tip Swabs for rapid streptococcal tests do not require transport media.

Materials needed include a tongue depressor, collection swab in a sterile tube containing transport media, such as a Becton Dickinson (Franklin Lakes, NJ) Culturette, and possibly a flashlight.

To obtain the specimen (Fig. 12–3):

1 Have the patient tilt the head back and open the mouth wide.
2 Remove the cap with its attached swab from the tube using sterile technique.
3 Gently depress the tongue with the tongue depressor.
4 Being careful not to touch the cheeks, tongue, or lips, swab the area in the back of the throat, including the tonsils and any inflamed or ulcerated areas.
5 Return the swab to the sterile tube and crush the ampule of transport media, making sure the released media are in contact with the swab (Fig. 12–4).
6 Label the specimen, and deliver it to the microbiology section.

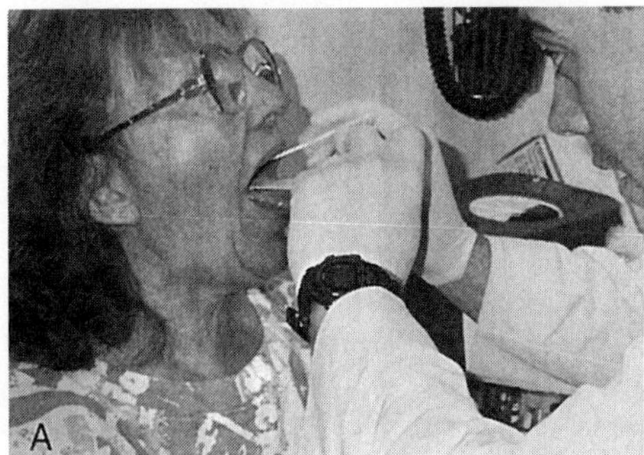

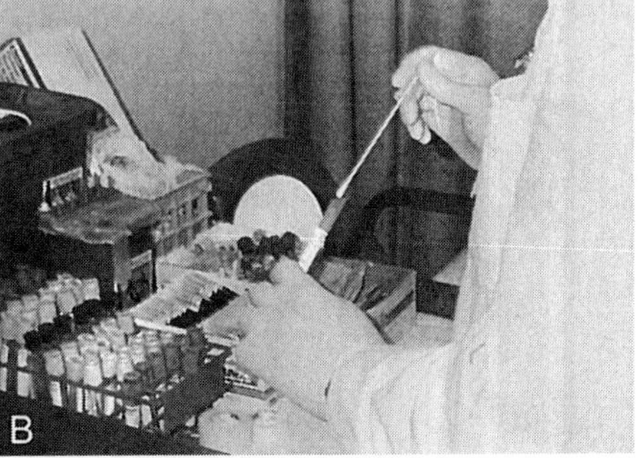

Figure 12–3 Throat culture collection. (*A*) Swabbing the back of the throat. (*B*) Returning the swab to its sterile tube.

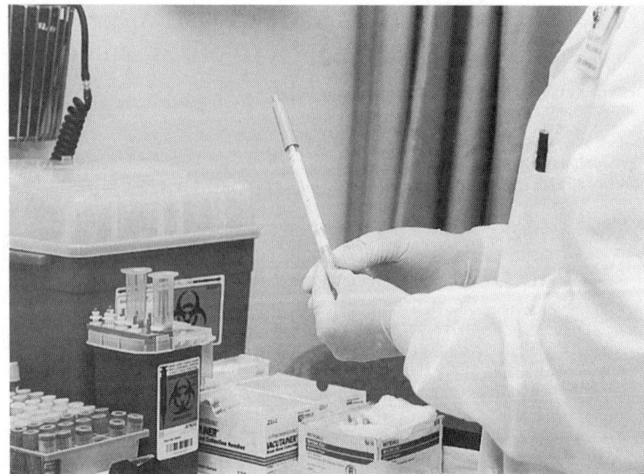

Figure 12–4 Phlebotomist crushing ampule of transport medium after specimen collection. (From Strasinger, SK, and Di Lorenzo, MS: Skills for the Patient Care Technician. FA Davis, Philadelphia, 1999, p. 247, with permission.)

Collection of Sweat Electrolytes

Measurement of the ***sweat electrolytes***, sodium and chloride, is performed to confirm the diagnosis of cystic fibrosis, a genetic disorder of the mucus-secreting glands. Because cystic fibrosis involves multiple organs, many clinical symptoms can lead the physician to suspect its presence. Symptoms usually appear early in life; therefore, sweat electrolytes are frequently collected from infants.

Specimen collection is time consuming and must be performed under very controlled conditions to ensure that the small amount of sample collected is not altered by contamination or evaporation.

Patients are induced to sweat using a technique called pilocarpine ***iontophoresis***, which is illustrated in Figure 12–5. ***Pilocarpine***, a sweat-inducing chemical, is applied to an area of the forearm or leg that has been previously cleansed with deionized water. The pilocarpine is then iontophoresed into the skin by the application of a mild electrical current provided by a device designed for pilocarpine iontophoresis. After iontophoresis, the area exposed to the pilocarpine is again thoroughly cleansed with deionized water and dried.

technical tip Be sure to use deionized water to cleanse the sweat collection area.

Several methods are available for collection of sweat for electrolyte analysis, including the use of preweighed gauze, filter paper pads, or coil collectors. The collection apparatus is placed on the stimulated area; covered securely with plastic if the collection material is gauze or filter paper; and allowed to remain for a specified length of time,

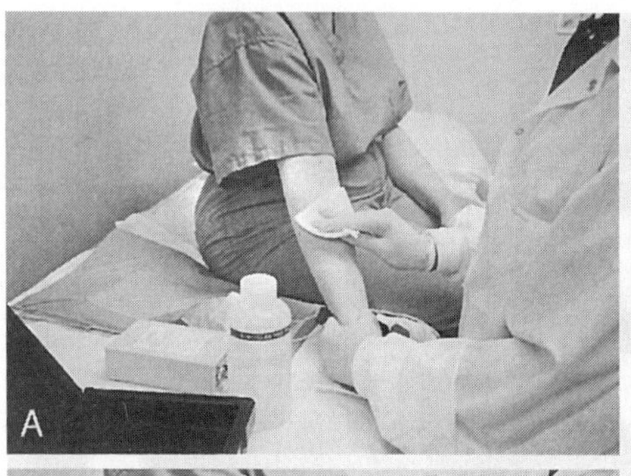

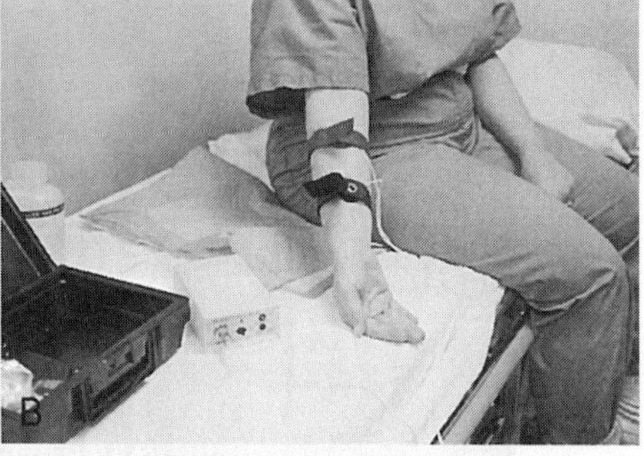

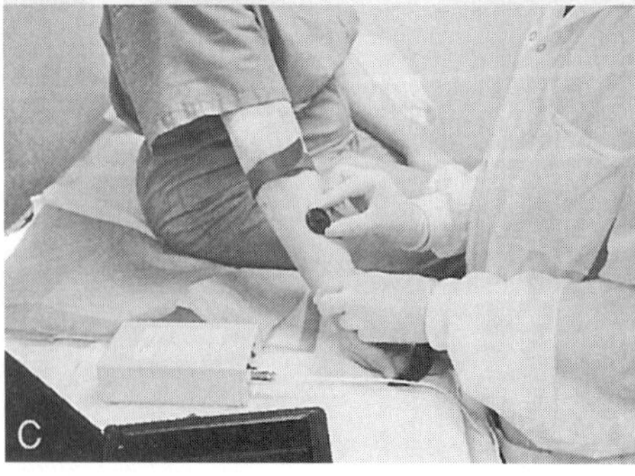

Figure 12–5 Sweat collection by means of pilocarpine iontophoresis. (*A*) Cleansing the collection site with distilled water. (*B*) Performing iontophoresis sweat stimulation. (*C*) Applying the sweat collection container.

usually 30 minutes. Regardless of the collection method used, it is essential that:

1 The collection apparatus is handled only with sterile forceps or powder-free gloves and not contaminated by use of the fingers.
2 The collection apparatus is tightly sealed during the collection period to prevent evaporation of the collected sweat.
3 The collected sweat is tightly sealed during transportation to the laboratory to prevent evaporation.

Phlebotomists may be required to perform sweat electrolyte collections or to assist personnel from the chemistry section with the collection. If the collection of sweat electrolytes is one of the phlebotomist's duties, the phlebotomist is usually required to notify the chemistry section when a collection is requested and to obtain collection materials (which may have to be preweighed) from the department.

Blood Donor Collection

Phlebotomists may be assigned to work in the blood donor collection station as a part of their routine duties, or they may obtain employment in a donor station. In the donor station, units of blood are collected to provide the blood bank with a supply of blood and blood components for transfusions. A unit of blood consists of 405 to 495 mL of blood mixed with 63 mL of anticoagulant. After collection, a unit of blood can be separated by centrifugation into its individual components, including red blood cells, white blood cells, platelets, plasma, and plasma proteins. Experienced phlebotomists are needed to perform donor unit collections. Blood donor collections are performed following guidelines established by the American Association of Blood Banks (AABB) and the Food and Drug Administration (FDA) for donor selection and unit collection and processing.

Donor Selection

Persons volunteering to donate blood must be interviewed and tested to ensure that the donation will not be physically harmful to them, as well as to determine that their blood is unlikely to cause an adverse condition in the recipient. Donor units are always tested with all available tests for bloodborne pathogens; however, exclusion of donors with possible exposure to these pathogens provides additional protection for the recipient.

Donor registration requires identification (including name, address, telephone number, date of birth, social security number, sex) and date of last donation (at least 8 weeks is required between donations). This information is needed in case the donor must be contacted in the future. Donors must also sign a consent form permitting the laboratory to draw the blood and test it for bloodborne pathogens.

Donors should be 17 years of age or older, weigh at least 110 pounds, and have a temperature of 99.5°F or lower, blood pressure no higher than 180/100 mm Hg, a pulse rate between 50 and 100, and a hemoglobin level of 12.5 g/dL or higher. The donor should also appear to be in good health.

Donors are asked an extensive list of questions regarding their previous medical history, medications currently being taken, and their social habits particularly related to bloodborne pathogen exposure. Persons performing this interview must be certain that all questions are fully understood by the donor and that the donor understands the importance of a truthful answer to the future health of the recipient. It is also required that all donors be given a private opportunity to indicate that after the unit is collected, it should not be used for transfusion. There are two boxes on the donor consent form, one giving permission to use the blood for transfusion and one denying permission to use the blood. A donor who for social reasons wants to donate blood but who knows the blood should not be used can check the "do not transfuse" box. The form is sealed until the unit is being processed. Another method is to provide the donor with two barcode labels (Use or Do Not Use), and the donor attaches the appropriate label to the collected unit. The unit is then scanned for acceptability during processing.

technical tip Be very careful to put donors at ease during the interview process.

Donor Collection

Units of blood are collected into sterile, closed systems consisting of one or more plastic bags connected to tubing and a sterile needle. Large-gauge needles (15 to 16 regular gauge or 17 gauge thin-walled) are used for collection of donor units, both to prevent hemolysis and to facilitate collection of the large amount of blood. Thin-walled needles provide a larger bore without increasing the diameter of the needle, so that there is less discomfort for the donor. The plastic bags fill by gravity and must be located below the collection site. They are frequently placed in an automatic mixing device that is also designed to stop when the unit reaches a weight that is consistent with the appropriate volume of blood. **Hemostats** may be applied to the tubing to start and stop the flow of blood into the bag.

A large vein, usually located in the antecubital area, is necessary to accommodate the large needle and supply the required amount of blood. A tourniquet or blood pressure cuff is used to facilitate vein selection. Aseptic site preparation is essential to prevent introduction of microorganisms into the unit of blood. Cleansing is a two-step process, beginning with a soap or dilute iodine scrub and followed by application of more concentrated iodine or chlorhexidine that is allowed to dry for 30 seconds.

Venipuncture is performed in the usual manner, and when blood appears in the tubing, the needle is securely taped to the donor's arm. Donors are encouraged to open and close their fists during the collection to speed the flow of blood. In contrast to routine venipuncture, hemoconcentration is acceptable in donor blood. After removal of the needle, donors are instructed to elevate the arm and apply firm pressure to the puncture site. The phlebotomist completes any required procedures such as transferring blood from the tubing into tubes for testing and discards the needle. Labels corresponding to those on the unit collection bag must be attached to all additional tubes.

Donors should not be left alone during the collection period and should be carefully observed for dizziness or nausea during and after the collection. They are usually offered fruit juice and a snack before they leave the donor station.

Additional Donor Collection

A specialized area of blood donation is ***apheresis***. Apheresis is performed to collect a specific blood component such as platelets or plasma. Under sterile conditions, donor blood is anticoagulated and sent directly to a specialized separation instrument (centrifuge). The desired component is removed, and the remainder of the blood is returned to the donor. Apheresis donors are able to donate more frequently than whole blood donors. Donors may be able to donate platelets every two weeks up to 24 times a year. Plasma may be donated every 28 days. Donors frequently have unusual blood components that can be necessary for specific patients or can be of value for the manufacture of certain blood bank reagents. Phlebotomists must receive additional training to perform apheresis procedures.

Patients scheduled for elective surgery may choose to donate units of their own blood to be transfused back to them during their surgery if blood is needed. This is referred to as an ***autologous donation*** and has become a common procedure because of the concern about transmission of bloodborne pathogens. Patients may donate as often as every 72 hours, providing they have their healthcare provider's approval and a hemoglobin level of at least 11.0 g/dL.

Phlebotomists may also perform a procedure called a ***therapeutic phlebotomy***. In this procedure, a unit of blood is collected from patients with conditions causing overproduction of red blood cells (polycythemia) or iron (**hemochromatosis**). Patients requiring therapeutic phlebotomy are not as healthy as routine blood donors and should be carefully monitored during the collection period. Frequently, therapeutic phlebotomy is performed in a designated area of the laboratory or in a hospital unit and not in the donor station.

Because of the requirements of additional personnel, equipment, documentation of compliance with the regulations imposed by the AABB and the FDA and the legal responsibilities, not all hospitals have donor stations. However, most hospitals do perform therapeutic phlebotomy.

Receiving and Transporting Specimens

Phlebotomists encounter a variety of specimens other than those they personally collect. When collecting blood in the hospital units, they are often asked to transport specimens back to the laboratory. Many inpatient and outpatient specimens are delivered to the central processing area, and phlebotomists must be knowledgeable about any special handling requirements, the laboratory sections that analyze the specimens, and the laboratory policy for accepting specimens. A procedure manual detailing specimen requirements should be present in the central processing area.

In addition to urine, fecal, and semen specimens, common specimens received in the laboratory that are not collected by phlebotomists include cerebrospinal, synovial, pleural, pericardial, peritoneal (ascitic), and amniotic fluids; and tissue specimens. It is extremely important that phlebotomists recognize that these specimens are collected using procedures that are more invasive than phlebotomy. Patients are subjected to more discomfort and possible complications. Therefore, specimens should be transported and delivered to the appropriate department with high priority.

technical tip Many nonblood specimens such as CSF must be analyzed immediately to prevent loss of glucose and cellular elements.

Cerebrospinal fluid (CSF) is delivered in tubes usually numbered 1 through 3, representing the order in which the specimen was collected. Tube No. 1 is designated for chemistry, tube No. 2 for microbiology, and tube No. 3 for hematology. It is important that tubes be delivered in this order because tube No. 1 is more likely to contain cells or microorganisms obtained during the punctures and not actually present in the CSF.

Specimens such as synovial (joint), pleural (chest), pericardial (heart), and peritoneal (abdominal) fluids are frequently collected in evacuated tubes corresponding to those used for similar tests performed on blood. Specimens with a large quantity of fluid designated for cytology may also be received.

Amniotic fluid collected from the fetal sac may be tested for the presence of bilirubin, to monitor hemolytic disease of the newborn; and lipids, to determine fetal lung maturity. In addition, it may be examined by the cytogenetics section for the presence of abnormal chromosomes. Specimens for bilirubin analysis must be protected from light in the same manner as blood specimens, and specimens for cytogenetic analysis should be delivered immediately for processing to preserve the limited number of cells present.

Tissue specimens are routinely received in a preservative solution and are processed by the histology section. Specimens that are not preserved must be immediately delivered to the histology section.

When delivering specimens to laboratory sections, phlebotomists should be sure to alert the technical personnel about the specimen. If specimens are delivered to sections where no personnel are present, as may be the case on evening and night shifts, the phlebotomist must be aware of specimen preservation requirements. This information should be available in the procedure manual or may be posted in the section; it varies with the type of specimen and the section to which it is delivered. For example, CSF specimens are refrigerated in hematology and left at room temperature in microbiology.

Specimens accepted by phlebotomists, either on the units or in the laboratory, must be accompanied by a requisition form containing appropriate information and must have a label containing information that correlates with the requisition form. Specimens should be transported in biohazard bags.

technical tip Always consult the procedure manual whenever you are unsure of a specimen handling procedure

In some hospitals, specimens are transported to the laboratory through a ***pneumatic tube system***. Delivery of specimens through a pneumatic tube system is a very efficient method because both personnel time and delivery time are saved. Specimens must be properly cushioned to prevent breakage and enclosed in leak-proof material. Gloves should be worn when removing specimens from the specimen container (Fig. 12–6).

Specimen Processing, Accessioning, and Shipping

In some laboratories, particularly in large hospitals, phlebotomists may be involved in centrifuging, ***aliquoting***, and assigning accession numbers or bar codes to specimens before their delivery to the laboratory sections. They may also process and package specimens sent to reference laboratories.

Universal precautions must be strictly followed when processing all specimens. In accordance with Occupational Safety and Health Administration (OSHA) regulations, protective apparel must include

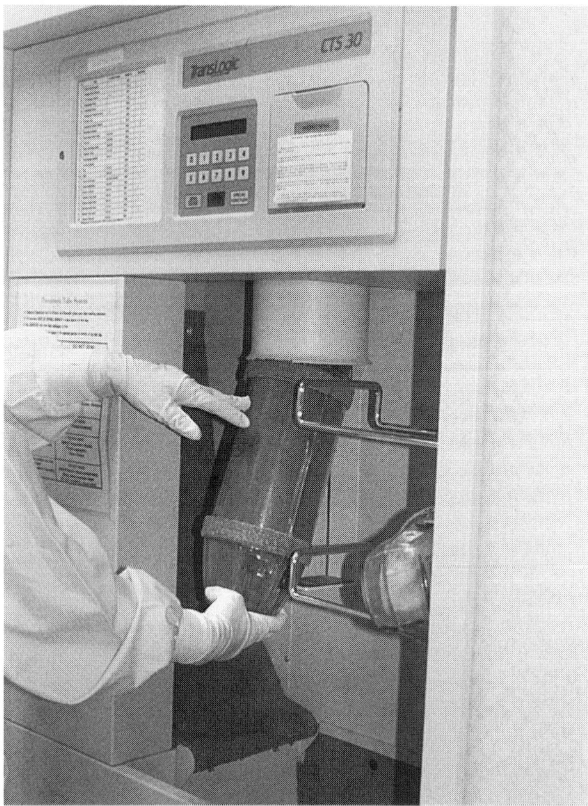

Figure 12–6 Loading specimens into a pneumatic tube system. (From Strasinger, SK, and Di Lorenzo, MS: Skills for the Patient Care Technician. FA Davis, Philadelphia, 1999, p. 252, with permission.)

gloves, fluid-resistant laboratory coats that are completely closed, and face shields with protective sides. Specimens must never be centrifuged in uncapped tubes.

Specimen processing involving centrifugation and aliquoting is primarily associated with laboratory tests performed on plasma and serum. Plasma is obtained by centrifugation of anticoagulated blood, and serum is similarly obtained from clotted blood. To prevent contamination of plasma and serum by cellular constituents, it is recommended that specimens be separated within 2 hours. Anticoagulated specimens can be centrifuged immediately after collection, and the plasma removed. Specimens collected without anticoagulant must be fully clotted before centrifugation. Clotting time can vary from 5 minutes, when clot activators are present, to an hour, for specimens from patients receiving anticoagulant therapy. Loosening clots from the side of the tube (rimming) before centrifugation is not recommended because it may cause hemolysis.

technical tip Blood specimens should be stored in an upright position while clotting.

In the accessioning area, there are a number of types of centrifuges available, including table models, floor models, and refrigerated models. The relative centrifugal force (**RCF**) of a centrifuge is expressed as gravity (*g*) and is determined by the radius of the rotor head and the speed of rotation (revolutions per minute [**rpm**]). Most laboratory specimens are centrifuged at 850 to 1000 g for 10 minutes. Improper use of the centrifuge can be dangerous, and the following rules of operation must be observed:

1 Tubes placed in the cups of the rotor head must be equally balanced. This is accomplished by placing tubes of equal size and volume directly across from each other. Failure to follow this practice will cause the centrifuge to vibrate and possibly break the tubes. A final check for balancing should be made just before closing the centrifuge lid.
2 A centrifuge should never be operated until the top has been firmly fastened down, and the top should never be opened until the rotor head has come to a complete stop. Should a tube break during centrifugation, pieces of glass and biohazardous aerosols will be sprayed from a centrifuge that is not covered.
3 Do not walk away from a centrifuge until it has reached its designated rotational speed and no evidence of excessive vibration is observed.
4 When a tube breaks in the centrifuge, immediately stop the centrifuge and unplug it before opening the cover. Don puncture-resistant gloves before beginning the cleanup. The cup containing the broken glass must be completely emptied into a puncture-resistant container and disinfected. The inside of the centrifuge must also be cleaned of broken glass and disinfected. Deposit any cleaning materials that may contain broken glass into a puncture-resistant container.

Specimen Aliquoting

Separation of serum and plasma from the cellular elements and specimen aliquoting require careful attention to detail so that specimens are placed in properly labeled tubes. Care must also be taken to prevent the formation of aerosols when stoppers are removed from evacuated tubes. As discussed in Chapter 5, stoppers should be covered with gauze and twisted rather than "popped" off. Specimens must never be poured from one tube to another, because this will produce aerosols. A Plexiglas shield should be used when aliquoting specimens (Fig. 12–7).

A variety of transfer systems is available. All systems are designed to prevent the formation of aerosols and to provide minimum contact with the specimen by laboratory personnel. Some automated instruments are equipped to sample directly from the sealed tube.

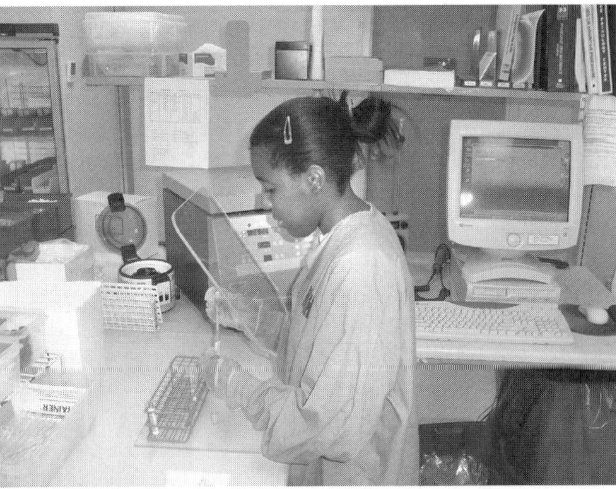

Figure 12–7 Blood specimen processing.

Specimen Shipping

Specimens collected from home healthcare or nursing home patients and specimens being transported between laboratories must be appropriately packaged for transport. The United States Department of Transportation regulates the interstate shipping of infectious substances and diagnostic specimens, and stipulates strict guidelines for packaging and labeling. Many of these requirements can apply to local specimen transport.

Specimens for local transport should be placed in securely closed, leak-proof primary containers (tubes and screw-top containers). The primary containers are enclosed in a secondary leak-proof container with sufficient absorbent material present to separate the specimens and absorb the contents of the primary containers in case of leakage or breakage. Containers should be labeled as biohazardous. Specimens can be kept cool by transporting them in Styrofoam containers using plastic refrigerant packs. Refrigerant packs should not be placed directly on or against specimen containers. Specimens that must remain frozen are packaged in carbon dioxide permeable containers with dry ice.

When preparing specimens for transport to reference laboratories, information provided by the reference laboratory regarding specimen stability, type of specimen, and volume required must be consulted. Many laboratories contract with a particular reference laboratory that may pick up specimens on a daily basis or provide specific packaging materials. Personnel preparing specimens for shipping must be sure all specimens are properly labeled. Appropriate requisition forms must accompany the specimens. They should be protected from accidental specimen contamination.

Specimens requiring refrigeration can be shipped in Styrofoam containers with refrigerant packs of ice enclosed in a leak-proof bag. Specimens that must remain frozen are packaged in containers with dry ice.

technical tip Most blood specimens should be kept cool when being transported between off-site locations.

Use of the Laboratory Computer

In recent years, computers have become an essential part of the laboratory. Phlebotomists are in frequent contact with the laboratory computer through the generation of requisitions and specimen labels, registration of outpatients, and the logging in of specimens personally collected or received from other locations. They should understand the basic components of computer systems, be able to enter and retrieve data, be willing to learn new applications as the laboratory computer system expands, and realize that computers are intended to increase the efficiency and accuracy of patient care.

Most people have some experience using micro or personal computers in school, the workplace, or at home. The differences between these computers and laboratory computers are primarily the amount of information that can be processed, the speed of processing, and the ability to transfer information to other computers. Therefore, the actual computer operated by a phlebotomist appears to be no different than a familiar school or home model, although it may be connected to a higher-powered mainframe computer for transfer and storage of data. Data can be transferred among the laboratory sections or other hospital departments and by computer-telephone-cable connections to outside agencies such as healthcare providers' offices. In many laboratories, employees are assigned computer mailboxes through which they can receive intralaboratory communications, that is, notification of meetings, telephone messages, and procedural changes.

Many application programs for laboratory use are currently available, and the decision to use a particular program is determined by the requirements of the laboratory. These laboratory information management systems (LIMS) or laboratory information systems (**LIS**) may be used only by the laboratory or may be integrated into a hospital-wide computer system. Companies that provide LIMS work closely with the laboratory staff to adapt the system to correspond with particular laboratory operations.

Phlebotomists first encounter a LIMS through the receipt of computer-generated requisitions and specimen labels. They must learn to recognize the information provided, to be sure that it corresponds with the required information discussed in Chapter 6, and to compare this information with the information on the specimen labels. Many computer-generated requisitions also provide the phlebotomist with the number and type of tubes to be collected.

Phlebotomists required to input or retrieve data with the computer are assigned a password that allows them to use the computer. The purpose of the password is to provide computer security so that patient data are available only to authorized personnel. Phlebotomists should understand that any computer transaction performed when their password has been used to enter the computer can be traced back to them; therefore, the password should not be given to other persons. New government regulations to protect the privacy of patient healthcare records (discussed in Chapter 14) have increased the importance of password protection.

Data are frequently entered or retrieved with computers with the help of codes, which can be numeric (1 = retrieve information) or memory-aiding abbreviations (**mnemonics**), such as typing *RI* to retrieve information. The method varies with the system in use. Another method of data entry is the use of bar codes, from which information can be scanned into the computer by a specially designed light source (this method has been used in retail stores for many years). The black and white stripes of varying width on a bar code correspond to letters and numbers, and are grouped together to represent patient names, identification numbers, and laboratory tests. As discussed earlier, use of bar code systems decreases the possibility of laboratory error caused by clerical mistakes.

New reimbursement requirements for Medicare and other third-party payers require documentation of the medical necessity of laboratory and other medical procedures. This documentation requires the use of standardized codes by both the healthcare provider and the department performing the tests or procedures. Patient conditions or symptoms are classified using the International Classification of Disease, 9th edition (**ICD-9**), which will continue to be updated. Healthcare providers ordering tests primarily on outpatients must provide the ICD-9 code on the request. Laboratory tests are also coded using Current Procedure Terminology (**CPT**) codes. For reimbursement purposes, the CPT code (laboratory test) should be consistent with the medical necessity of the ICD-9 code (patient diagnosis). Depending on the institution, phlebotomists may need to enter CPT codes into the computer, particularly when drawing from outpatients.

Additional computer duties for phlebotomists may include generation and retrieval of collection lists and schedules, posting of patient charges, computing monthly phlebotomy workloads, and retrieving information for personnel in healthcare providers' offices (Fig. 12–8). Because of the variety of laboratory information systems available, the

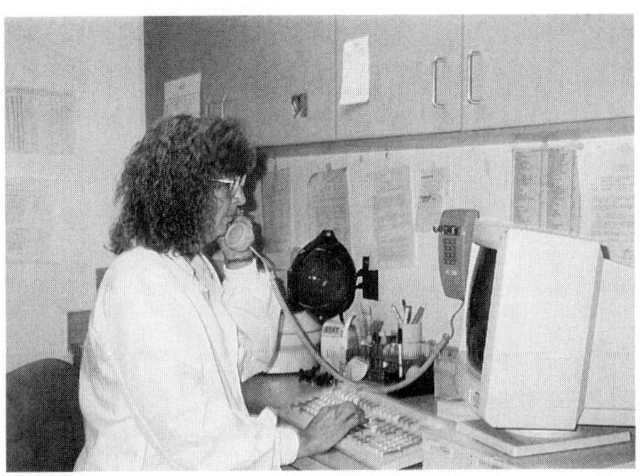

Figure 12–8 Phlebotomist using a laboratory computer.

major learning requirement of a technically trained phlebotomist (or other laboratory worker) when entering a new job is usually the operation of the computer system. This can only increase as laboratories expand their computer applications.

Bibliography

Harmening, DM: Modern Blood Banking and Transfusion Practices. FA Davis, Philadelphia, 1999.

Henry, JB: Clinical Diagnosis and Management by Laboratory Methods. WB Saunders, Philadelphia, 1996.

National Committee for Clinical Laboratory Standards Approved Standard C34-A2: Sweat Collection: Sample Collection and Quantitative Analysis. NCCLS, Wayne, PA, 2000.

Strasinger, SK, and Di Lorenzo, MS: Urinalysis and Body Fluids, ed. 4. FA Davis, Philadelphia, 2001.

Study Questions

1. If a urine specimen cannot be delivered to the laboratory within 2 hours, how should the specimen be stored?

____

2. State the specific type of specimen a patient should be instructed to collect for the following tests.

   a. Urine culture

   ____

   b. Quantitative fecal fat

   ____

   c. Routine urinalysis

   ____

   d. Ova and parasites

   ____

   e. Follow-up urinalysis

   ____

   f. Quantitative urine creatinine

   ____

3. Name a specimen and test that patients collect on filter paper.

____

4. Why should a patient begin and end a timed urine collection period with an empty bladder?

____

5. True or False. A patient delivers a semen specimen for fertility studies to the laboratory in a condom. He should be given a sterile container and told to collect another specimen in 3 days. Explain your answer.

____

6. What information (other than patient ID) must be placed on the requisition that accompanies a semen specimen?

____

7. Describe the areas that should be swabbed when collecting a throat culture.

____

8. Name three areas that should be avoided when collecting a throat culture.

   a. ______________________________

   b. ______________________________

   c. ______________________________

9. Sweat electrolytes are collected to confirm the diagnosis of

   ______________________________.

10. List three collection errors that could produce falsely elevated sweat electrolytes.

   a. ______________________________

   b. ______________________________

   c. ______________________________

11. The name of the technique used for collection of sweat electrolytes is

   ______________________________.

12. State the purpose of:

   a. An autologous donation

   ____

   b. A therapeutic phlebotomy

   ____

   c. Apheresis

   ____

13. State the reason for the following parts of the donor selection process.

   a. Identification information

   ____

   ____

   b. Physical examination

   ____

   ____

   c. Medical and social history

   ____

   ____

14. Place a "Q" for qualify or a "D" for disqualify in front of the following results of a donor selection process.

a. ______________________ Weight: 220 pounds

b. ______________________ Hemoglobin: 11.0 g/dL

c. ______________________ Rehabilitated heroin user

d. ______________________ Blood pressure: 160/90 mm Hg

e. ______________________ Temperature: 100°F

15. Why do the following procedures in the collection of donor blood differ from those of routine venipuncture?

a. Cleansing the site

____

____

b. Needle gauge

____

____

c. Clenching and unclenching of donor's fist

____

____

16. CSF specimens labeled No. 1, No. 2, and No. 3 are delivered to the laboratory. What section should they be delivered to? Indicate the specimen least affected by outside contamination.

a. ______________ No. ______________

b. ______________ No. ______________

c. ______________ No. ______________

17 Match the following specimens with the area of the body from which they were collected.

Specimen		**Body Area**
a. ______________	Ascitic fluid	1. Heart
b. ______________	Synovial fluid	2. Lymph node
c. ______________	Pericardial fluid	3. Joint
d. ______________	Pleural fluid	4. Abdomen
		5. Chest

18. State a special handling requirement for amniotic fluid to be tested for hemolytic disease of the newborn.

____

19. List two reasons why a specimen delivered to the central processing area would be unacceptable.

    a. ____

    b. ____

20. What protective apparel must be worn when processing body fluid specimens?

____

21. True or False. Specimens collected in light blue stopper tubes must be allowed to sit for 30 minutes before centrifugation. Explain your answer.

____

22. List two factors that determine the RCF of a centrifuge.

    a. ____

    b. ____

23. State three causes of aerosol production when processing specimens.

    a. ____

    b. ____

    c. ____

24. What is the purpose of placing a primary specimen container into a secondary container before transporting the specimen from a patient's home to the laboratory?

____

25. Name two advantages of a LIMS.

    a. ____

    b. ____

26. Given the following tubes and spaces in a centrifuge rotor head, show how you would balance the centrifuge by placing the numbers of the appropriate tubes in the space on the rotor head.

____

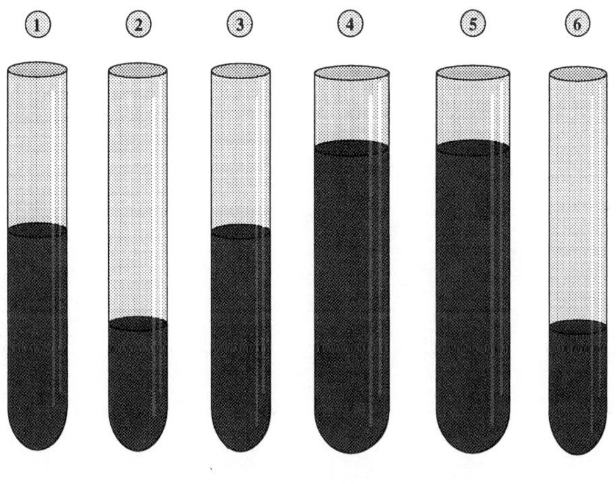

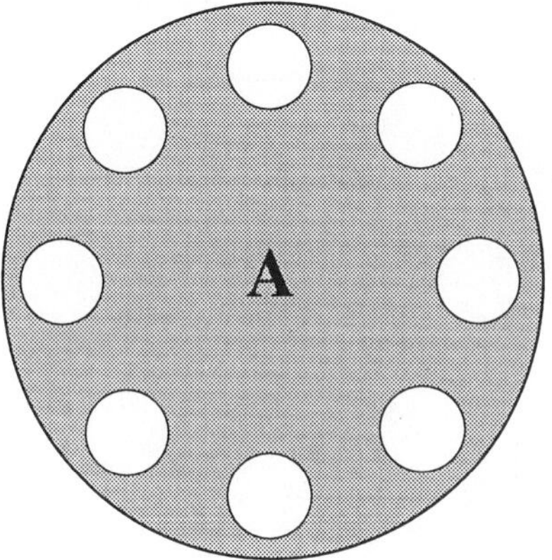

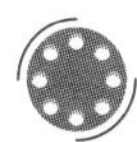

Clinical Situations

1. A patient delivering a 24-hour urine specimen to the laboratory mentions that he or she did not save a small amount of urine voided while visiting a neighbor.

   a. What should the patient be told?

   ____

   b. How would this affect the test result?

   ____

2. What should a phlebotomist do in the following situations?

   a. An unwitnessed urine drug collection has a temperature of 30°C.

   ____

   b. A table model centrifuge begins to noticeably vibrate.

   ____

c. A specimen of pleural fluid is received in a lavender stopper tube.

____

3. A supervisor counsels a phlebotomist because two computer entry errors on the previous day were traced back to the phlebotomist. The phlebotomist states that he/she did not use the computer that day.

   a. How could this have occurred?

   ____

   b. How could it be avoided?

   ____

4. A phlebotomist delivers Tube No. 1 of a CSF specimen to the hematology department and Tube No. 3 to the chemistry department.

   a. Will the hematology result be affected? Explain your answer.

   ____

   ____

   b. Will the chemistry result be affected? Explain your answer.

   ____

Chapter 13

Point-of-Care Testing

Chapter Outline

Regulation of Point-of-Care Testing

Quality Control

Procedures

- Blood Glucose
- Transcutaneous Bilirubin Testing
- Hemoglobin
- Urinalysis
- Occult Blood
- Pregnancy Testing
- Strep Tests
- Whole Blood Immunoassay Kits
- Blood Coagulation Testing
- Cholesterol
- Arterial Blood Gas and Electrolyte Analyzers
- Future Applications

Learning Objectives

Upon completion of this chapter, the reader will be able to:

1. Define point-of-care testing (POCT), identify the synonyms associated with POCT, and state various locations performing POCT.
2. Discuss the advantages of POCT.
3. State the regulations required for POCT and the qualifications required for healthcare personnel to perform testing.
4. Explain the POCT quality control procedures for CLIA '88 compliance.
5. Describe the tests and instrumentation commonly used in POCT.

Key Terms

Calibration
Control
Critical value
Point-of-care testing
Proficiency testing
Quality control
Reagent
Shift
Trend
Turn-around time

Point-of-care testing (**POCT**), often referred to as alternate site testing, near-patient testing, or ancillary testing, is the performance of laboratory tests at the patient's bedside or nearby rather than in a central laboratory. POCT uses portable devices or simple reagent test kits different from those used in the central laboratory. POCT is frequently performed at the bedside of a hospitalized patient and is particularly beneficial to patient care in the critical care or intensive care unit, operating room, emergency department, or neonatal intensive care unit. Other POCT models include satellite laboratories, mobile carts that go from room to room, physician offices, ambulatory clinics, health maintenance organizations, ambulances or helicopters, nursing homes, workplace screenings, dialysis centers, and home settings.

Factors that have motivated the practice of POCT include the increased acuteness of inpatient illnesses that require a faster ***turn-around-time*** (TAT) of results and the decreased length of hospital stays that require the increased performance of procedures and care on an outpatient basis. TAT is defined as the time from when the healthcare provider orders the test until the result is returned to the healthcare provider. The shorter the TAT, the sooner the healthcare provider can treat the patient. In critical care units, the TAT of stat tests is of the utmost importance in providing the best possible patient care.

POCT is well suited to the concept of patient-focused care, which brings the caregivers to the patient rather than taking the patient to the service. The immediate availability of test results provides convenience to both the patient and the healthcare provider by decreasing the time required for diagnosis and treatment, resulting in faster patient recovery. This streamlined workflow provides more effective healthcare provider-patient interaction because the clinical signs, symptoms, and test results can be evaluated immediately for patient treatment, reducing follow-up visits for patients. Quick and accurate test results enable the patient to be treated on the spot, thereby improving patient outcomes.

The growing popularity and scope of POCT is a result of the rapidly evolving technology. Small, hand-held, user-friendly instruments provide mobility, low maintenance, ease of use, cost effectiveness, compliance with the Clinical Laboratory Improvement Amendments of 1988 (CLIA '88), and most important, reliable test results when properly used. Most tests require only a drop of whole blood obtained by dermal puncture using a single lancet versus collecting a tube of blood using venipuncture equipment. This feature not only decreases the specimen acquisition cost but also is an advantage for geriatric or pediatric patients in whom **iatrogenic** anemia is a concern. Another advantage of POCT is the decreased chance of preanalytical errors that occur with specimen labeling, transporting, and processing.

There are many tests available from a variety of reputable manufacturers, and new POCT procedures and instruments are continuously being developed. The importance of proper instrument maintenance and ***calibration***, ***quality control*** (**QC**), and **documentation** is the same for all instruments and procedures. Healthcare professionals performing POCT must be trained to collect the specimen correctly and understand the quality assurance (**QA**) criteria involved in performing laboratory tests. Persons performing POCT include phlebotomists, nurses, physicians, residents, medical students, respiratory therapists, medical assistants, rescue workers, perfusionists, patient care technicians, medical technologists, and patients. Medical technologists perform the least number of POCTs, but the laboratory is often responsible for administering the POCTs program. CLIA '88 regulates the qualifications for healthcare personnel authorized to perform POCT.

Regulation of Point-of-Care Testing

The CLIA '88 encompasses all laboratory testing and requires every testing site examining "specimens derived from the human body for the purpose of providing information for the diagnosis, prevention or treatment of disease, or impairment of or assessment of health" to be regulated. All testing sites are subject to CLIA '88 and must be licensed based on the test complexity model regardless of the number of tests performed or whether there is a charge for the test.

The Center for Medicare and Medicaid Services (CMS), formerly known as the Health Care Financing Administration (HCFA), administers CLIA '88 and requires CLIA certification for reimbursement of laboratory tests. CMS grants deemed status to agencies that have demonstrated equivalency with CLIA '88 standards. These agencies include the Commission on Laboratory Assessment (COLA), which is popular with physician office laboratories; the Joint Commission on the Accreditation of Healthcare Organizations (JCAHO), and the College of American Pathologists (CAP), which primarily serves larger laboratories.

Under CLIA '88, all clinical laboratories, regardless of location, size, or type, must meet standards based on the complexity of the tests that they perform. Test complexity is determined by the testing characteristics such as stability of the reagent, preparation of the reagent, operational steps, calibration, and QC. Complexity also depends on the degree of knowledge, training, experience, troubleshooting, and interpretation required in the testing process. The complexity level of the highest complexity test performed determines the level of certification required. The Food and Drug Administration (FDA) has the responsibility for categorizing tests and classifying testing devices and systems. Three levels of testing complexity were defined in the original regulation: waived, moderate complexity, and high complexity. Laboratories performing moderate or high complexity testing must meet requirements for ***proficiency testing***, patient test management, QC, QA, and personnel. The major differences in regulatory requirements between moderate and high complexity testing are in the QC and personnel standards. Most POCT is in the waived or moderate complexity categories.

Waived tests are defined as simple laboratory examinations and procedures that are cleared by the FDA for home use; employ methodologies that are so simple and accurate as to render the likelihood of erroneous results negligible; or pose no reasonable risk of harm to the patient if the test is performed incorrectly. Waived tests are considered easy to perform and interpret, require no special training or educational background, and require only minimum QC. This category has been greatly expanded from the original eight tests that were listed as meeting these criteria in 1988 (Table 13–1). Table 13–2 lists the current CLIA '88 waived tests. This list continues to grow as new test kits and instrumentation are developed. To perform waived testing, the organization must obtain a Certificate of Waiver from the CMS and follow manufacturers' directions for the testing process. Many waived tests, such as glucose monitoring and pregnancy tests, are available over the counter to all consumers.

TABLE 13-1
Original CLIA '88–Waived Tests

Blood glucose
Dipstick or tablet reagent urinalysis
Erythrocyte sedimentation rate (nonautomated)
Fecal occult blood
Hemoglobin by copper sulfate (nonautomated)
Ovulation tests
Spun hematocrit
Urine pregnancy tests

technical tip Tests are continually being developed and added to the waived test category. For an up-to-date listing of waived tests, refer to *www.cms.hhs.gov/clia*

The first CLIA '88 modification created a new certificate category for provider-performed microscopy (**PPM**) procedures. The new category included certain procedures that can be performed in conjunction with any waived test and includes clinical microscopy procedures only.

The tests within this new category can be performed only by physician's assistants, nurse practitioners, physicians, and dentists during a patient's examination. In addition, laboratories performing these tests must meet the moderate complexity requirements for proficiency testing, patient test management, QC, and QA as required by the accreditation agency. CLIA '88 PPM tests are listed in Table 13–3.

Moderate complexity tests are more difficult to perform than are waived tests and require documentation of training in testing principles, instrument calibration, and QC. Many laboratory tests in chemistry and hematology have been assigned to this category. Facilities performing moderate complexity tests are subject to proficiency testing and on-site inspections. In institutions with CAP, JCAHO, and COLA accreditation, waived tests also must adhere to most of the moderate complexity test standards. In most hospitals and large institutions, the clinical laboratory administers the training, proficiency testing, and monitoring of QC. Persons performing POCT may

TABLE 13-2
Current CLIA '88–Waived Tests

Alanine aminotransferase (ALT[SGPT])	*Helicobacter pylori*
Alcohol, saliva	Hemoglobin by copper sulfate, HemoCue
Amines	Infectious mononucleosis antibodies (mono)
Amphetamines	Influenza A/B
Bladder tumor–associated antigen	Ketones
Cannabinoids (THC)	Lactic acid (lactate)
Catalase, urine	**Luteinizing hormone (LH)**
Cholesterol	Lyme disease antibodies
Cocaine metabolites	Methamphetamines
Collagen type I crosslink, N-telopeptides (NXT)	Microalbumin
Creatinine	Morphine
Erythrocyte sedimentation rate (nonautomated)	Nicotine and/or metabolites
Estrone-3 glucuronide	Opiates
Ethanol (alcohol)	Ovulation test (LH)
Fecal occult blood	pH
Fern test, saliva	Phencyclidine (PCP)
Follicle-stimulating hormone (FSH)	Prothrombin time (PT)
Fructosamine	Semen
Gastric occult blood	Spun hematocrit
Gastric pH	Streptococcus, group A
Glucose	Triglyceride
Glycosylated hemoglobin (HGB A1C)	Urine dipstick
HCG, urine pregnancy test	Vaginal pH
HDL cholesterol	

be required to demonstrate testing competency on a periodic basis.

High complexity tests require sophisticated instrumentation and a high degree of interpretation by the testing personnel. Personnel performing high complexity tests must have formal education with a degree in laboratory medicine. Most tests performed in microbiology, immunology, immunohematology, and cytology are in this category. They are not performed as POCT.

TABLE 13-3
CLIA '88 PPM Tests

Fecal leukocyte examination
Fern test
Potassium hydroxide (KOH) preparation
Nasal smear for eosinophils
Pinworm examination
Qualitative semen analysis
Urine sediment examination
Wet mounts (vaginal, cervical, skin, or prostatic secretions)

Laboratories performing moderate or high complexity tests must be inspected every 2 years. Waived and PPM laboratories are not subject to routine inspection, although a certain number are inspected to ensure compliance or when a complaint has been filed. Inspections must be announced and are done within the first 2 years of certification. CAP performs an initial inspection for sites seeking CAP accreditation, and every 2 years thereafter. When requested, JCAHO accepts CAP and COLA inspections and reinspects waived testing as part of hospital accreditation. CMS has state inspectors who inspect testing sites seeking only CLIA accreditation. CLIA inspection standards are the federal standards of CLIA '88 and are listed in the Federal Register. Requirements of each agency follow CLIA regulations, but other requirements may differ. Each testing site must decide on an accrediting agency and follow its standards. CLIA '88 regulations include patient test management assessment, QC assessment, proficiency testing assessment, comparison of test results, relationship of patient information to patient test results, personnel assessment, communications, complaint investigation, QA review with staff, and QA records.

Patient test management includes methods of patient preparation, proper specimen collection, sample identification, sample preservation, sample transportation, sample processing, and accurate result reporting. The testing site must have and follow written procedures for these methods so that specimen integrity and identification are maintained from the pretesting through the post-testing process.

QC must include records of the date, results, testing personnel, lot numbers, and expiration dates for reagents and controls. These must be retained for 2 years. It is recommended that records be reviewed daily, as well as monthly, in order to detect trends, shifts, unstable test systems, or operator difficulties.

All laboratories performing moderate or high complexity testing must enroll in an approved proficiency-testing program. This program involves three events per year, with five challenges per analyte in the survey material. All survey samples are tested in the same manner as patient specimens. No communication with other laboratories is permitted.

Personnel assessment includes education and training, continuing education, competency assessment, and performance appraisals. Each complexity level has its own requirements and is identified per CLIA requirements.

Each new employee must have documentation of training during orientation to the laboratory. This is a checklist of procedures and must include date and initials of the person doing the training and of the employee being trained.

CLIA mandates continuing education, although no minimum hours are given. A record of all applicable continuing education sessions should be maintained. The personnel file must include a certificate of the education level of each employee performing laboratory testing.

Competency assessment as mandated by CLIA must be done for each employee for each procedure twice the first year of employment and then annually. Methods for assessing competency include direct observation, review of QC records, review of proficiency testing records, and written assessments. Performance appraisals are done according to institution protocol and include standards of performance linked to the job description. The standards may include evaluation of organizational and communication skills and attitude.

The laboratory must maintain patient test records for 2 years, blood banking for 5 years, and pathology/cytology for 10 years. Other records that must be kept include QC, reagent logs, proficiency testing, competency assessment, education and training, equipment maintenance, service calls, documentation of problems, complaints, and communications, inspection files, and certification records.

Quality Control

QC of testing procedures is part of a much larger system referred to as QA, the purpose of which is to provide overall quality patient care. QA includes written policies and documented actions that are used to evaluate the entire testing process from test ordering and specimen collection through reporting and interpreting of results. QC procedures are performed to ensure that acceptable standards for **accuracy** and **precision** are being met during the process of specimen testing to provide reliable results. QC includes internal and external QC, proficiency testing, calibration or calibration verification, and equipment maintenance. Performance and monitoring of QC are a major part of POCT, performed to verify that instrumentation is functioning properly and has been accurately calibrated, that ***reagents*** are stable and are reacting appropriately, and that the testing is being performed correctly (methodology and standards of performance). The person performing patient testing must be the person performing the QC. However, QC does not verify the integrity of the patient specimen. Collection procedures discussed in previous chapters must be followed.

QC is performed at scheduled times, such as at the beginning of each shift and before testing patient samples, and it must always be performed if an instrument is dropped or if test results are questioned by the healthcare provider. Laboratory guidelines depend on the accrediting agency and the manufacturer's recommendation. POCT procedures or instruments may include electronic ***controls***, calibration verification, optical checks, procedural controls, and external manufactured controls. Commercial controls are manufactured specimens with known values, and they are available in several strengths, such as abnormal low, normal, and abnormal high ranges, or positive and negative depending on the test being performed. The concentration of controls should be at medically significant levels and be as much like the human specimen as possible. At least two levels of assayed controls are used to evaluate daily performance of instruments. Many waived tests have internal procedural controls that indicate that the test was performed correctly and that it was completed.

Documentation of QC includes dating and initialing the material when it is first opened and recording the manufacturer's lot number and the expiration date each time a control is run and the test result obtained (Fig. 13–1). Controls are plotted on QC charts, usually Levy-Jennings charts, which indicate the mean and the control range. Results should fall within the range of two standard deviations (± 2SD) 95% of the time, and the values should be evenly distributed on either side of the mean, confirming precision and accuracy. Two consecutive values cannot fall outside of the two standard deviations, and no value should exceed three standard deviations. Controls should be plotted at the time of testing and in the order of measurement. Separate charts are required for each test and each level of control. Some POCT instruments have QC data management software that does this automatically (Fig. 13–2). These instruments can be programmed to lock out all patient testing if a control value falls outside the established control ranges and if QC has not been performed within the allotted time frame. Six sudden consecutive values on one side of the mean indicate a ***shift*** that may be caused by a malfunction of the instrument or a new lot number of reagents. A gradual increase or decrease for six consecutive values indicates a ***trend*** that may be caused by a gradual deterioration of reagents or deterioration of instrument performance. QC charts provide a visual display of statistical information that monitors shifts or trends in the testing procedure or instrument (Fig. 13–3).

Patient results must not be reported if QC is out of control. Patient results are reported with reference and interpretive ranges. There must be written procedures for handling abnormal control and patient results. Corrective action for abnormal control results or errors in reporting patient results must be taken and documented. Individuals performing the testing must be identified on the patient report. Various POCT instruments require that an operator use a unique personal identification number, which allows all QC testing to be identified and monitored. Instrument maintenance checks and function checks must be performed and documented. A designated supervisor reviews all patient results, QC, and instrument maintenance results.

technical tip Patient test results can never be reported if the QC test results are not in range. The problem must be resolved and the test repeated.

Procedures

CLIA '88 requires that laboratories performing POCT follow manufacturer's guidelines; therefore, testing personnel must read the entire **package insert** or procedure manual before performing the test. The information in package inserts includes specimen collection and handling, safety precautions regarding biologic, chemical, electrical, and mechanical hazards; instrument maintenance and calibration; reagent storage requirements; acceptable control ranges; specimen requirements; procedural steps; interpretation of results and normal values; and sources of error. Manufacturers also provide training materials and assistance in troubleshooting technical problems.

Areas in which POCT is performed are required to maintain a procedure manual that is readily available to all testing personnel. The procedure manual contains the information provided in the package inserts from the instrumentation, reagents, and controls for each procedure. It also contains site-specific information, such as the location of supplies, instructions for reporting and recording results, and the protocol to follow when critically low or high test results (***critical values***) are encountered. Training for personnel performing POCT includes reading both the package inserts and the procedure manual thoroughly, and demonstrating an understanding of the information. It is important to understand that POCT procedures vary among manufacturers; therefore, package inserts and procedures in the procedure manual are not interchangeable.

This chapter provides a general overview of some of the commonly performed POCT procedures and does not include all of the material that would be found in the package inserts or a procedure manual. It also does not include all of the many currently available tests and instruments.

Test Strip Lot # ________________ Control Code: __________________ Exp. Date: __________
Low Control Lot # ____________ Low Control QC Range: ________________ Exp. Date: __________
High Control Lot # ____________ High Control QC Range: ________________ Exp. Date: __________

DATE	PATIENT NAME (Or use patient label)	PATIENT ID	DOCTOR	PATIENT RESULT	LOW CONTROL	HIGH CONTROL	TECH

Reviewed by: ________________________________ **Date:** ______________

Figure 13–1 SureStep® Whole Blood Glucose Patient/Quality Control Log. (Courtesy of Brenda L. M. Franks, MT[ASCP], POCT Coordinator, Nebraska Methodist Hospital, Omaha, NE.)

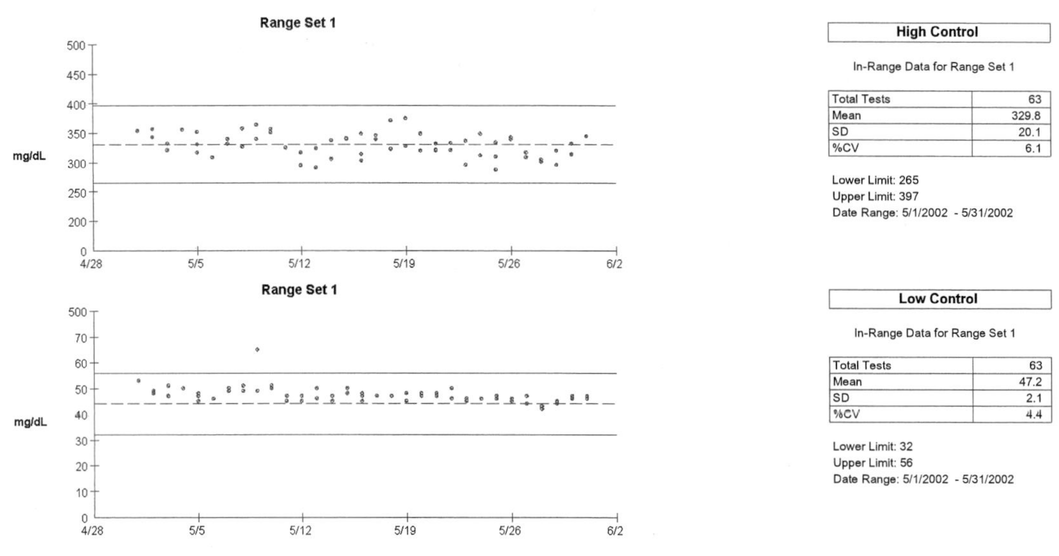

Figure 13–2 LifeScan DataLink Data Management System® Trend Graph Report. (Courtesy of Lifescan, Milpitas, CA.)

Blood Glucose

Measurement of blood glucose is performed as POCT primarily to monitor persons with diabetes mellitus to determine whether their diet and insulin dosage are maintaining an acceptable level of glucose in the body. Testing may also be performed in an outpatient setting to screen persons for the presence of diabetes mellitus. Normal values for blood glucose vary slightly among testing procedures and are higher when serum or plasma, instead of whole blood, is tested in the clinical laboratory. POCT must be performed on whole blood; however, most of the newer bedside glucose meters report a plasma equivalent result. It is important to know what type of result the glucose meter reports so that the glucose results are interpreted correctly. POCT glucose normal values are approximately 60 to 115 mg/dL in a fasting blood sugar. Levels below 60 mg/dL are termed hypoglycemic, and increased levels are termed hyperglycemic. The phlebotomist should be aware of the established critical value levels for blood glucose and notify the appropriate personnel immediately when they are encountered.

Many varieties of blood glucose POCT instrumentation are available, and the specific manufacturer's instructions for each instrument must be followed. The methodology may be photometric (Lifescan SureStep®) or electrochemical (Roche Comfort Curve) and use different reagents in the test strip. The SureStep® (LifeScan, Inc., Milpitas, CA), Accucheck II (Boehringer Mannheim Diagnostics, Indianapolis, IN), and ONE TOUCH II (Life Scan, Inc., Milpitas, CA) employ dry reagent technology using a special reagent test strip (Fig. 13–4). A glucose oxidase reaction occurs between the blood and reagents in the test strip, resulting in the formation of a blue color. The intensity of the blue color formed correlates with the concentration of glucose in the sample.

The reagent test strips must be stored in tightly closed containers and protected from heat, and they should not be used if they appear discolored or are past their expiration date. Care must be taken not to

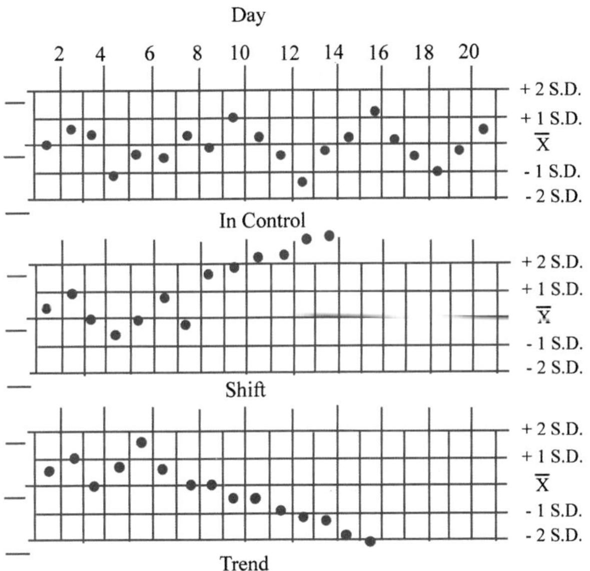

Figure 13–3 Levy-Jennings charts showing in-control results, trend, and shift. (From Strasinger, SK, and Di Lorenzo, MS: Urinalysis and Body Fluids, ed. 4. FA Davis, Philadelphia, 2001, p. 115, with permission.)

contaminate the testing area by rubbing it against the patient's skin or touching the pad before collection. Each container of test strips has a code number. The analyzer code number must be set to match the code number of the reagent strip container.

Whole blood obtained by dermal puncture is preferred, but some instruments can use blood samples collected in citrate, heparin, or ethylenediaminetetraacetic acid (EDTA) anticoagulant tubes. The appropriate area of the reagent strip is covered with a drop of blood and is inserted into the instrument. Applying too small a drop of blood to the test strip may cause falsely decreased values, and too much blood may falsely elevate results. The level of blood glucose is measured, and the results are displayed on a screen. Error codes appear if the sample did not completely cover the test area.

The HemoCue® Glucose 201 Analyzer (HemoCue, Inc., Mission Viejo, CA) analyzes arterial, venous, and capillary whole blood specimens. HemoCue® technology uses dual wavelength photometry and specially designed cuvettes containing freeze-dried reagents instead of a test strip. Five microliters of blood is drawn into the disposable cuvette by capillary action, where it mixes with the freeze-dried reagents. The plasma equivalent result is displayed on completion of the reaction. (Fig. 13–5).

technical tip If incorrect amounts of blood are applied to the test strip, use a new strip because the meter cannot accurately read glucose results when blood is reapplied to the original test strip.

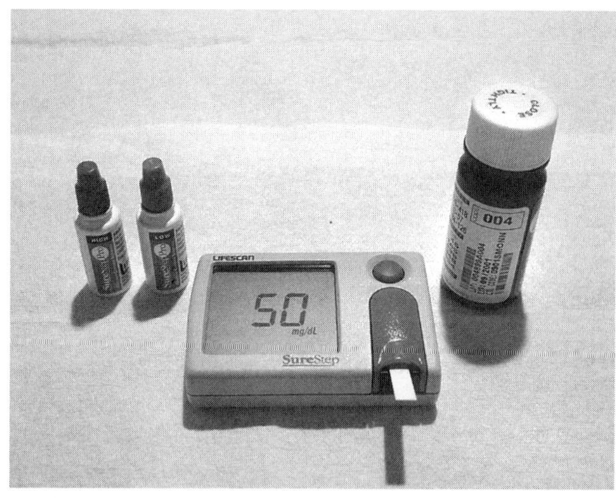

Figure 13–4 SureStep® glucose meter.

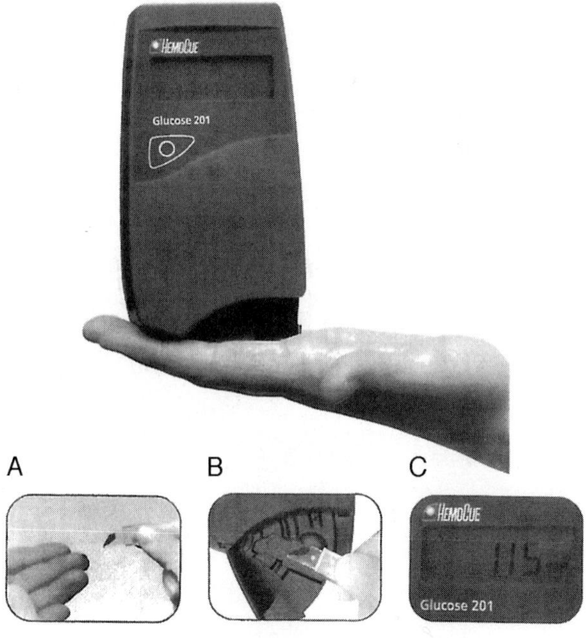

Figure 13–5 HemoCue® Glucose 201 Analyzer and test procedure. (*A*) Fill the cassette. (*B*) Place the filled cassette into the instrument. (*C*) Read the result. (Courtesy of HemoCue, Inc., Mission Viejo, CA.)

The phlebotomist must know about possible sources of test error, understand and perform daily maintenance and QC of the instrument and the QC of the reagent strips, and document all actions taken. Some of the POCT glucose instruments have software capability to store data such as user identification number, patient identification number, calibration and QC results, and patient results for CLIA compliance.

Transcutaneous Bilirubin Testing

As discussed in Chapter 9, newborns are frequently tested to detect and monitor increased levels of bilirubin (**hyperbilirubinemia**). In addition to hemolytic disease of the newborn (HDN) and premature birth, a variety of other risk factors for hyperbilirubinemia exist. However, these factors may not be considered in healthy-appearing, nonjaundiced infants. Of particular concern is the failure to visually detect jaundice in infants with dark skin.

The JCAHO has released a sentinel event alert (see Chapter 14) that addresses hyperbilirubinemia in the healthy newborn, recommending that risk assessment criteria be established. The JCAHO suggests implementation of earlier neonatal bilirubin testing on patients determined to be at risk by noninvasive transcutaneous bilirubin (**TcB**) testing or capillary serum bilirubin testing.

Noninvasive TcB testing is ideally suited to provide increased monitoring of infants who do not appear jaundiced but who may have risk factors associated with hyperbilirubinemia. TcB testing is performed at the patient bedside, using a portable, hand-held Bilichek® meter (Respironics, Inc., Murrysville, PA) (Fig. 13-6). The test is complete in less than 1 minute, which facilitates excellent TAT for neonatal bilirubin testing. The noninvasive technology also eliminates most infection control issues associated with capillary punctures, including wound care, lancing devices, blood exposure, and biohazard disposal.

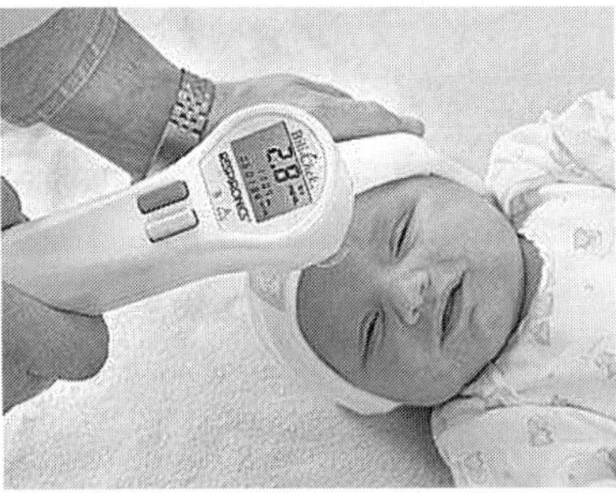

Figure 13-6 Bilichek® being performed on an infant. (Courtesy of Respironics, Inc., Murrysville, PA.)

The Bilichek® noninvasively directs white light into the skin of the newborn and measures the intensity of the specific wavelength that is returned. The Bilichek® measures the intensity of more than 100 wavelengths of reflected light. The intensity of the reflected light is converted to absorbance units/optical density for analysis. Interfering components in the skin are subtracted from the known spectral properties of the normal skin by the instrument before displaying the bilirubin concentration. When the disposable tip is placed on the Bilicheck® meter, the instrument initiates a self-test for integrity and an electronic check. After a successful calibration, the protective covering and calibration material are removed from the tip. The unit is activated and the tip is pressed flat against the infant's forehead. The indicator light will change from amber to green when proper pressure is applied. On completion of five measurements, a tone sounds and the test results are displayed with the current time and date.

TcB testing is approved for use on newborns of 27 to 42 weeks' gestational age, 0 to 20 days postnatal age, and 950 to 4995 g infant weight. The test is not affected by skin pigment and is appropriate for use on all races. Testing is not indicated for newborns who have received an exchange transfusion. A dermal puncture should be performed for closer monitoring of the bilirubin level.

technical tip Transcutaneous bilirubin measurements are performed only on the forehead of an infant. Avoid areas with bruising, birthmarks, hematomas, or excessive hair.

Hemoglobin

The primary function of the red blood cell (RBC) protein hemoglobin (Hgb) is to transport oxygen to all cells in the body. A decrease in the number of RBCs or the amount of Hgb in the cells (anemia) results in a decrease in the amount of oxygen reaching the cells. Normal values for Hgb vary with age and gender, with values for adult women ranging between 12 and 15 g/dL and for adult men between 14 and 17 g/dL. Measurement of Hgb is one of the most frequently performed screening tests in all healthcare settings and also provides a means to monitor patients known to have anemia.

Varieties of POCT analyzers that measure Hgb include instruments that provide Hgb concentration as part of a larger test menu that may analyze glucose and electrolytes, as well as instruments designed only to measure Hgb. The HemoCue® Hemoglobin System is designed to measure Hgb specifically (HemoCue®, Inc., Mission Viejo, CA) (Fig. 13–7) using arterial, venous, or capillary whole blood specimens. A fresh capillary or anticoagulated whole blood sample is placed into a microcuvette and inserted into the instrument. The Hgb measurement is determined photometrically using a dry reagent system. The reagents in the microcuvette lyse the RBCs to release hemoglobin, which is converted to azide methemoglobin by sodium nitrite and sodium azide to produce a color reaction. A dual wavelength photometer reads the absorbance of the reaction and corrects the hemoglobin value for lipemia and leukocytosis.

The HemoCue® hemoglobin analyzer is available with data management systems that can transfer QC and patient data to a LIS. Expanded analyzer functions include bar coding, linearity checks, proficiency testing, and more control levels for compliance with regulatory agencies.

technical tip Fill the cuvette with the blood in a continuous process without bubbles, making sure that the drop of blood is big enough to fill the cuvette completely.

Urinalysis

A routine urinalysis consists of a physical and chemical examination of urine and a microscopic examination when indicated. The microscopic portion of the urinalysis is not a part of POCT and should not be performed by phlebotomists.

Urine is a readily available and usually easy-to-collect specimen that contains information about many of the body's major functions. It is important to obtain a patient history before testing urine, because ingestion of highly pigmented foods, medications, and vitamins can interfere with results. Information regarding collection and specimen types can be found in Chapter 12. Urine should be tested within 2 hours of collection.

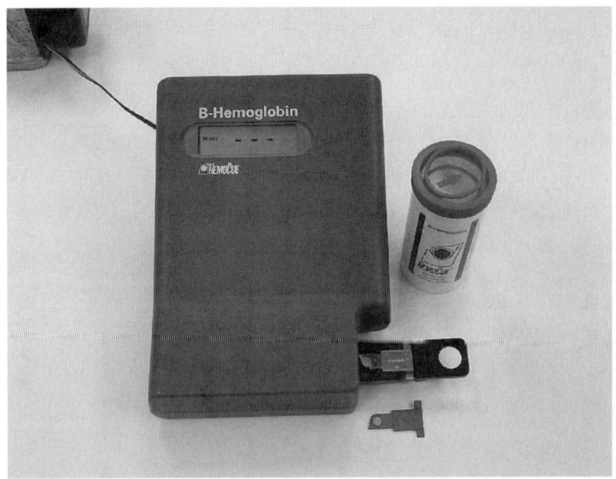

Figure 13–7 HemoCue® B Hemoglobin Analyzer, cassettes, and control.

Physical examination of urine describes the color and clarity of the specimen. Abnormal colors and increased turbidity can be indications of pathologic conditions. Normal urine color is yellow, and the intensity of the color is related to the concentration. A dilute urine is pale yellow, and a concentrated (first morning) urine is dark yellow. Common color descriptions of normal urine include pale yellow, light yellow, yellow, dark yellow, and amber, and may vary among institutions. If there are no interfering substances, red or brown-black urine is abnormal and could indicate a disease process. Amber urine that produces yellow foam when shaken is also abnormal, if there are no interfering substances, and could indicate a disease process associated with liver disease.

Normal urine is usually clear; however, normal substances such as epithelial cells may increase the turbidity. Describing clarity also varies from one facility to another. Common terms related to appearance include clear, hazy, cloudy, and turbid. A cloudy or turbid appearance in a fresh specimen may be cause for concern.

Routine chemical examination of urine is performed using plastic strips containing reagent-impregnated test pads that test for specific gravity, pH, glucose, bilirubin, ketone, blood, protein, urobilinogen, nitrite, and leukocytes. A color-producing chemical reaction occurs when the reagent pads come in contact with urine. The color reaction can be read visually by comparing the strip against a color chart on the container (Fig. 13–8) or

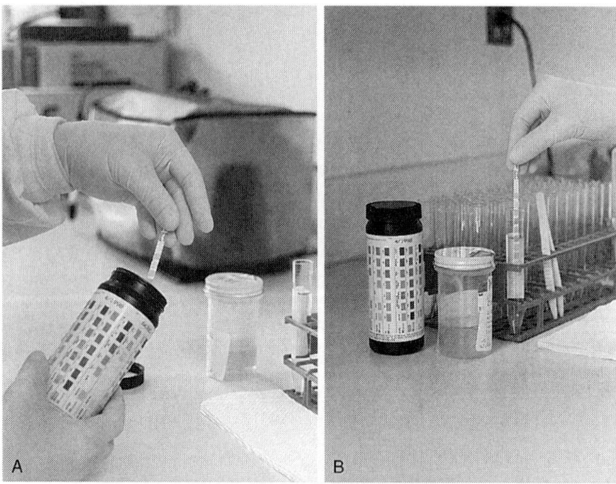

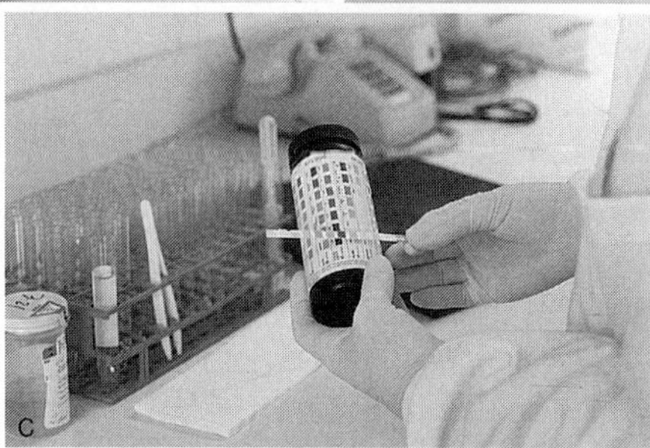

Figure 13–8 Chemical examination of urine. (*A*) Removing reagent strip from container. (*B*) Dipping reagent strip into specimen. (*C*) Comparing reagent strip color reactions. (From Strasinger, SK, and Di Lorenzo, MS: Skills for the Patient Care Technician. FA Davis, Philadelphia, 1999, p., 266, with permission.)

by inserting the strip into an automated instrument such as the Ames Clinitek® 50 (Miles, Inc., Elkhart, IN) that reads the strip and prints the results (Fig. 2–12).

Correct handling and storage of reagent strips is critical for obtaining accurate results. Strips are stored at room temperature in their original opaque bottles that contain a desiccant to protect them from exposure to excess light, moisture, and chemical contamination. Containers should be uncapped only long enough for a strip to be removed. When performing the test, strips should be briefly and completely dipped into the urine. They should not be left in the specimen because reagents will wash out of the pads, causing false-negative results. Failure to read the reactions within the time frame specified by the manufacturer will also produce inaccurate results. Table 13–4 summarizes routine chemical testing of urine.

Occult Blood

The purpose of occult blood testing is to detect gastrointestinal bleeding that is not visible to the naked eye. Detection of occult blood is a valuable aid in the early diagnosis of colorectal cancer. Test kits for occult blood consist of a packet containing filter paper areas impregnated with guaiac reagent on which small amounts of feces are placed, positive and negative control areas, and a bottle of color developing reagent (Fig. 13–9). The specimen can be collected and tested at the patient setting, or the packets can be sent home with the patient to collect the specimen and return the packet. Hgb present in the stool sample reacts with hydrogen peroxide in the color-developing reagent to release oxygen, which then reacts with the guaiac reagent to produce a blue color (Fig. 13–10). Test kits are available from several manufacturers, and it is important not to combine materials from different kits. Specimens should be collected following instructions provided by the test kit manufacturer. Contamination of the specimen with urine or toilet water should be avoided.

technical tip Results of a routine urinalysis can be seriously affected if the urine is not tested within 2 hours of collection or preserved by refrigeration.

Test kits for fecal occult blood must be sensitive enough to detect a very small amount of blood; therefore, they are highly subject to interference by diet and medications. A patient's diet should exclude red meat and certain vegetables that are sources of peroxidase and may cause false-positive results. Patients should be instructed to avoid the following items 72 hours before testing: red meat, turnips, radishes, melons, horseradish, alcohol, high doses of vitamin C, and excessive amounts of vitamin C-enriched foods. Aspirin and other nonsteroidal anti-inflammatory drugs that may cause gastrointestinal irritation should be avoided 7 days before testing.

technical tip Manufacturers' instructions for occult blood specimens must be followed strictly and stressed to patients.

TABLE 13-4
Summary of Chemical Testing by Reagent Strip

Test	Principle	Possible Reaction Interference: False-Positive Tests	Possible Reaction Interference: False-Negative Tests	Correlations with Other Tests
pH	Double-indicator system	None	Runover from the protein pad may lower	Nitrite Leukocytes Microscopic
Protein	Protein error of indicators	Highly alkaline urine, quaternary ammonium compounds (antiseptics), detergents	High salt concentration	Blood Nitrite Leukocytes Microscopic
Glucose	Glucose oxidase, double sequential enzyme reaction	Peroxide, oxidizing detergents	Ascorbic acid, 5-HIAA, homogentisic acid, aspirin, levodopa, ketones, high specific gravity with low pH	Ketones
Ketones	Sodium nitroprusside reaction	Levodopa, phthalein dyes, phenylketones		Glucose
Blood	Pseudoperoxidase activity of hemoglobin	Oxidizing agents, vegetable and bacterial peroxidases	Ascorbic acid, nitrite, protein, pH below 5.0, high specific gravity, captopril	Protein Microscopic
Bilirubin	Diazo reaction	Lodine Pigmented urine Indican	Ascorbic acid, nitrite	Urobilinogen
Urobilinogen	Ehrlich's reaction	Ehrlich-reactive compounds (Multistix), medication color	Nitrite, formalin	Bilirubin
Nitrite	Greiss's reaction	Pigmented urine on automated readers	Ascorbic acid High specific gravity	Protein Leukocytes Microscopic
Leukocytes	Granulocytic esterase reactions	Oxidizing detergents	Glucose, protein, high specific gravity, oxalic acid, gentamycin, tetracycline, cephalexin, cephalothin	Protein Nitrite Microscopic
Specific gravity	pK change of polyelectrolyte	Protein	Alkaline urine	None

Pregnancy Testing

Pregnancy testing is based on the detection of **human chorionic gonadotropin** (HCG) hormone in urine or serum. HCG is produced by cells of the placenta and, depending on the sensitivity of the test kit, can be detected approximately 10 days after conception. False-negative results are obtained if not enough HCG has been produced to be detected at the time of testing. It is also important to perform urine pregnancy testing on a first-morning specimen to achieve maximum concentration. Cloudy urine specimens should be centrifuged or allowed to settle before testing to avoid interference with the test reaction.

No special instrumentation is required for pregnancy testing, and a variety of commercial test kits are available. Most pregnancy testing kits use monoclonal antibodies that react with different regions of the HCG molecule. Antibodies to HCG molecules

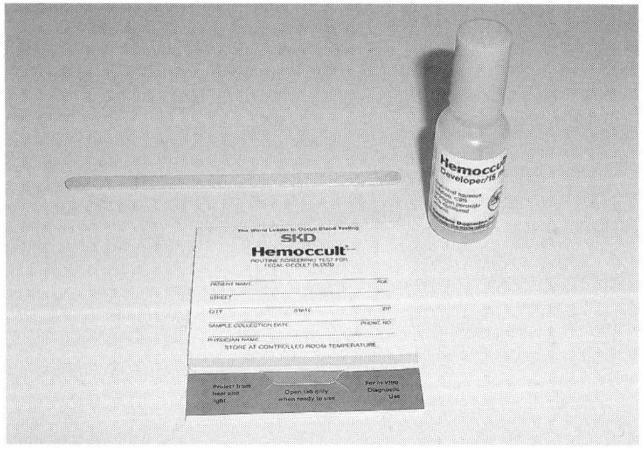

Figure 13–9 Hemoccult® fecal occult blood test kit.

are impregnated on a permeable membrane, and urine is added. If HCG is present in the urine, the antibodies will bind it on the membrane. Another reagent with enzyme-linked antibodies to a second region of the HCG molecule is added, thereby sandwiching the HCG molecules between the membrane-bound antibodies and the enzyme-linked antibodies in the reagent. The intensity of color is directly proportional to the amount of enzyme that was specifically bound to the membrane, which, in turn, is proportional to the amount that was present in the sample. The placement of the original antibody on the membrane determines the shape of the color reaction, such as a plus or minus sign, line, or circle. Areas to be used as positive and negative controls are also included on the test kit membranes. An example of the ICON® II HCG urine assay is shown in Figure 13–11. Reagents, timing, and methodology vary with each manufacturer's kit, and the directions must be followed exactly. Never mix components from different kits.

technical tip Package inserts indicate the sensitivity of the HCG assay and list interfering substances.

Strep Tests

Symptoms of a sore throat are an indication to test for group A streptococcus (strep throat). Although only a small percentage of children and adults with sore throat symptoms have positive results for group A streptococcus, complications of untreated positive infections are serious; therefore, all symptomatic patients are usually tested.

Detection of group A streptococci using a rapid test kit can be accomplished in a matter of minutes as opposed to the 1 or 2 days required when using conventional culture methods. Rapid tests work well when a high number of bacteria are collected on the throat swab. Fewer numbers of bacteria reduce the accuracy of the rapid tests, and it is common policy

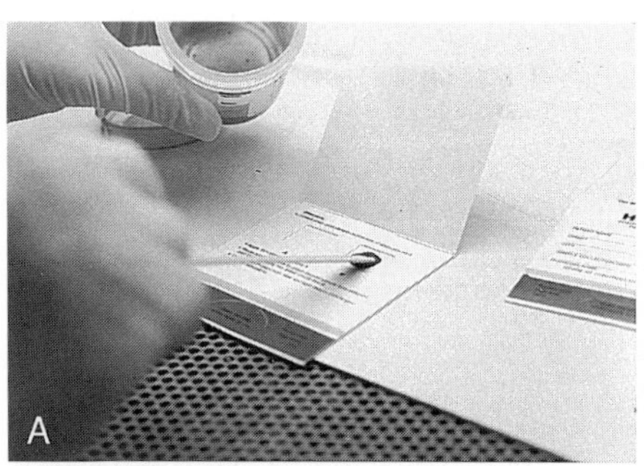

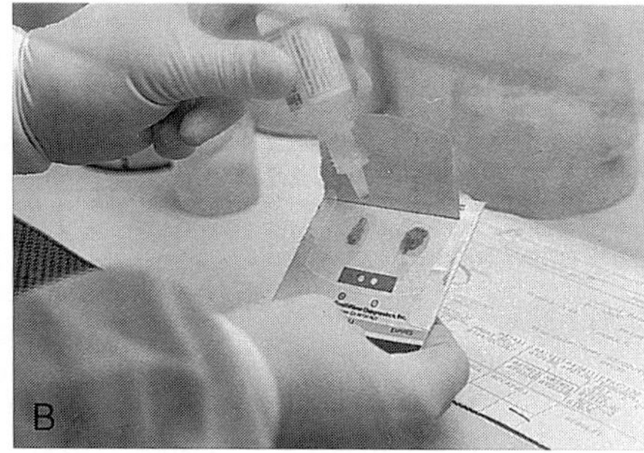

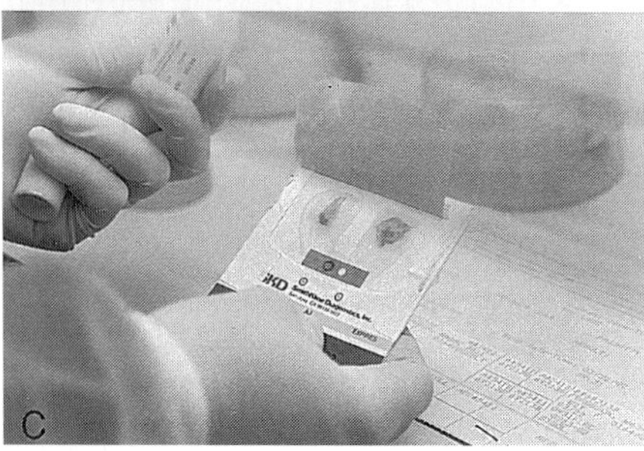

Figure 13–10 Fecal occult blood testing. (*A*) Applying stool sample to test slide. (*B*) Adding color developer to sample on test card. (*C*) Reading test and controls. (From Strasinger, SK, and Di Lorenzo, MS: Skills for the Patient Care Technician. FA Davis, Philadelphia, 1999, p. 269, with permission.)

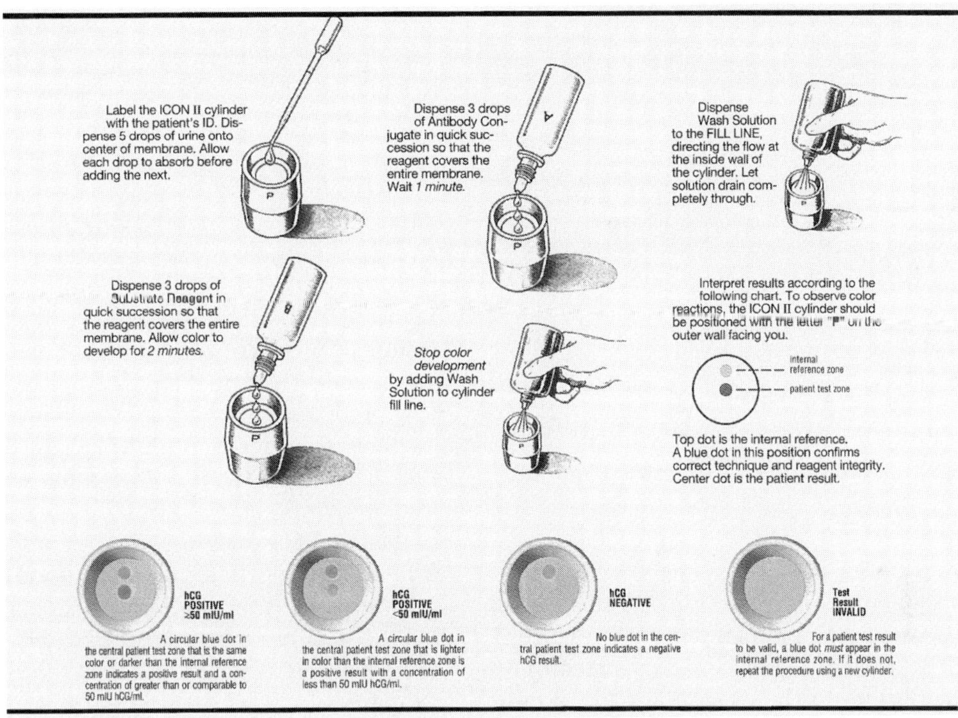

Label the ICON II cylinder with the patient's ID. Dispense 5 drops of urine onto center of membrane. Allow each drop to absorb before adding the next.
Dispense 3 drops of Antibody Conjugate in quick succession so that the reagent covers the entire membrane. Wait 1 minute.
Dispense Wash Solution to the FILL LINE, directing the flow at the inside wall of the cylinder. Let solution drain completely through.
quick succession so that the reagent covers the entire membrane. Allow color to develop for 2 minutes.
Stop color development by adding Wash Solution to cylinder fill line.
Interpret results according to the following chart. To observe color reactions, the ICON II cylinder should be positioned with the
outer wall facing you.
internal reference zone
patient test zone
Top dot is the internal reference. A blue dot in this position confirms correct technique and reagent integrity. Center dot is the patient result.
hCG POSITIVE ≥50 mIU/ml
A circular blue dot in the central patient test zone that is the same color or darker than the internal reference zone indicates a positive result and a concentration of greater than or comparable to 50 mIU hCG/ml.
hCG POSITIVE <50 mIU/ml
A circular blue dot in the central patient test zone that is lighter in color than the internal reference zone is a positive result with a concentration of less than 50 mIU hCG/ml.
hCG NEGATIVE
No blue dot in the central patient test zone indicates a negative hCG result.
Test Result INVALID
For a patient test result to be valid, a blue dot must appear in the internal reference zone. If it does not, repeat the procedure using a new cylinder.

Figure 13–11 Pregnancy testing procedure. (Courtesy of Beckman Coulter, Inc., Fullerton, CA.)

to perform a throat culture on patients with negative results on rapid tests. Therefore, it may be necessary to collect two throat swabs: one for the rapid test, and one to hold for possible culture. Specimens should be collected from the throat using a swab that does not have a cotton or calcium alginate tip and does not have a wooden shaft. When swabbing the throat, the procedures discussed in Chapter 12 should be followed.

Group A streptococcus tests employ various methodologies and different reagents. The QuickVue® In-Line® One-Step Strep A test (Quidel, San Diego, CA) is a CLIA '88–waived test that uses a lateral flow immunoassay in which the antigen extraction takes place in the test cassette. The swab is placed in the cassette. The extraction solution is mixed and added to the test cassette. Bacterial antigens are extracted from the swab within the testing device using a mild acid solution. The extracted solution flows onto a test strip by capillary action and flows through a label pad consisting of anti-group A streptococcus antibodies. If the extracted solution contains group A streptococcus antigen, the antigen will bind to the antibody on the test label and will then bind additional color-producing anti-group A streptococcus antibody on the membrane. Results are read at 5 minutes, and the test result pattern is compared with the interpretation chart. The test line indicates a positive or negative patient result, and the control line indicates that the reagents were mixed and added properly, that the proper volume of fluid entered the test cassette, and that capillary flow occurred (Fig. 13–12).

Whole Blood Immunoassay Kits

In addition to the kits for pregnancy and group A streptococcus testing, a large variety of CLIA '88–waived kits are available for detection of abnormal whole blood components. Complete kits include reaction cassettes or cards, color developer, positive and negative controls, and detailed instructions. Depending on the test methodology, the color developer and controls may be impregnated into the reaction cassettes or cards, or added by the person performing the test. The previously described group A streptococcus test is an example of a kit in which the controls are included in the test cassette.

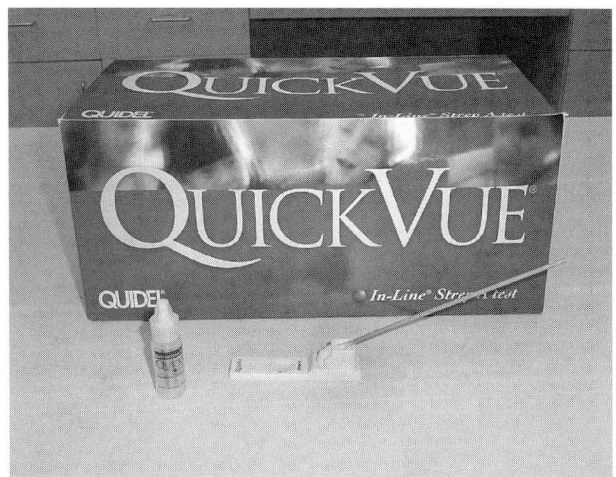

Figure 13–12 QuickVue® In-Line® Strep A test kit: Test cassette, swab, and extraction reagent.

To avoid using the wrong reagents, it is important that all components of a kit be stored in their designated box. Kits contain enough reagents to perform a specified number of tests, and reagents from a different kit should not be used. Many kits require refrigeration and must be allowed to warm to room temperature before use. All kits contain a package insert that provides information concerning the stability, sensitivity, and storage of reagents; specimen collection guidelines; sources of error; and detailed step-by-step instructions. It is essential that all instructions be followed strictly.

All immunoassay kits use the same basic principle— that is, the appearance of a color reaction when antigens and antibodies combine. The color, size, and shape of the reaction will vary among kits and manufacturers. In addition, some procedures are designed to detect antibodies in the patient's blood and others are designed to detect antigens in blood and body substances. Antibodies are produced by the body when a foreign substance (antigen) enters the body. Detection of antibodies is often used to diagnose bacterial and viral infections caused by microorganisms that are difficult to culture or obtain on a swab. Antigen testing is used to identify substances produced by the body in specific conditions or bacteria that can be obtained on a swab. The previously discussed pregnancy and group A streptococcus tests are examples of antigen testing by immunoassay. Reagent antibodies known to be specific for HCG or group A streptococcus antigens are used to detect their presence.

technical tip When working for a different organization, do not assume that you will be using the same immunoassay procedures. Read the directions.

Three frequently used immunoassays detect the antibodies present in infectious mononucleosis (**IM**) and gastrointestinal disorders caused by *Helicobacter pylori* and the antigen troponin T present in a myocardial infarction (MI). Several different manufacturers produce kits for the detection of these substances. The actual kit used is a matter of laboratory preference.

IM is an acute, self-limiting infection caused by the Epstein-Barr virus. Symptoms include fatigue, swollen lymph glands, sore throat, and enlargement of the liver. The diagnosis can be confirmed by detection of unique heterophile antibodies formed in response to the infection. The manufacturer's instructions must be followed closely to ensure that only the heterophile antibodies specific for IM are detected.

Helicobacter pylori is the causative agent of several gastrointestinal disorders, of which the most common are duodenal and gastric ulcers. The rapid detection of antibodies specific for *H. pylori* in the blood of a patient with symptoms of gastrointestinal pain alerts the healthcare provider to prescribe antibiotics. Early treatment prevents the bacteria from causing additional damage to the gastrointestinal tract.

Early diagnosis of a MI can be critical to patient survival. Troponin T is a protein specific to heart muscle and is only released into the blood after an MI. It can be detected within 4 hours of damage to the heart and remains elevated for 14 days. Troponin T is one of the earliest markers present in MI, and the ability to detect it by rapid immunoassay is a valuable diagnostic aid. The test is well suited for use in outpatient settings and the emergency room.

Blood Coagulation Testing

Several POCT instruments are available to monitor blood coagulation therapy and clotting deficiencies in patients. The anticoagulant heparin is administered intravenously to patients to prevent the formation of clots after certain surgeries and clinical procedures that can initiate the clotting process such as cardiac catheterization, hemodialysis, and coronary angioplasty. Heparin is a fast-acting anticoagulant that must be monitored closely because too much heparin can produce internal hemorrhaging and too little heparin may lead to clot formation. An oral anticoagulant, Coumadin, is frequently given to outpatients at risk for clot formation. The prothrombin time (PT) test is used to monitor Coumadin. The activated partial thromboplastin time (APTT) test is used to monitor heparin therapy. The activated clotting time (ACT) also monitors heparin therapy.

Depending on the manufacturer, POCT instruments for coagulation testing are capable of providing a combination of PT, APTT, and ACT results or only PT results. The type of instrument chosen depends on the needs of the POCT site. As mentioned previously, surgical areas must be able to monitor heparin therapy, and therefore an instrument that performs an APTT or ACT is required. In contrast, outpatient sites are monitoring Coumadin therapy and need only to perform a PT.

The ProTime® Microcoagulation System (International Technidyne Corporation, Edison, NJ.) is a complete system for PT testing consisting of the ProTime® instrument, a three-channel reagent cuvette with built-in QC, and the Tenderlett Plus LV sample collection system. It is a CLIA '88–waived test that performs PTs from fingerstick whole blood and displays the results as the PT result in seconds or the more standardized **International Normalized Ratio (INR)**. ProTime® runs two levels of QC with each patient's sample (Fig. 13–13).

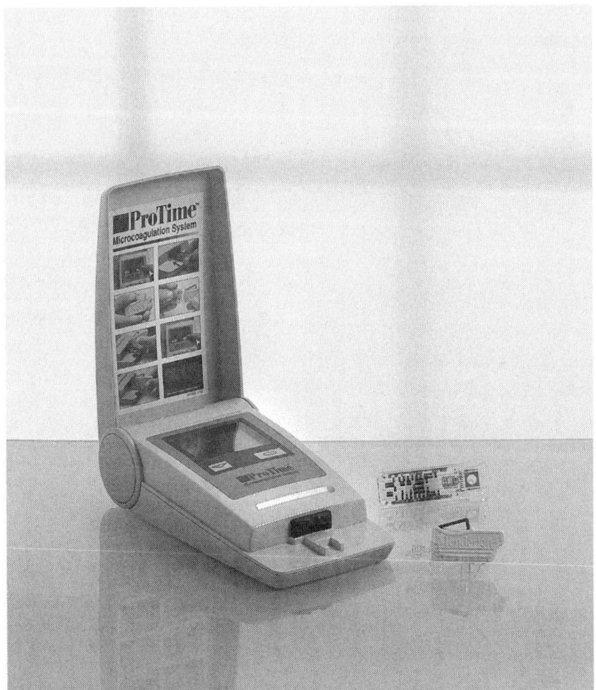

Figure 13–13 ProTime® Microcoagulation System. (Courtesy of International Technidyne Corporation, Edison, NJ.)

technical tip The INR standardizes PT results between different reagent manufacturers. The INR should be reported for patients taking Coumadin for at least 2 weeks.

The CoaguChek® system (Roche Diagnostics, Indianapolis, IN) performs a PT using a drop of fingerstick whole blood applied to a test strip containing dried thromboplastin reagent and tiny iron particles. The sample, dried reagent, and iron particles move through alternating magnetic fields that cause the iron particles to move. The endpoint is reached when a clot forms and stops the iron particles from moving. The analyzer displays both the PT and INR result (Fig. 13–14).

The HEMOCHRON® Jr. Signature Whole Blood Microcoagulation System (International Technidyne

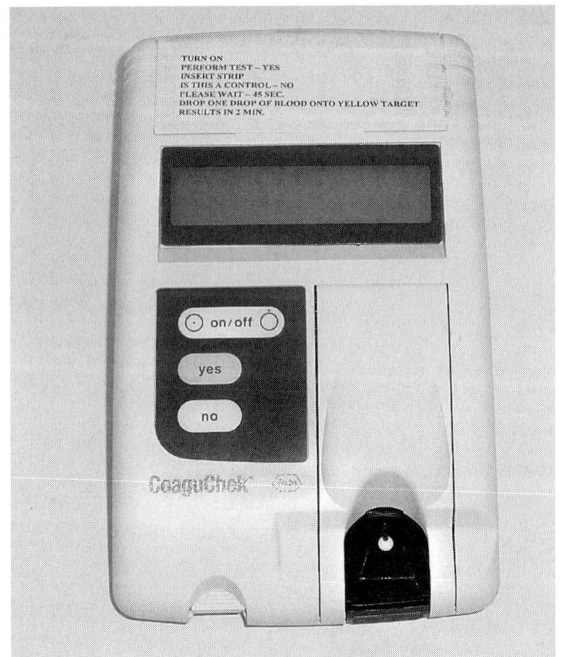

Figure 13–14 CoaguChek® system.

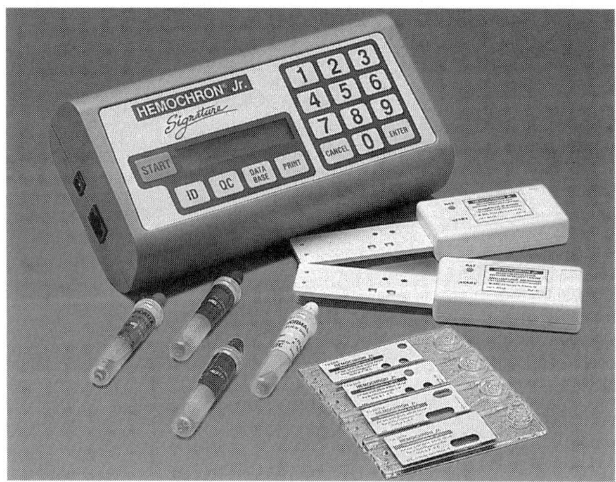

Figure 13–15 HEMOCHRON® Jr. Signature Whole Blood Microcoagulation System. (Courtesy of International Technidyne Corporation, Edison, NJ.)

Corporation, Edison, NJ.) is a POCT instrument that performs ACT, APTT, and PT tests using one drop of whole blood per test. Specific cuvettes containing dried reagents for each test are placed into the instrument, blood is added, and the timing begins. The timing stops when a clot is detected and the result is displayed. The instrument has data management capabilities to identify, store, and print both patient and QC results (Fig. 13–15).

technical tip POCT coagulation tests often specify that the first drop of blood obtained by dermal puncture be used for testing.

Cholesterol

Cholesterol is a lipid manufactured by the body for use in cell membranes and as a precursor to steroid hormones. It is found in high concentrations in animal fats; therefore, additional cholesterol enters the body through ingestion. When excessive amounts of cholesterol are ingested or produced by the body, the increased cholesterol circulating in the blood adheres to the walls of the blood vessels, resulting in blockage of blood flow and subsequent coronary artery disease.

Normal values for cholesterol vary with age. The ideal value is less than 200 mg/dL, but it may be as high as 240 mg/dL in persons over age 50 years. Studies show that lowering cholesterol to acceptable levels reduces the risk of developing coronary heart disease. The studies also suggest that increases in high-density lipoprotein (HDL) reduce coronary heart disease risk. The National Institutes of Health has recommended aggressive efforts to identify and treat those at risk for coronary heart disease. Several POCT instruments are available that can perform cardiac risk profiles from a single drop of whole blood.

The Cholestech LDX® (Cholestech Corporation, Hayward, CA) analyzer measures total cholesterol, HDL cholesterol, and triglycerides using a cassette containing dry reagents capable of performing an enzymatic reaction when blood is added to the cassette (Fig. 13–16). Estimated low-density lipoprotein (LDL) cholesterol, very-low-density lipoprotein **(VLDL)** cholesterol, and a total cholesterol/high-density lipoprotein **(TC/HDL)** ratio are calculated using the measured values. Each cassette has a magnetic stripe containing calibration information; therefore, no operator calibration is required. The analyzer is designed to go into a locking mode if QC testing is not within acceptable limits. The operator must then contact a technical service representative at Cholestech, Inc.

technical tip Hold the cassette by the short sides only. Do not touch the black bar or the brown magnetic stripe.

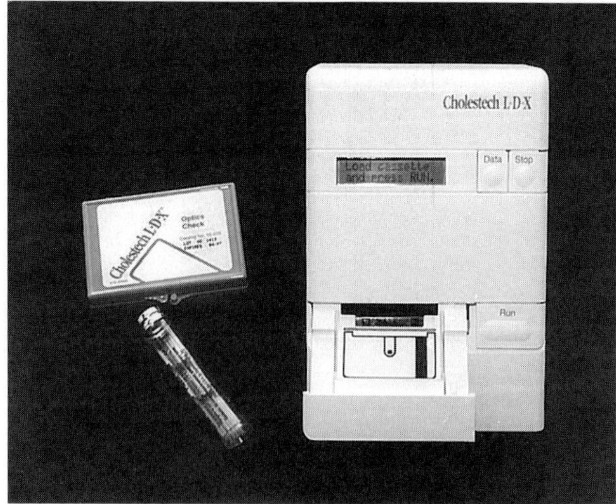

Figure 13–16 Cholestech LDX® with optics cassette and capillary tubes. (From Strasinger, SK, and Di Lorenzo, MS: Skills for the Patient Care Technician. FA Davis, Philadelphia, 1999, p. 274, with permission.)

Arterial Blood Gas and Electrolyte Analyzers

Arterial blood gases (ABGs) and electrolyte testing are used for the stat analysis of a critical patient population because delayed results would significantly affect patient care. ABGs include the pH, the partial pressure of carbon dioxide (Pco_2), and the partial pressure of oxygen (Po_2) in the blood. Electrolytes commonly measured are sodium (Na^+), potassium (K^+), chloride (Cl^-), bicarbonate ion (HCO_3^-), and ionized calcium (iCa^{++}). POCT for electrolytes uses small instruments located in emergency rooms, operating rooms, and intensive care and critical care units.

ABGs are obtained to determine if the patient is well oxygenated and to determine the acid-base status of the patient. Electrolytes maintain osmotic pressure, proper pH, regulation of heart and other muscles, and oxidation-reduction potential; and participate as catalysts for enzymes. Disturbance of K^+ homeostasis causes muscle weakness and affects heart rate. Sodium maintains normal distribution of water through osmotic pressure. Ionized calcium is the active form of calcium and is useful in evaluation of renal function and endocrine disorders during cardiac surgery and in neonatology.

The IRMA® SL Series 2000 Point-of-Care Diagnostics Blood Analyzer system (Diametrics Medical, Inc., St. Paul, MN) measures blood gas values for pH, Pco_2, and Po_2, the electrolytes Na^+, K^+, Cl^-, and iCa^{++}, and the hematocrit, and calculates the HCO_3^- and O_2 saturation ($SO_2\%$) parameters. These analytes are measured with a single-use analytical cartridge containing reagents and electrodes for the determination of each analyte or group of analytes. Cartridges are automatically calibrated when inserted into the instrument. A small sample of blood is injected into the system's sensor cartridge and a test is performed in 2 minutes. Results are displayed on a screen and a hard copy can be printed (Fig. 13–17).

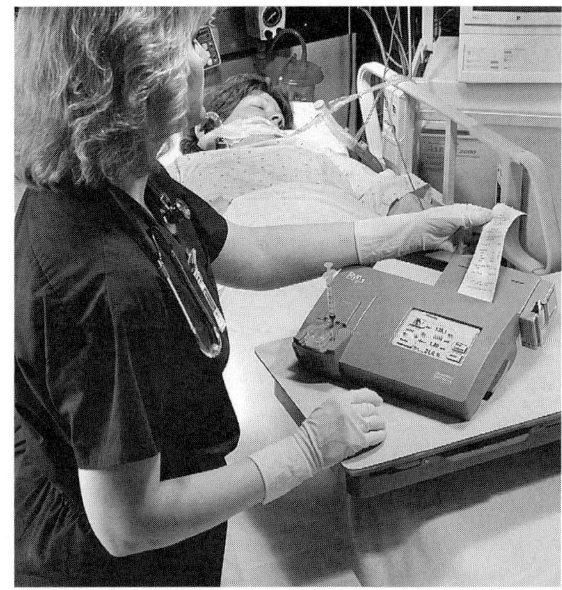

Figure 13–17 IRMA® SL Series blood analysis system. (Courtesy of Diametrics Medical Inc., St. Paul, MN.)

The hand-held i-STAT® Portable Clinical Analyzer (i-STAT Corporation, Princeton, NJ) measures ABGs (pH, Pco_2, and Po_2), electrolytes (Na^+, K^+, Cl^-, and HCO_3^-), blood urea nitrogen (BUN), glucose, and hematocrit (Hct) values using capillary blood. (Fig. 13-18).

The Stat Profile pHOx® Plus L Analyzer (Nova Biomedical, Waltham, MA) uses optical and electrode technology to measure pH, Pco_2, Po_2, $SO_2\%$, Hct, Hb, glucose, Na^+, K^+, iCa^{++}, and Cl^-. It provides an automated QC system for POCT with

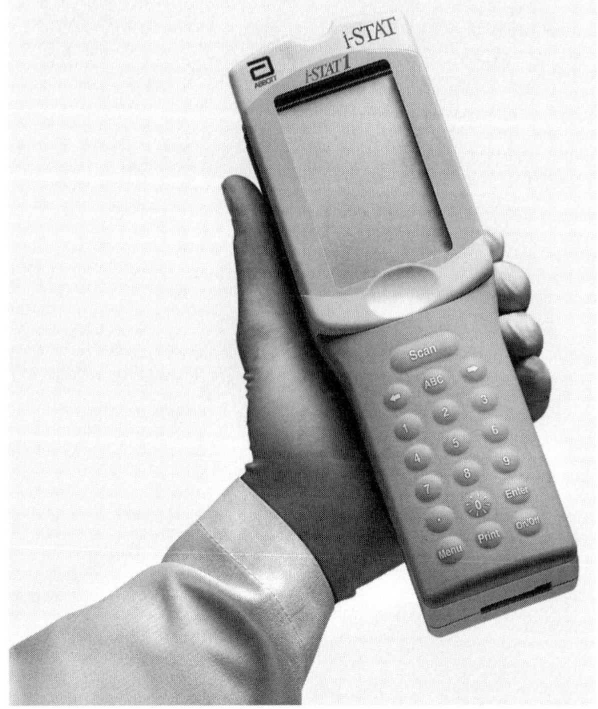

Figure 13–18 i-STAT® Portable Clinical Analyzer (PCA). (Courtesy of i-STAT Corporation, Princeton, NJ.)

controls that are analyzed automatically on a preset schedule or on demand. Out-of-range results can be followed by an optional system shut down. A single snap-in reagent pack contains all required blood gas and chemistry reagents, plus a self-sealing waste container. The 10-test menu requires 100 μL of whole blood, and a blood gas panel requires 40 μL of arterial blood (Fig. 13–19).

Future Applications

The evolving technologic advances have allowed POCT to expand to all areas of laboratory analysis with techniques for noninvasive sample collection and the use of nonblood specimens, including saliva, for analysis. With the increased POCT demand, manufacturers are being challenged to develop automated devices for all procedures to document complete compliance and capture billing revenue. With the approval of the National Committee for Clinical Laboratory Standards POCT 1-A communication standard, manufacturers must develop sophisticated data management systems to integrate data from the various POCT devices to the core laboratory. Data management systems will be able to collect data in one central database, allowing various test results to be easily correlated and available.

The advancements in technology coupled with improved instrument connectivity will continue to facilitate the rapid expansion of POCT to provide clinically relevant information accurately and rapidly.

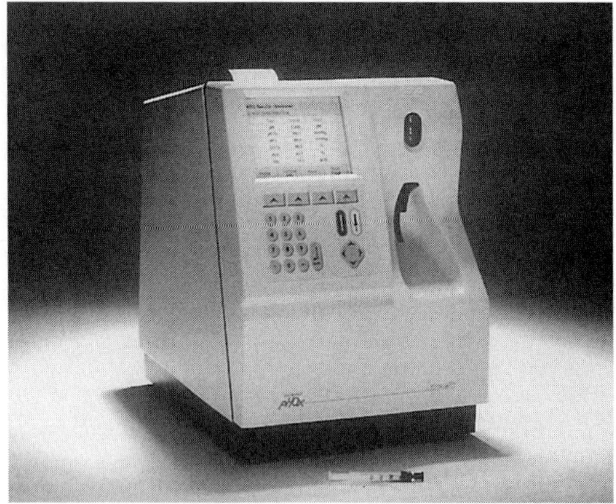

Figure 13–19 STAT Profile pHOx® Plus L analyzer. (Courtesy of Nova Biomedical, Waltham, MA.)

Bibliography

Di Lorenzo, MS, et al: Basic Laboratory Methods for Allied Health Professionals. UNMC Division of Medical Technology, School of Allied Health Professions, 2002.

Henry, JB (ed): Clinical Diagnosis and Management by Laboratory Methods, ed. 19. WB Saunders. Philadelphia, 1996.

Laboratory Improvement Laboratory Accreditation Checklists (Checklist 30): *http://www.cap.org./html/ftpdirectory/checklistftp.html*

NCCLS: Point-of-Care Connectivity: Approved Standard, NCCLS document POCT 1-A. NCCLS, Wayne, PA 2001.

Rubaltille, FF., Gourley, GR., Loskamp, N., Modi, N., Roth-Kleiner, M., Sender, A., Vert, P.: Transcutaneous bilirubin measurement: A multicenter evaluation of a new device. Pediatrics 107:(6), 2001. p. 1264-1271.

Strasinger, SK, and Di Lorenzo, MS: Skills for the Patient Care Technician. FA Davis, Philadelphia, 1999.

Strasinger, SK, and Di Lorenzo, MS: Urinalysis and Body Fluids, ed. 4. FA Davis, Philadelphia, 2001.

What's New With CLIA'88, JCAHO, & CAP: http://www.westgard.com

Study Questions

1. State the two categories of laboratory testing that may be performed by a phlebotomist according to CLIA '88 guidelines.

   a. ______________________________

   b. ______________________________

2. Define POCT and name three different settings in which POCT is performed.

   a. The definition of POCT is

   ______________________________.

   b. Setting 1

   ____

   c. Setting 2

   ____

   d. Setting 3

   ____

3. Name three advantages of POC testing:

   a. ______________________________

   b. ______________________________

   c. ______________________________

4. Define QC and explain why it is required before any patient testing.

   ____

   ____

5. The most common POCT performed in the hospital and at home is

   ______________________________.

6. A fasting blood sugar (FBS) of 40 mg/dL is considered (a) normal (b) abnormal. (Circle one.) What would you do if you obtained the above result on a patient specimen?

   ____

7. Give a reason why the Bilichek® cannot be used to perform a bilirubin test on an infant.

   ____

8. Describe the primary function of hemoglobin.

   ____

9. Why does the HemoCue® read the absorbance of the reaction at two different wavelengths?

____

10. The physical examination of urine includes visually examining the specimen for:

 a. ____

 b. ____

11. A phlebotomist has been assigned to test 10 urine specimens chemically. He or she removes 10 strips from the container and proceeds with testing. What is wrong with this scenario?

____

12. Urine should be analyzed within ______________________ of collection.

13. The Hemoccult® is a slide card test for ______________________. List three things patients should avoid before having this test performed.

 a. ____

 b. ____

 c. ____

14. Pregnancy test kits are designed to detect the presence of ______________________ .

15. What is the purpose of the final wash solution step in the Beckman Coulter ICON® II pregnancy test kit?

____

16. Strep throat is caused by the presence of ______________________ .

17. Why would two throat swabs be collected from a patient who is symptomatic for strep throat?

____

18. True or False. Immunoassay kits can be used to detect the presence of either antigens or antibodies.

____

19. The most desirable blood cholesterol level is ______________________ mg/dL.

20. High blood cholesterol levels have been shown to increase the risk of

____ .

21. What is the purpose of the magnetic stripe found on each testing cassette used with the Cholestech LDX®?

____

22. Explain what has happened if the Cholestech LDX® instrument goes into a locking mode and does not allow the user to continue with the procedure.

____

23. What is the purpose of heparin therapy?

____

24. Name three clinical procedures that may require a patient to be placed on heparin therapy.

a. _______________

b. _______________

c. _______________

25. Name two tests to monitor heparin therapy.

a. _______________

b. _______________

26. Name the test that is used to monitor Coumadin therapy and a bedside instrument used to measure this analyte.

a. Test: _______________

b. Instrument: _______________

27. What chemistry tests can be performed on an i-STAT® or IRMA® POCT blood analyzer?

a. _______________

b. _______________

c. _______________

d. _______________

e. _______________

f. _______________

g. _______________

h. _______________

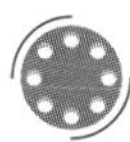

Clinical Situations

1. A phlebotomist performs daily bedside glucose tests on an inpatient using a POCT glucose meter. Daily results for the patient were:

Day 1 - 100 mg/dL

Day 2 - 105 mg/dL

Day 3 - 98 mg/dL

Today the phlebotomist gets a result of 48 mg/dL. The patient states no change in diet or routine in the past 24 hours.

a. What should the phlebotomist do?

____

b. What three things could be a cause of an incorrect glucose value?

1. ______________________________
2. ______________________________
3. ______________________________

2. A phlebotomist performed the daily morning QC on the glucose meter. The results were:

Abnormal low = 50 mg/dL

Abnormal high = 200 mg/dL

The range for the abnormal low is 33 to 57 mg/dL; the abnormal high range is 278 to 418 mg/dL.

a. Can the phlebotomist report patient results?

____

b. What actions are required by the phlebotomist?

____

c. What is a possible cause of any discrepancy?

____

3. An outpatient urine specimen was delivered to the clinic at 8:00 A.M. and placed on the counter in the laboratory. The phlebotomist finished the blood collections at 11:30 A.M. and then performed the urinalysis on this specimen. The results were:

COLOR: Yellow	PROTEIN: Negative	BILIRUBIN: Negative
CLARITY: Cloudy *	GLUCOSE: Negative	UROBILINOGEN: Normal
SP. GRAVITY: 1.020	KETONES: Negative	NITRITE: Positive *
pH: 9.0 *	BLOOD: Negative	LEUKOCYTE: Negative

* Significant results

a. What could be a possible cause for the abnormal results?

____

b. What should have been done with this specimen?

____

4. Indicate whether each of the following actions is acceptable or unacceptable POCT technique by placing an "A" or a "U" in front of the action. Explain why an action is unacceptable.

   a. ____________________ A phlebotomist is performing microscopic analysis of urine.

   ____

   b. ____________________ A phlebotomist records the lot number and expiration date of a control on the QC log sheet.

   ____

   c. ____________________ Transcutaneous bilirubin testing is performed on an infant who does not appear jaundiced.

   ____

   d. ____________________ A phlebotomist performs a urine pregnancy test using a cartridge from one test kit and color developer from a different manufacturer's kit.

   ____

   e. ____________________ When performing a QuickVue® In-Line® Strep A test, the phlebotomist adds 5 drops of extraction solution to the cassette.

   ____

   f. ____________________ The phlebotomy supervisor requires that phlebotomists performing immunoassay tests memorize the instructions.

   ____

   g. ____________________ A phlebotomist reports a PT result in seconds and as the INR.

   ____

   h. ____________________ A stat laboratory in the operating room is equipped with CoaguChek® and an i-STAT®.

   ____

NAME ____________________

Evaluation of Blood Glucose Determination

RATING SYSTEM 2 = SATISFACTORILY PERFORMED 1 = NEEDS IMPROVEMENT
0 = INCORRECT/DID NOT PERFORM

_______ 1. Turns on instrument

_______ 2. Verifies that "Code Key" inserted in monitor matches lot number of test strips and documents results

_______ 3. Performs two levels of QC

_______ 4. Verifies that QC is acceptable and documents results

_______ 5. Understands and follows monitor display throughout procedure

_______ 6. Correctly removes one test strip from container

_______ 7. Recaps container

_______ 8. Collects capillary specimen from patient according to procedure in Chapter 9

_______ 9. Applies appropriate-sized drop of blood to the test strip

_______ 10. Correctly inserts test strip into the instrument within the specified time frame

_______ 11. Visually reads result from monitor and documents results

_______ 12. Disposes of biohazardous materials according to OSHA guidelines

_______ 13. Follows monitor directions for additional testing and/or appropriate instructions for turning off monitor

TOTAL POINTS _______

MAXIMUM POINTS = 26

Comments:

NAME ____________________

Evaluation of Hemoglobin Determination Using the HemoCue® System

RATING SYSTEM 2 = SATISFACTORILY PERFORMED 1 = NEEDS IMPROVEMENT 0 = INCORRECT/DID NOT PERFORM

______ 1. Turns on instrument

______ 2. Correctly pulls out cuvette holder into insertion position

______ 3. Performs photometer check with photometer cuvette and documents results

______ 4. Removes cuvettes needed for testing from container

______ 5. Recaps container

______ 6. Performs QC and documents results

______ 7. Performs dermal puncture according to procedure in Chapter 9

______ 8. Correctly touches blood to tip of cuvette in one step, allowing blood to fill test area completely without creating air bubbles

______ 9. Correctly removes any excess blood without touching cuvette opening

______ 10. Positions filled cuvette correctly into cuvette holder

______ 11. Pushes cuvette holder into its inner position

______ 12. Understands and follows monitor display throughout procedure

______ 13. Correctly reads and documents patient results

______ 14. Disposes of biohazardous materials according to OSHA guidelines

______ 15. Follows directions for additional testing and/or appropriate instructions for turning off monitor

TOTAL POINTS ______

MAXIMUM POINTS = 30

Comments:

NAME ______________________________

Evaluation of Urinalysis (Physical Determination)

RATING SYSTEM 2 = SATISFACTORILY PERFORMED 1 = NEEDS IMPROVEMENT 0 = INCORRECT/DID NOT PERFORM

__________ 1. Prepares to observe urine by assuring specimen is in clear container with lid

__________ 2. Positions container in a good light source

__________ 3. Examines color visually by looking down through container against a white background

__________ 4. Documents color of urine specimen according to facility guidelines

__________ 5. Places lid on container

__________ 6. Swirls container to completely mix specimen

__________ 7. Examines clarity visually by holding specimen container in front of a light source

__________ 8. Documents clarity of urine specimen according to facility guidelines

TOTAL POINTS __________

MAXIMUM POINTS = 16

Comments:

NAME ______________________________

Evaluation of Urinalysis (Chemical Determination)

RATING SYSTEM 2 = SATISFACTORILY PERFORMED 1 = NEEDS IMPROVEMENT
0 = INCORRECT/DID NOT PERFORM

__________ 1. Verifies and documents lot number and expiration date of test strips

__________ 2. Removes one test strip from container at a time

__________ 3. Recaps container

__________ 4. Visually checks test strip for discoloration

__________ 5. Performs QC and documents QC results

__________ 6. Mixes patient urine specimen

__________ 7. Dips test strip completely, but briefly, into patient specimen

__________ 8. Correctly removes excess urine from strip without causing carryover onto adjacent test pads

__________ 9. Visually compares any color changes to test pads under a good light source at specified timing intervals

__________ 10. Documents results

__________ 11. Disposes of biohazardous materials according to OSHA guidelines

TOTAL POINTS __________

MAXIMUM POINTS = 22

Comments:

NAME ______________________

Evaluation of Fecal Occult Blood Determination

RATING SYSTEM 2 = SATISFACTORILY PERFORMED 1 = NEEDS IMPROVEMENT 0 = INCORRECT/DID NOT PERFORM

_________ 1. Opens front of slide card

_________ 2. Visually examines test areas for discoloration

_________ 3. Correctly applies thin smear of stool to cover both test areas

_________ 4. Closes slide card by inserting cover into flap

_________ 5. Allows card to sit for 3 to 6 minutes

_________ 6. Opens back of slide card

_________ 7. Correctly applies two drops of developer onto each test area

_________ 8. Waits 1 minute and visually examines slide card for color reaction

_________ 9. Correctly applies one drop of developer onto the positive and negative controls area of slide card

_________ 10. Waits 10 seconds and visually examines control area for color reaction

_________ 11. Documents results of patient and performance monitor

_________ 12. Disposes of biohazardous materials according to OSHA guidelines

TOTAL POINTS _________

MAXIMUM POINTS = 24

Comments:

NAME ____________________

Evaluation of Cholesterol Determination Using the Cholestech LDX®

RATING SYSTEM 2 = SATISFACTORILY PERFORMED 1 = NEEDS IMPROVEMENT 0 = INCORRECT/DID NOT PERFORM

_______ 1. Turns on instrument

_______ 2. Correctly performs optics check using optics cassette and documents acceptability

_______ 3. Correctly removes cassette from package and does not touch the black bar or magnetic stripe

_______ 4. Places cassette on flat surface

_______ 5. Prepares Cholestech LDX® capillary tube by inserting plunger into end with red mark

_______ 6. Correctly performs self-test on instrument

_______ 7. Understands and follows instrument display throughout procedure

_______ 8. Performs dermal puncture according to procedure in Chapter 9

_______ 9. Correctly fills capillary tube to black mark in one step without creating air bubbles

_______ 10. Gently pushes plunger of capillary tube and applies blood sample to test well of cassette within 5 minutes of collection

_______ 11. Keeps cassette level

_______ 12. Correctly places cassette into analyzer drawer

_______ 13. Performs test run according to procedure

_______ 14. Documents results

_______ 15. Disposes of biohazardous material according to OSHA guidelines

_______ 16. Follows instrument directions for additional testing and/or turning off instrument

TOTAL POINTS _______

MAXIMUM POINTS = 32

Comments:

NAME ______________________________

Evaluation of INR (PT) Whole Blood by CoaguChek®

RATING SYSTEM 2 = SATISFACTORY 1 = NEEDS IMPROVEMENT
0 = INCORRECT/DID NOT PERFORM

_________ 1. Turns on instrument

_________ 2. Removes test strips and controls from refrigerator and allows to warm at room temperature for 30 minutes

_________ 3. Verifies that the lot number of the test strips matches the Code Chip installed in the analyzer

_________ 4. Performs the electronic QC using the Electronic Quality Control Cartridge (EQC)

_________ 5. Performs QC using Level 1 and 2 CoaguChek® Liquid QC

_________ 6. Verifies that QC is acceptable and documents results

_________ 7. Understands and follows monitor display throughout procedure

_________ 8. Correctly removes test strip and inserts the test strip into the analyzer, printed side up

_________ 9. Uses test strip within 4 minutes of opening the foil pouch

_________ 10. Performs dermal puncture following procedure in Chapter 9

_________ 11. Does NOT wipe away the first drop of blood

_________ 12. Applies the FIRST DROP of blood directly from the finger to the yellow sample target area of the test strip

_________ 13. Visually reads result from the monitor and documents results

_________ 14. Disposes of biohazardous materials according to OSHA guidelines

_________ 15. Follows monitor directions for additional testing and/or appropriate instructions for turning off monitor

TOTAL POINTS _________

MAXIMUM POINTS = 30

Comments:

NAME ______________________________

Generic Evaluation of Test Kit Performance

RATING SYSTEM 2 = SATISFACTORY 1 = NEEDS IMPROVEMENT
0 = INCORRECT/DID NOT PERFORM

__________ 1. Removes the test kit from the refrigerator and allows the reagents to warm to room temperature, if required

__________ 2. Checks the expiration date of the kit

__________ 3. Washes hands and puts on gloves

__________ 4. Performs the test following the manufacturer's directions

__________ 5. Interprets the test results according to the provided interpretation chart

__________ 6. Records results

__________ 7. Cleanses work area and disposes of biohazardous materials according to OSHA guidelines

__________ 8. Removes gloves and washes hands

TOTAL POINTS __________

MAXIMUM POINTS = 16

Comments:

Chapter 14

Quality Phlebotomy and Legal Issues

Chapter Outline

Learning Objectives

Upon completion of this chapter, the reader will be able to:

1. Discuss the interactions of quality control (QC), quality assurance (QA), continuous quality improvement (CQI), and total quality management (TQM) and their differences.
2. Discuss forms of documentation used in the phlebotomy department.
3. List the information contained in a procedure manual and describe how the manual is used by the phlebotomist.
4. Discuss the role of variables in the development of a QA program.
5. Differentiate among preanalytical, analytical, and postanalytical variables related to the phlebotomist's scope of practice.
6. Discuss the role of the phlebotomist in controlling preanalytical, analytical, and postanalytical variables.
7. Define HIPAA and describe its association with phlebotomy.
8. State the primary goals of TQM and CQI.
9. Relate phlebotomy to the four areas of TQM.
10. State the four dimensions of performance and relate them to phlebotomy.
11. Define PDMAI and PDCA.
12. Define and give examples of sentinel events.
13. Describe the role of the phlebotomist in preventing sentinel events.
14. Differentiate between medical ethics and medical law.
15. Explain how the Patient's Bill of Rights affects the phlebotomist.
16. Define the legal terms associated with tort law, confidentiality, malpractice, patient consent, and professional liability insurance.
17. Give examples of how phlebotomists could be involved in medical malpractice litigation.
18. State the goals of a risk management program.

Key Terms

Analytical variables	*Informed consent*	*Postanalytical variables*	*Root cause analysis*
Continuous quality improvement	*Invasion of privacy*	*Preanalytical variables*	*Sentinel event*
Documentation	*Malpractice*	*Procedure manual*	*Total quality assurance*
Ethics	*Negligence*	*Quality assurance*	*Variable*
Incident report			

Throughout the previous chapters, many of the aspects of providing quality patient care have been discussed in relation to phlebotomy techniques. These procedures provide the quality control (QC) needed to ensure that acceptable standards are being met while the procedures are being performed. This QC is a part of the laboratory's overall program of ***quality assurance*** **(QA)**. In this chapter, it is appropriate to review these QC procedures, combine them with additional information, and discuss their interactions in laboratory QA, the institutional processes of ***total quality management*** **(TQM)** and ***continuous quality improvement*** **(CQI)**, and the prevention of medical errors. The actions of the phlebotomist in these programs are critical to their success.

Quality Assurance

QA is the program through which the laboratory guarantees quality patient care by providing accurate and reliable test results in an appropriate and timely manner. The Joint Commission on Accreditation of Healthcare Organizations (JCAHO) requires a planned systematic process for the monitoring and evaluation of the quality and appropriateness of patient care services and the resolving of identified problems. The phlebotomy department is a central part of the laboratory QA program because of its close contact with patients and other hospital personnel. The quality of laboratory testing is absolutely dependent on the quality of the specimens received.

Documentation of a QA program requires:

- Written policies and procedures covering all aspects of service
- Evidence of compliance with standards of good practice and achievement of expected outcomes
- Collection of data (metrics) to monitor and evaluate the program
- Evidence of work being performed efficiently and in the best interests of the patient
- Actions taken to resolve problems

In the phlebotomy department, documentation is provided in a variety of ways. These include a detailed procedure manual present in the department, identification of variable factors associated with the performance of phlebotomists, policies developed to provide guidelines to control and monitor these variables, **laboratory reference manuals** (floor books) provided to nursing units and outreach locations, and continuing education records for all members of the department.

Procedure Manual

For each test or procedure performed, the ***procedure manual*** provides the principle and purpose, specimen type and method of collection, equipment and supplies needed, standards and controls, step-by-step procedure, specific procedure notes, limitations and variables of the method, corrective actions, method validation, normal values, and references. The procedure manual documents the intention of the laboratory to comply with the standards of good practice to achieve expected outcomes.

The procedure manual must be present in the department at all times. Phlebotomists should not hesitate to refer to the manual when unfamiliar requests are encountered. It is the responsibility of the phlebotomy supervisor to enter all policy and procedure changes into the manual, notify personnel of the changes, and document an annual review of the entire manual.

Variables

Identification of ***variables*** provides the basis for development of procedures and policies in the department. Variables can be divided into three groups:

1 *Preanalytical variables:* Processes that occur before testing of the sample
2 *Analytical variables:* Processes that occur during the testing of the sample
3 *Postanalytical variables:* Processes that affect the reporting and interpretation of test results

Phlebotomists are primarily involved with preanalytical variables, which include the ordering, collection, transportation, and processing of specimens. Their actions in these areas affect the quality of the analytical results obtained in the various laboratory sections. They continue to be involved in the postanalytical phase because the timeliness of collection affects the amount of time required to report the test results. Their duties may also include delivery of reports to the units and computer entry or retrieval of results.

Preanalytical Variables

ORDERING OF TESTS

This is a joint effort between the phlebotomy department and the personnel who generate the requests for laboratory tests. The laboratory must facilitate test ordering by providing a laboratory reference manual, floor book, or a computerized medical information system. Information contained in the manual should include:

- Laboratory schedules for collection of routine specimens. These may be called "sweeps" and are scheduled to correspond with the primary times that patient specimens are requested. Examples of scheduled sweeps are the early morning, when patients are in a basal state, and late morning and afternoon, when physicians have completed their patient visits. Unit personnel need to understand that whenever possible issuing test requisitions to the laboratory at these times increases not only the efficiency of the phlebotomy department but also the entire laboratory, because tests can then be performed in batches. Computerized medical information systems organize unit requisitions into scheduled times. The laboratory can then access the patient list (Fig. 14–1).
- A list of laboratory tests including the type of specimen required, specimen handling procedures, normal values, and any pertinent patient preparation or scheduling requirements. Personnel may be referred to additional instructions provided separately in the laboratory reference manual. Instructions can also be included on computer-generated requisitions. For example, the appearance of "clean-catch" under the heading of special instructions on a requisition form for a urine culture prompts personnel collecting the specimen to check the manual for additional information.
- Any changes or additions to laboratory policies affecting personnel in the unit. These should be promptly added to the manual, and all personnel should be notified of the changes.

As discussed in previous chapters, requisition forms must contain the required patient information and request the tests actually ordered by the healthcare provider. Errors in requisitioning include generation of duplicate requisitions and the missing of tests, either by the person transferring the healthcare provider's orders to the requisition or by the phlebotomist when organizing or reading the requisitions. The discovery of a missed test by personnel on the unit frequently causes a routine test to be ordered stat. A test overlooked by the phlebotomist may cause the patient to undergo a second, unnecessary venipuncture.

Monitoring of specimen ordering can include records of:

- The number of incomplete requisitions
- The number of duplicate requisitions
- The number of missed tests
- Delays in the collection of timed tests
- The number of stat requests by hospital location
- The time between test requests and collection
- The number of unit collected specimens rejected
- Turnaround time (TAT) (the amount of time between the ordering of a test and the reporting of the test results)
- Healthcare provider complaints

Evaluation of these records may then be used to determine the need for additions or changes to the laboratory reference manual; for in-service continuing education presentations to personnel ordering tests in order to reduce the number of errors or decrease the number of stat requests; to justify

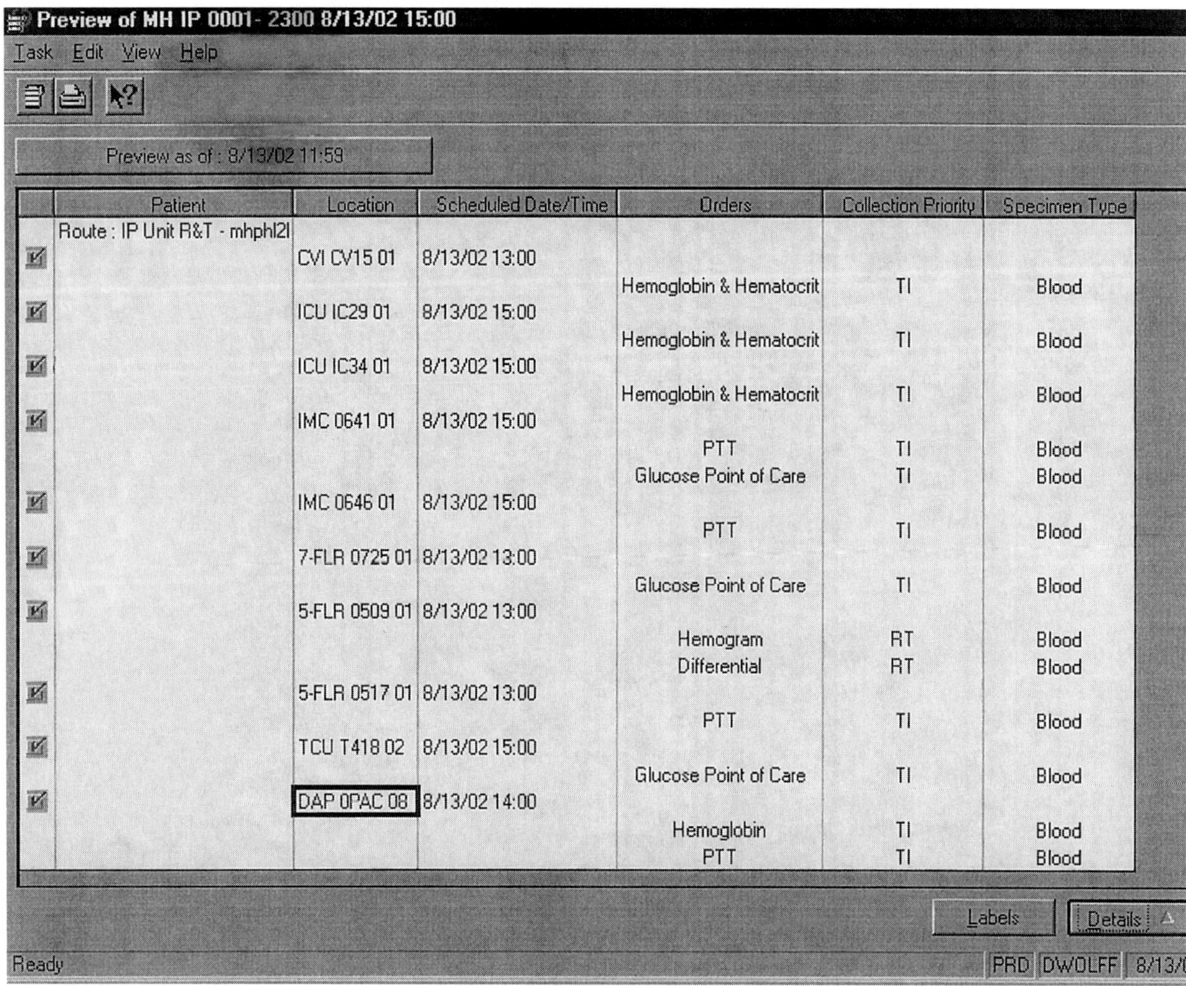

Patient	Location	Scheduled Date/Time	Orders	Collection Priority	Specimen Type
Route : IP Unit R&T - mhphl2l					
	CVI CV15 01	8/13/02 13:00			
			Hemoglobin & Hematocrit	TI	Blood
	ICU IC29 01	8/13/02 15:00			
			Hemoglobin & Hematocrit	TI	Blood
	ICU IC34 01	8/13/02 15:00			
			Hemoglobin & Hematocrit	TI	Blood
	IMC 0641 01	8/13/02 15:00			
			PTT	TI	Blood
			Glucose Point of Care	TI	Blood
	IMC 0646 01	8/13/02 15:00			
			PTT	TI	Blood
	7-FLR 0725 01	8/13/02 13:00			
			Glucose Point of Care	TI	Blood
	5-FLR 0509 01	8/13/02 13:00			
			Hemogram	RT	Blood
			Differential	RT	Blood
	5-FLR 0517 01	8/13/02 13:00			
			PTT	TI	Blood
	TCU T418 02	8/13/02 15:00			
			Glucose Point of Care	TI	Blood
	DAP 0PAC 08	8/13/02 14:00			
			Hemoglobin	TI	Blood
			PTT	TI	Blood

Figure 14–1 Example of a computerized phlebotomy collection list. (TI = timed; RT = routine). [Courtesy of Diane Wolff, MLT (ASCP) Phlebotomy Team Leader, Nebraska Methodist Hospital, Omaha, NE.]

additional phlebotomists or changes in staffing schedules to provide faster specimen collection; and for additional training of phlebotomists who are missing tests or collecting specimens inefficiently.

A sample error/corrective action worksheet is shown in Figure 14–2.

PATIENT IDENTIFICATION

Failure to identify a patient properly is the most serious error in phlebotomy and can result in injury or death to the patient. Identification of errors may be discovered in the laboratory, before the patient is harmed, through an analytical QA procedure known as the **delta check**. A delta check is a comparison between a patient's previous test results and the current results. Variation of results outside of established parameters alerts laboratory personnel to the possibility of an error. Documentation of errors in patient identification can result in suspension or dismissal of a phlebotomist. Identification of patients using bar code technology could provide a solution to problems with patient identification.

PHLEBOTOMY EQUIPMENT

Ensuring the sterility of needles and puncture devices and the stability of evacuated tubes, anticoagulants, and additives is essential to patient safety and specimen quality. Providing needle safety devices and needle disposal containers as specified by the Occupational Health and Safety Administration (OSHA) is essential for phlebotomist safety.

Disposable needles and puncture devices are indi-

Month/year ________/____

Core Laboratory
Errors/Corrections

				Origin of Error - place a check mark in one box																Check one								
				Collection				Processing			Mis-info			Tech sec.			Result rpt			Discov		When						
Error by: Initials	Recorded by: Initials	Date	Major Error/Incident rpt	Patient Identification	Specimen Identification	Specimen Integrity	Document Status	Aliquot ID	Requisition/Order	Specimen Processing	Nursing	Respiratory Therapy	Client	Performance	Interpretation	Math	Entry (tech)	Transcription (tech)	Clerical Personnel	By Lab	Non-lab	Immediately	Same Shift	After Shift	nrbc	Other non-error	Comments	Patient Name, Test
			/																									
			/																									
			/																									
			/																									
			/																									
			/																									
			/																									
			/																									
			/																									
			/																									
			/																									
			/																									
			/																									
			/																									
			/																									
			/																									
			/																									
			/																									
			/																									
			/																									

Figure 14–2 Samples of errors and corrections documentation form. (From The Department of Pathology, Nebraska Methodist Hospital, Omaha, NE, with permission.)

vidually packaged in tightly sealed sterile containers. Phlebotomists should not use puncture equipment if the seal has been broken. Visual inspection for nonpointed or barbed needles detects manufacturing defects.

Manufacturers of evacuated tubes must ensure that tubes, anticoagulants, and additives meet the standards established by the National Committee for Clinical Laboratory Standards (NCCLS). These standards specify the acceptable concentrations to provide quality specimens. The expiration date of the evacuated tubes should be checked each time a new package of tubes is opened, and outdated tubes should not be used. For the most economical management of phlebotomy supplies, packages of tubes should be stored in groups by lot number, and lots with the shortest expiration dates should be placed in the front of the storage area.

technical tip Donate expired evacuated tubes to your local phlebotomy teaching program for use on artificial arms.

Defects in the manufacturing of evacuated tubes are possible and, when present, frequently affect an entire lot of tubes. QC procedures that can be used when a new lot of tubes is opened include checking for the following items: a vacuum by measuring the amount of water drawn into the tube, the presence of small clots in anticoagulated tubes, the visual appearance of additives, the stability of tubes and gel during centrifugation, and stopper integrity and ease of stopper removal. Results of these checks are documented, and testing may need to be repeated if problems with tube integrity develop later. Manufacturers must be notified when defects are discovered.

SAFETY DEVICES

Documentation of phlebotomist involvement in the selection of safety equipment is required by the Needlestick Safety and Prevention Act (see Chapter 3).

PATIENT PREPARATION

Numerous variables in patient preparation can affect specimen quality, and the phlebotomist cannot be expected to control and monitor all variables. However, phlebotomists should be aware of the most critical variables, such as fasting before glucose testing and abstaining from aspirin before a bleeding time test. Any discrepancies should be reported to the nursing staff or a supervisor. Phlebotomists should also be alert for noticeable unusual circumstances and should note this information on the requisition form. Special patient preparation procedures must be included in the laboratory reference manual or floor book. Patient variables that may affect test results are discussed in Chapter 7.

Monitoring and evaluation of QA in patient preparation must be done jointly by the laboratory, nursing staff, and healthcare providers.

TOURNIQUET APPLICATION

Application of the tourniquet for longer than 1 minute increases the concentration of large molecules such as bilirubin, lipids, protein, and enzymes, and may produce a slight hemolysis that affects potassium levels. Investigation of an increase in unacceptable potassium results should include documentation of the length of tourniquet application time.

SITE SELECTION

QA is affected by the choice of a puncture site. A site may be located in an area where specimen contamination may occur or patient safety may be compromised.

Sites to be avoided because of the possibility of specimen contamination include:

- Hematomas
- Edematous areas
- Arms adjacent to mastectomies
- Arms receiving intravenous fluids

Sites to be avoided to prevent injury to the patient include:

- Burned and scarred areas
- Arms adjacent to mastectomies
- Arms with fistulas and shunts
- The back of the heel
- Previous dermal puncture sites
- Arteries for routine testing

Errors in site selection are detected by delta checks, test results that are markedly affected by intravenous fluids, and reports from patients and nursing staff. Documentation of counseling, retraining, or dismissal of phlebotomists associated with poor choices in site selection should be available.

CLEANSING THE SITE

Blood culture contamination is the most frequently encountered variable associated with improper cleansing of the puncture site. The microbiology department maintains records of contaminated blood cultures. Increases in contamination rates are investigated and documented. Corrective action documentation could include in-service training of personnel collecting blood cultures. Failure to remove iodine from the patient's arm after specimen collection will generate patient complaints. Use of iodine for dermal puncture collections falsely elevates bilirubin, phosphorus, and uric acid levels.

PERFORMING THE PUNCTURE

Variables in phlebotomy technique affect both specimen quality and patient safety. Errors affecting specimen quality include collection in the wrong tube, failure to mix the specimen adequately, failure to follow the correct order of draw or fill, and excessive dilution of dermal puncture specimens with tissue fluid.

The patient's impression of the laboratory quality is heavily influenced by phlebotomy technique. Painful probing, hematomas, unsuccessful attempts, repeat draws because of poor specimen quality, and excessive and inappropriately located heel punctures generate reports from patients, nursing staff, and healthcare providers.

technical tip Phlebotomists should remember how often patients tell them about previous bad experiences and strive to not become another bad memory for the patient.

Documentation of poor technique affecting patients or specimen quality is frequently made in the form of an ***incident report*** generated by a nursing or laboratory supervisor. Incident reports describe the incident and the problem caused, document the corrective action taken, and become a part of an employee's permanent record.

DISPOSAL OF PUNCTURE EQUIPMENT

The availability of and the proper use of sharps containers and activation of venipuncture safety devices is essential to quality performance by phlebotomists. Accidental punctures with contaminated sharps must be reported immediately to a supervisor. A protocol that includes immediate and follow-up testing and counseling for the affected employee must be in place and followed (see Chapter 3).

Documentation of excessive accidental punctures can lead to changes in the type of equipment used or to disciplinary action against employees who are not following acceptable disposal procedures.

TRANSPORTATION OF SPECIMENS

Variables in the transportation of specimens include the method and timing of delivery to the laboratory and the use of special handling procedures discussed in previous chapters.

Specimen quality can be compromised when red blood cells are hemolyzed because of excessive vibration during delivery of tubes to the laboratory. Tubes should be placed in an upright position in racks provided in the phlebotomy tray. This method permits uniform clotting and prevents tubes from hitting against each other, thereby eliminating excessive vibration and the possibility of breakage.

Many hospitals have pneumatic tube systems running between the units and support areas. These systems increase the timeliness of specimen delivery to the laboratory. However, they must be carefully monitored to ensure that specimens are not hemolyzed or broken during transit. The most frequently affected tests are potassium, lactic dehydrogenase, plasma hemoglobin, and acid phosphatase. To transport laboratory specimens, the system should be designed to avoid sharp turns, provide a soft landing, and use containers that can be equipped with shock-absorbent lining materials. Records of unacceptable specimens must be maintained and evaluated to verify satisfactory performance of the pneumatic tube system.

Phlebotomists' duties include timely delivery of specimens to the laboratory. Tests such as lactic acid should be analyzed within 15 minutes. This procedure requires the ability to organize the workload efficiently and to adapt to emergency situations. Documentation of the time between the delivery of a requisition to the laboratory and the arrival of the specimen in the laboratory can be obtained by computer entry or by using a time-stamping machine (Fig. 14–3). These data can then be evaluated to determine the need for possible changes in phlebotomy staffing patterns.

SPECIMEN PROCESSING

Variables associated with specimen processing include the length of time between collection and processing or testing, centrifugation time and speed, contamination, evaporation, storage conditions, and labeling.

No more than 2 hours should elapse between specimen collection and separation of serum or plasma from the cells, and less time is recommended for potassium, ammonia, adrenocorticotropic hor-

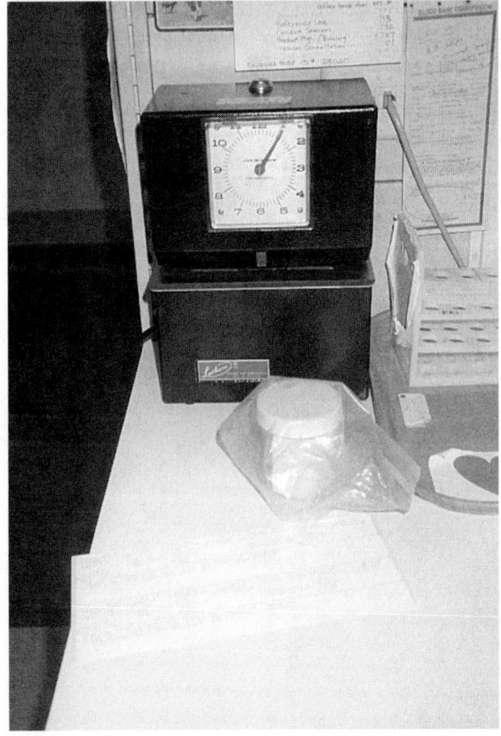

Figure 14–3 A time-stamping machine to document the time and date of specimen delivery.

mone (ACTH), and cortisol determinations. When delays in separation are longer than 2 hours, the most noticeable changes are decreased glucose concentrations and increased potassium and lactic dehydrogenase concentrations. Serum or plasma does not have to be removed after centrifugation from tubes containing separator gel if a tight gel seal is present. Blood smears from ethylenediaminetetraacetic acid (EDTA) anticoagulated blood also should be made within 2 hours of blood collection.

Documentation of centrifuge calibration and maintenance is required for accreditation. Centrifuges are routinely calibrated every 3 months using a **tachometer** to confirm revolutions per minute at various settings. This information can then be converted into relative centrifugal force using nomograms provided by the centrifuge manufacturer. Marked changes in the calibration may indicate the need to replace the centrifuge brushes, or problems with the bearings. Procedure manuals should include specifications for centrifuge speed, type, and time for each specimen. Failure to perform centrifuge calibration routinely or to follow the specifications stated in the procedure manual can affect specimen quality resulting from incomplete separation of liquid and formed elements, cellular damage caused by use of excessive speed or time, and deterioration of chemical elements if special requirements such as the use of a refrigerated centrifuge are needed.

technical tip Always check the centrifuge for proper balancing of tubes before operating.

Poor technique during specimen processing can seriously alter specimen composition by causing contamination or evaporation. All specimens left uncovered for extended periods of time are subject to external contamination and fluid evaporation. Small aliquots are particularly affected by evaporation, and specimens for blood gases, lactic acid, ammonia, and alcohol are severely affected if they are uncovered for even short periods of time. Aliquots of serum or plasma may contain red blood cells if separation is not carefully performed. Very serious interference with test results will occur if specimens collected in different anticoagulants or additives are combined.

technical tip Contamination of specimens caused by powdered gloves may falsely increase calcium levels.

The temperatures of refrigerators and freezers used for specimen storage must be monitored, either continually with automatic temperature recorders or daily by recorded checks of thermometer readings. Documentation of temperature readings or recording charts and centrifuge calibration and maintenance must be available for accreditation reviews.

technical tip Specimens should not be stored in self-defrosting freezers because they may be thawed and refrozen during defrosting cycles.

When aliquoting specimens into different tubes, particular attention must be paid to labeling, to ensure that specimen numbers are correctly transferred. Computer-generated labels often include additional labels for this purpose.

Errors in specimen processing can occur when personnel are not trained to prioritize specimens. This can include failure to differentiate between tests designated stat and routine; rejection of specimens because of minor paperwork discrepancies that could be easily resolved; rejection of critical specimens such as cerebrospinal fluid without seeking assistance to resolve the problem; and general overestimation of one's knowledge and ability to make decisions.

Documentation in the specimen processing area should include not only technical processing instructions but also instructions for contacting a designated supervisor when nontechnical situations arise. Records must be kept of any corrective actions taken.

technical tip A specimen should never be rejected or arbitrarily classified as a lower priority than requested without consulting a supervisor.

Analytical Variables

Phlebotomists must be aware of analytical values when performing point-of-care testing (POCT). As discussed in Chapter 13, variables in the testing process are best controlled by strictly following the procedure instructions, consistently using all available controls, and performing all required instrument calibration .

Postanalytical Variables

Reporting of test results to the appropriate healthcare providers in an efficient and accurate manner is essential to quality patient care. Reports may be handwritten and delivered, telephoned, or electronically transmitted. Phlebotomists can be involved in all forms of reporting.

WRITTEN REPORTS

Written reports are usually recorded on the original requisition form. The form may consist of several carbon copy sheets to provide records for the patient's chart, the billing office, and the laboratory. Forms must be designed to provide adequate patient identification, specimen information, collection information, room for reporting, test reference ranges, additional comments, and the initials of the person performing the test. Phlebotomists may be involved with the physical delivery of reports to the patient area, which could include placement in the patient's chart. They also may be required to enter data from the written record into a computer system. The quality of patient care can be severely affected by a delay in delivery of results, failure to place the reports in the correct location, and errors in the transfer of written reports to the computer.

TELEPHONE (VERBAL) RESULTS

The telephone is frequently used to transmit results of stat tests and critical values. Depending on the institutional computer capability, calls requesting additional results may be received from personnel on hospital units and healthcare providers. When telephoning results, be sure that they are being reported to the appropriate person (ideally the actual healthcare provider). Always document the time of the call and the name of the person receiving the results.

technical tip To ensure the accuracy of telephoned results, ask the recipient to repeat the results.

ELECTRONIC RESULTS

Electronic transmission is now the most common method for reporting results. Many laboratory instruments, including those used for POCT, have the capability for the operator to generate and transmit reports directly from the instrument to the designated healthcare provider. It is essential that the operator carefully review results before transmittal.

As mentioned previously, results also may be manually entered into the laboratory computer system and then transmitted to the healthcare providers. An additional electronic method of reporting is to fax results to designated areas. Computer transfer is rapidly replacing this method, but it is still in use for transmission of results to off-site areas.

Documentation of the reporting of results is essential and required by accrediting agencies. Permanent records of all reported results must be available. A method to verify the actual reporting of results also must be available and used by all employees.

THE HEALTH INSURANCE PORTABILITY AND ACOUNTABILITY ACT OF 1996

The Health Insurance Portability and Accountability Act of 1996 (**HIPAA**) legislation encompasses a variety of healthcare issues, not all of which directly affect the laboratory. Primary goals of the legislation are to:

- Protect workers with pre-existing conditions from losing health insurance when changing jobs
- Provide easier detection of fraud and abuse
- Reduce paperwork by requiring electronic data transactions
- Guarantee the privacy of individual health information

In addition to developing approved methods of data transmission, healthcare workers are most affected by the requirement to guarantee privacy of individual health information. The release of patient test results now falls under the HIPAA. In general, release of patient information, even between healthcare providers, must be kept to the minimum required for care, and written patient consent to release the information must be obtained. Standards for complying with HIPAA continue to be developed. Phlebotomists can expect to encounter continually evolving methods and regulation of data transfer.

Total Quality Management

Laboratory QA is part of the institutional TQM and CQI programs. QA is designed to maintain an established level of quality; TQM and CQI strive to develop methods to improve the standard of healthcare continually.

TQM is based on a team concept involving personnel at all levels to achieve a final outcome of customer satisfaction. TQM applies principles of management and graphic and statistical analysis of data to implement changes identified by the CQI program to increase customer satisfaction. TQM is based on the assessment of the quality and performance of infrastructure (physical, personnel, and management), processes, outcomes, and customer satisfaction. Infrastructure relates to the general workplace environment. Process is the method by which patient care is delivered and includes QC. Outcomes are primarily concerned with patient status after treatment. The five Ds described in Table 14–1 are patient outcomes to be avoided. In addition to the patients, the laboratory has other customers that TQM is designed to satisfy. These include the patient's families and guests, physicians, and other healthcare providers, both inside and outside the institution.

The focus of CQI is to improve patient outcomes by providing continual quality healthcare in a constantly changing healthcare environment by improving worker performance. The level of performance in healthcare is the degree to which what is done is effective and appropriate for the individual patient and the degree to which it is available in a timely manner. The dimensions of performance can be broken down into four categories:

1 Doing the right things wrong
2 Doing the wrong things right
3 Doing the wrong things wrong
4 Doing the right things right

Table 14–2 relates the dimensions of performance to an area of phlebotomy. The goal of CQI is to ensure that the right things are done right all the time.

Standards from the JCAHO address the concepts of TQM and CQI by requiring documentation that effective, appropriate patient care is being provided and demonstrated by positive patient outcomes. Areas included in the standards are availability of services, timeliness, continuity of care, effectiveness and efficiency of services, safety of services provided, and respect and care by the personnel providing the care. The JCAHO requires that organizations have a systematic plan for implementing CQI. An example of this is the JCAHO 10-step process shown in Table 14–3. Another recommendation of the JCAHO for improving organizational performance is the PDMAI (Plan, Design, Measure, Assess, and Improve)

TABLE 14–1
Relationship of TQM to Phlebotomy Infrastructure

Physical:	Distance between patients and the laboratory Availability of safety equipment Specimen transport methods
Personnel:	Number of phlebotomists Employment requirements/training
Management:	Phlebotomy staffing patterns Availability of supervisors
Process:	Venipuncture technique Dermal puncture technique Quality control of equipment
Outcomes:	Patient receives efficient diagnosis and treatment based on test results Dissatisfaction from repeat punctures Discomfort from a hematoma Disability caused by nerve damage from vigorous probing Disease from unsterile technique Death from patient or sample misidentification
Customer Satisfaction:	Patient praises phlebotomist's technique Physician appreciates rapid turn-around-time of results Nurse criticizes delayed collection of stat test

TABLE 14-2
Examples of Phlebotomy Performance Dimensions

Doing the right thing wrong:
Correctly applying a tourniquet and leaving it on for 5 minutes
Doing the wrong thing right:
Applying the tourniquet too tightly for no longer than 1 minute
Doing the wrong thing wrong:
Applying the tourniquet too tightly and leaving it on for 5 minutes
Doing the right thing right:
Applying the tourniquet correctly for no longer than 1 minute

approach, which provides standards for performance (PI.1 to PI.5).

- Plan (PI.1): The institution has a planned, systematic, hospital-wide approach to process design and performance measurement, assessment, and improvement.
- Design (PI.2): New processes are designed well.
- Measure (PI.3): The organization has a systematic process in place to collect data.
- Assess (PI.4): The institution uses a systematic process to assess collected data.
- Improve (PI.5): The institution systematically improves its performance.

Another widely used improvement plan is the Plan-Do-Check-Act (PDCA) strategy:

- Plan: Identify customers and their expectations; analyze current process, focusing on areas for improvement; and generate solutions.
- Do: Design and institute a trial run of the improvement and collect and analyze data.
- Check: Evaluate the results and draw a conclusion as to the effect of the change.
- Act: Standardize the change by developing procedures and policies for personnel and customers.

TABLE 14-3
JCAHO 10-Step Process

1. Appoint responsibility.
2. Outline the scope of care.
3. Identify key aspects of care.
4. Devise indicators.
5. Define thresholds of evaluation.
6. Collect and organize data.
7. Evaluate data.
8. Develop a corrective action plan.
9. Assess actions and document improvement.
10. Communicate relevant information.

As the laboratory member with the most direct patient (customer) contact, the phlebotomist plays a central role in TQM and CQI. Phlebotomists should think about how often they hear people characterize a hospital stay by describing their experience with blood collection and always strive to make this a positive experience. Phlebotomists can also become valuable members of TQM and CQI planning teams.

Preventing Medical Errors

In November 1999, the National Academy of Sciences' Institute of Medicine (IOM) issued a report entitled "To Err is Human: Building a Safer Health System." The report stimulated considerable public and governmental concern by stating that the majority of adverse medical events were caused by preventable medical errors. Healthcare institutions, accrediting agencies, and government agencies are placing increased emphasis on the designing of safe medical practices. The IOM report stresses that most of the medical errors are system related and are not caused by individual negligence or misconduct. Therefore, in keeping with the CQI dimensions of performance, systems should be designed to make it easy to do the right thing and hard to do the wrong thing.

The JCAHO has issued a new standard referred to as "***Sentinel Event*** Policies and Procedures" requiring reporting of sentinel events. A sentinel event is defined as any unanticipated death or major permanent loss of function not related to the natural course of the patient's illness or underlying condition. Reportable events are suicide during institutional care, infant abduction or discharge to the wrong family, rape during institutional care, hemolytic transfusion reactions from major incompatibilities, and surgery on the wrong patient or body part. Sentinel events must be reported to the JCAHO within 45 days of the event. The report must include a ***root cause analysis*** and an action plan. Acceptable root cause analyses identify basic or causal factors that underlie variation in performance and focus primarily on systems and processes rather than individual performance. As the JCAHO analyzes sentinel event reports, it periodically publishes lists of specific sentinel event causes to alert the healthcare community of areas to evaluate in their institutions. Refer to the mention of a sentinel event in Chapter 13.

A significant number of sentinel events involve incorrect patient identification. This problem directly affects the phlebotomist and serves to stress again the importance of this first step in any phlebotomy procedure. Action plans addressing these events recommend the use of bar code technology as discussed in Chapter 6 and illustrated in Figure 14–4. When electronic identification is not possible, the JCAHO recommends the use of two forms of patient identification, neither of which uses the patient's room number. Identification methods can include the patient's wrist identification band, asking the patient to state his or her name, and verification by a primary healthcare giver. Of equal concern to the phlebotomist should be the impro-per labeling of specimens delivered to the labora-tory and in particular the blood bank, because this can be the root cause of a hemolytic transfusion reaction.

Ethical and Legal Aspects of Phlebotomy

Principles of right and wrong, called the code of ethics, provide the personal and professional rules of performance and moral behavior as set by members of a profession. Medical ***ethics*** or bioethics focus on the patient to ensure that all members of a healthcare team possess and exhibit the skill, knowledge, training, professionalism, and moral standards necessary to serve the patient. Professional agencies such as the American Society of Clinical Pathologists (ASCP), American Society for Clinical Laboratory Science (ASCLS), and the National Phlebotomy Association (NPA) have developed codes of ethics for laboratory personnel. Phlebotomists are expected to follow this code by performing the duties specified in their job description, adhering to established standards of performance, and continuing to improve their knowledge and skills.

Patient's Bill of Rights

A document published by the American Hospital Association called the **Patient's Bill of Rights** specifies what the patient has a right to expect during medical treatment. A patient's rights and dignity must be protected in the process of providing quality care. The document addresses the following 12 areas:

1. Patients have the right to considerate and respectful care.
2. Patients have the right to obtain from their healthcare provider complete current information about their diagnosis, treatment, and prognosis in terms that patients can be reasonably expected to understand.
3. Patients have the right to receive from a healthcare provider the information necessary to give informed consent before a procedure. The information should include knowledge of the proposed procedure, with risks and probable duration of incapacitation. In addition, the patient has a right to information about medically significant alternatives.
4. Patients have the right to refuse treatment to the extent permitted by law and to be informed of the medical consequences of their action.
5. Patients have the right to privacy in their medical care. Case discussion, consultation, examination, and treatment should be conducted discreetly. Those not directly involved with a patient's care must have the patient's permission to be present.
6. Patients have the right to expect that all communication and records pertaining to their care be treated as confidential.
7. Patients have the right to expect the hospital to make a reasonable response to their request for services and to provide evaluation, service, and referral as indicated.
8. Patients have the right to obtain information as to any relationship of their hospital with other healthcare and educational institutions, insofar as their care is concerned, and to the professional relationship among individuals who are treating them.
9. Patients have the right to be advised if the hospital proposes to engage in or perform human experimentation affecting their care

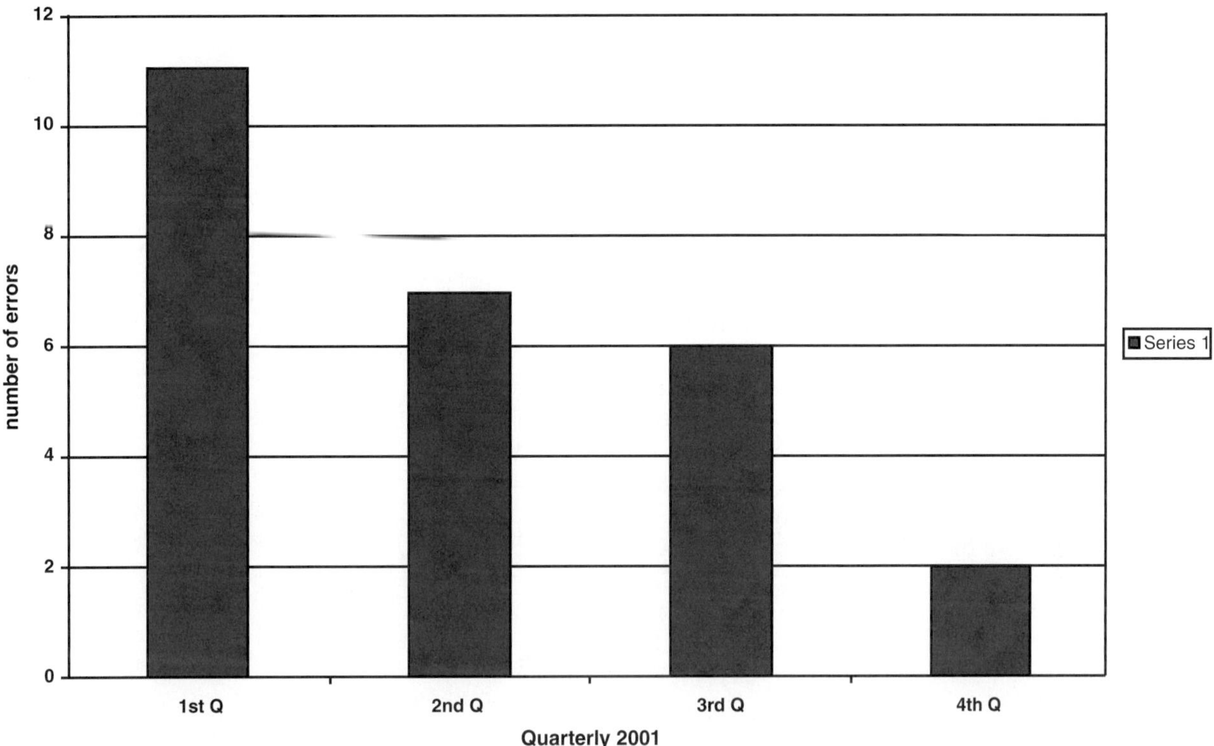

Figure 14–4 Evaluation of an improvement plan. [Courtesy of Diane Wolff, MLT (ASCP), Phlebotomy Team Leader, Nebraska Methodist Hospital, Omaha, NE.]

or treatment. Patients have the right to refuse to participate in research projects.

10 Patients have the right to expect continuity of care, including future appointments and instructions on continuing healthcare requirements after discharge.

11 Patients have the right to examine and receive an explanation of their bill, regardless of the source of payment.

12 Patients have the right to know what hospital rules and regulations apply to their conduct as a patient.

The phlebotomist is directly involved with several sections of the Patient's Bill of Rights, including:

1 Patients may be difficult to deal with because they are afraid to be in the hospital or are angry because they have just received an unfavorable diagnosis. However, the phlebotomist must still treat them with respect and consideration.

2 Notice that it is the healthcare provider, not the phlebotomist, who must provide information concerning the purpose of test procedures. When questioned, phlebotomists should refer the patient to the healthcare provider. In addition, laboratory test results are reported only to healthcare providers or their designated representatives and are never given to patients or their family members.

3 The patient has the right to refuse to have blood drawn. If the patient still refuses after you have explained the procedure and explained that it was requested by the healthcare provider to provide treatment, do not forcibly obtain the sample. Notify the nursing staff or the healthcare provider of the patient's refusal and note this information on the requisition form.

4 The patient's condition and laboratory test results are confidential and must not be discussed with anyone who is not directly

involved with the patient's care or testing. Do not discuss patient information in elevators or in the cafeteria where bystanders may overhear it.

Legal Issues

Failure to respect patients' rights can result in legal action initiated by the patient or the patient's family. Medical law regulates the conduct of members of the healthcare professions. It differs from ethics, which are recommended standards, by being legally required conduct. **Litigation** initiated because of illegal actions can be at the local, state, or national level and can result in criminal or civil prosecution. Penalties may include revocation of professional licenses, monetary fines, or imprisonment.

A **criminal lawsuit** is an action initiated by the state for committing an illegal act against the public welfare and can be punishable by imprisonment. A **civil lawsuit** is a court action between parties seeking monetary compensation for an offense. In a law-suit, the person who brings the lawsuit or action is the plaintiff, and the healthcare worker or institution against whom the action or lawsuit is filed is the defendant.

Tort Law

A wrongful act committed by one person against another that causes harm to the person or his or her property is called a **tort**. Torts are classified as intentional and unintentional. Assault and battery, defamation, and invasion of privacy are considered intentional torts, whereas negligence and malpractice are considered unintentional torts.

The threat to touch another person without his or her consent and with the intention of causing fear of harm is termed **assault**. The actual harmful touching of a person without his or her consent is called **battery**. These charges could be initiated against a phlebotomist who forcibly tries to collect a sample from a patient who refuses to have blood drawn.

Defamation is spoken or written words that can injure a person's reputation. Libel is false defamatory writing that is published, whereas slander is false and malicious spoken word.

Patients have the right to be left alone and the right to be free from unwanted exposure to public view. Entering a patient's room without asking permission may be considered a physical intrusion and an ***invasion of privacy***. Release of confidential information is considered an invasion of privacy. Other examples of invasion of privacy would be using a patient's laboratory requisition for classroom instruction purposes without removing the identification criteria or releasing patient information to a local newspaper or television reporter.

Confidentiality

The right to privacy of information is termed confidentiality. Healthcare professionals are required by law to keep confidential any information communicated in the treatment of a patient. This information includes patient or healthcare provider communications, the patient's verbal statements, or the patient's chart or laboratory results. All information acquired through the care of a patient must be kept confidential and given only to health professionals who have a medical need to know. Laboratory results may be given only to the healthcare provider, and the patient must give permission to release the test results. Phlebotomists collect specimens for employee or athlete drug or alcohol screening, as well as screening for human immunodeficiency virus (HIV) or other sexually transmitted diseases. Care must be taken that this information not be discussed where it can be overheard by unauthorized people. Special consideration is given to the confidential nature of information about patients who have positive test results for HIV. All 50 states require that acquired immunodeficiency syndrome (AIDS) cases be reported, without the patient's consent, to the Centers for Disease Control and Prevention (CDC) or to their state's health department. However, the patient's name is not reported.

With the use of computers in healthcare, confidentiality and accessibility must be addressed. HIPAA has mandated that healthcare professionals become familiar with information security standards, and ensure that policies exist to control access to and release of patient-identifiable health information.

Malpractice

Medical ***malpractice*** is misconduct or lack of skill by a healthcare professional that results in injury to the patient. ***Negligence***, which is defined as failure to give reasonable care by the healthcare provider, must be proven. Reasonable care requires that the healthcare professional understand and practice a specific "standard of care," which essentially means that they perform their duties with the same skill and knowledge as other workers with the same training and experience would. State statutes; licensing requirements; and regulatory and professional organizations such as the American Hospital Association, JCAHO, and OSHA establish these standards. Four factors must be proven to claim negligence. They are the following:

1 Duty: Indicates that there was an established standard of care and proof that it was not followed.
2 Breach of Duty: The plaintiff (patient) must show what actually happened and that the defendant (phlebotomist) failed to perform. It has to be proven that the defendant knew or should have known that this failure could cause harm.
3 Causation: Indicates that the breach of duty directly caused the injury and that no other factors could have contributed.
4 Damages: Actual physical, emotional, or financial injury had to occur to the plaintiff (patient) because of the negligent act.

Examples of medical malpractice that could involve the phlebotomist include the following:

- Failure to raise a bedrail that has been lowered during the phlebotomy procedure, resulting in the patient falling out of bed
- Performing an unauthorized arterial puncture, producing an arteriospasm or excessive bleeding
- Failure to follow OSHA required standard precautions, causing transmission of an infectious disease
- Performing a venipuncture at an excessive angle or from a nonoptimal location, causing permanent nerve damage
- Misidentification of a patient or specimen, resulting in inappropriate treatment or death

Patient Consent

Informed consent is the voluntary agreement to allow touching, examination, or treatment by medically authorized personnel. Informed consent requires that the healthcare professional explain what the medical procedure is; how it is to be performed, including possible risks; and the expected results. The healthcare provider should also explain alternative procedures and the consequences if treatment is not given. The procedure must be explained in nontechnical terms and in the patient's native language. An interpreter may be necessary to ensure comprehension. Vital to consent is the patient's belief that the healthcare professional is competent to perform the procedure. Healthcare professionals may be legally liable for failing to offer information to patients and for not obtaining informed consent. Consent may be obtained orally or in writing, or expressed by nonverbal behavior. For blood collection, the phlebotomist must explain the procedure that will be used to collect the blood specimen, stressing that the patient's healthcare provider ordered the test. The patient expects that the phlebotomist is competent in blood collection procedures and gives consent to collect the blood samples by extending the arm or rolling up the sleeve. Written consent is necessary for more invasive procedures. Figure 14–5 is an example of a written consent form that a patient would be required to sign before any diagnostic or therapeutic procedure. Phlebotomists often assist the physician when a bone marrow biopsy is performed. It might be the phlebotomist's responsibility to ensure that the consent form is signed before the procedure. A patient has the right to refuse medical treatment, and this decision should be documented in the medical record.

Blood collection in minors requires consent of their parents or legal guardians. A legally responsible person must give consent for patients who cannot communicate, persons who are mentally incompetent, patients in shock or trauma, demented patients, or those under the influence of drugs or alcohol. A legal guardian who can give consent may have to be appointed by the courts.

Implied Consent

Implied consent exists when emergency procedures must be performed to save a person's life or prevent permanent impairment to the patient. The law implies consent for treatment for these patients without consent from the responsible party. Implied consent is a state statute, and the limitations vary from state to state.

Consent for Testing for Human Immunodeficiency Virus

State legislation requires informed consent be obtained before HIV testing is performed. The laws

AUTHORIZATION FOR AND CONSENT TO SURGERY OR SPECIAL DIAGNOSTIC OR THERAPEUTIC PROCEDURES

Patient's Name: ____________________

Proposed operation(s) or Procedure(s): ____________________

____

I have been advised by my physician(s) that the operation(s) or procedure(s) listed above may be beneficial in the diagnosis or treatment of my condition; therefore,

I authorized and direct ____________________, M.D. and associates or assistants of his choice, if any, to perform the operation(s) or procedure(s) listed above and to do any other procedure that he may deem necessary during the above operation. I also authorize the use of such services involving anesthesia, radiology, pathology and the like, as may be advisable for my well-being.

The nature and purpose of the operation(s) or procedure(s) have been explained to me by my physician(s) and no guarantees or assurance has been made as to the results that may be obtained. I have been advised that these surgical operations and special diagnostic or therapeutic procedures all involve risks or serious complications from both known and unknown causes. I understand that, except in cases of emergency or exceptional circumstances, these operations and procedures are not performed unless the patient has had an opportunity to discuss them with his physician. Each patient has the right to consent or refuse to consent to any proposed operation or special procedure.

I understand that body parts, organs, or other human tissues may be removed as a necessary part of this procedure. Except as noted below, I relinquish any claim to these tissues and authorize the physician(s) or hospital to dispose of these tissues in their discretion, or to preserve these tissues for use in scientific research, education, treatment of other persons, or the development of new medical products or procedures. Exceptions (if any): ____________________

____

MY SIGNATURE BELOW CONSTITUTES MY ACKNOWLEDGEMENT THAT I HAVE READ AND AGREED TO THE FOLLOWING:

(1) That the proposed operation(s) or procedure(s) has been satisfactorily explained to me and that I have all of the information that I desire; and

(2) That I hereby give my authorization and consent.

Patient's Signature: ____________________

Witness: ____________________

Date: __________ Time: __________ A.M. __________

I, the physician, discussed the operation(s)/procedure(s) listed above including the risks, benefits, and alternatives, with the patient/parent/legal guardian prior to the operation(s) procedure(s) ____________________

Physician signature

100020626 Rev. 11/98

Figure 14–5 Example of a patient consent form. [Courtesy of Diane Wolff, MLT (ASCP), Phlebotomy Team Leader, Nebraska Methodist Hospital, Omaha, NE.]

dictate what type of information must be provided to the patient. The patient must have an explanation of the test and its purpose, possible uses of the test, the limitations of the test, and the meaning of the test results. In some states an accidental needlestick is considered a significant exposure to the healthcare worker, and HIV testing can be ordered by a healthcare provider without patient consent. In this situation, the HIV results are not entered into the patient's chart.

Medical Records

Medical records must be kept on each patient to document a patient's medical history. The records include medications, prescriptions, diagnostic procedures, and test results. The primary purposes of a medical record are the following:

- To provide a plan for managing patient care
- To document communication between the healthcare provider and others involved in patient care
- To document total healthcare from birth to death
- To provide documentation of patterns in the patient's illness and treatment
- To serve as a legal document for evidence in litigation and to protect the legal interests of the patient, hospital, and healthcare workers
- To provide clinical data for peer review and medical research, education, and statistics
- To assist in billing, utilization review, TQM, and CQI

A good medical record must be accurate, complete, and concise. The initials or name of every healthcare worker that performed a diagnostic procedure, collected blood specimens, or performed laboratory tests on a patient is documented in a patient's record. Without a medical record, it would be impossible for a phlebotomist to remember every patient from whom he or she had collected a blood specimen. This is why it is important that the requisition or computer label be properly documented with the phlebotomist's initials, as well as the date and time. Document all actions completely on the patient's chart or in the computer stating unusual circumstances, such as deviations from standard practice, possible reason for a hematoma, patient refusal to have blood collected, patient not fasting, location of intravenous (IV) or indwelling lines, or any other problems associated with the blood collection.

With the efficiency of computers, patient test results can be quickly transmitted to the patient's record. Before releasing results, always double-check that they have been entered into the computer accurately. If a result has been entered incorrectly and is on the patient's record, follow the institution's policy for correcting the result on the patient's chart or in the computer.

Tips for documentation in a patient's record include the following:

- Write in ink.
- Record phlebotomist's initials and complete date and time of specimen collection.
- Use standardized medical abbreviations.
- Document your actions and the patient's actions completely.
- Never erase an error; draw a single thin line through the error and initial it.
- Do not delete errors in computer test results. Enter the correct test result online with a comment indicating a data entry error.

Statute of Limitations

State legislatures establish the statute of limitations that restricts the time allowed for an individual to initiate any type of legal action. These are established to force legal action while patient records are available and the persons involved can remember the facts of the case. The statute of limitations begins:

- At the time when the negligent act was allegedly committed
- When the patient discovered or should have discovered the alleged negligence
- When the care, treatment, or healthcare provider-patient relationship ended

The statute of limitations varies from state to state, ranging from 1 to 6 years depending on the offense.

Respondeat Superior

The Latin phrase *respondeat superior*, "let the master answer," establishes that employers are responsible for their own acts of negligence as well as their employees' acts. Institutions are responsible for ensuring that their employees perform only those tasks that are within the scope of their knowledge and training. However, this does not diminish the responsibility of the employee. Both the institution and the employee can be found liable if injury occurs to the patient because of the employee's actions. Professional liability should be a concern for all healthcare workers.

Malpractice Insurance

All healthcare workers should carry malpractice insurance. Liability insurance can be purchased at a reduced rate through professional organizations. Most institutions have policies covering all workers, and the phlebotomist should confirm this coverage at the time of employment. The phlebotomist who works independently for insurance companies or home healthcare agencies should be covered by personal malpractice insurance.

By consistently practicing good patient care, the phlebotomist can avoid the trauma of a lawsuit. Guidelines to preventing a lawsuit include the following:

- Obtain informed consent before collecting specimens.
- Perform within the scope of training and education.
- Comply with state statutes and federal regulations (OSHA and JCAHO regulations).
- Adhere to standard blood collection techniques as determined by NCCLS guidelines, procedure manuals, and package inserts.
- Practice aseptic phlebotomy techniques.
- Correctly use personal protection equipment including safety devices and containers.
- Practice standard precautions.
- Keep patient information confidential.
- Practice good communication skills and genuine caring for the patient.
- Accurately record information concerning patients.
- Relay patient reports to the proper supervisor.
- Document incidents immediately and report them to a supervisor.
- Document any deviations from the standard care of practice.
- Avoid unethical criticism of other healthcare professionals.
- Regularly participate in continuing education to maintain proficiency.
- Ensure that continuing education records are maintained.

Risk Management

The potential for injury exists in the healthcare profession, and the phlebotomist should be aware of these risks and the precautions necessary to minimize them. Risk is inherent with every venipuncture. Risk management departments develop policies to protect patients and employees from preventable injuries and the employer from financial loss. Risk management programs must identify the risk; determine policies and procedures to prevent the risk; educate employees, patients, and visitors; and evaluate changes that may be necessary for improvement.

Various tools are available to identify risks and determine methods for reducing risk and the financial loss incurred by paying for the occurrences after they have happened. One commonly used tool in the phlebotomy department is the incident report. The employee who detects the incident describes both the incident and the corrective action taken. Each step of the follow-up should be clearly documented. This form is used to investigate the occurrence and is signed by the employee's supervisor and reviewed by the QA coordinator (Fig. 14–6).

New policies and procedures are continually being developed and instituted as incidents are investigated. Effective communication and education in the new policies must be available for employees for successful implementation.

The Pathology Center at Methodist Hospital
PATHOLOGY INCIDENT REPORT

PART 1. TO BE COMPLETED BY EMPLOYEE DETECTING OCCURRENCE

Date of incident ________ Time of incident ________

Employee initiating report ________ Date of report ________

Patient Name ________ Patient ID ________ Room Number ________

Description of occurrence. Include any attachments, pertinent details, any supporting evidence or documentation, and immediate corrective action taken. Attach additional pages if necessary.

Immediate Corrective Action ________

Employee signature (or initials)

Forward to Team Leader or Employee for additional comments

Page 1 of 2

The Pathology Center at Methodist Hospital

PART 2. TO BE COMPLETED BY EMPLOYEE (If different than employee initiating report)
(Forward to Team Leader)
Additional Comments

Signature/Date ________

Part 3. To be completed by Team Leader (Forward to Service Leader)
Patient Condition : Changed ________ Unchanged ________
Physician Notifed? Y N Name ________ Time ________ Date ________

Corrective Action Taken (if additional to immediate corrective action)

Team Leader signature/date

PART 4: Classification of Incident (To be completed by Service Leader or Quality Assurance Coordinator)

Pathology Incident	Methodist Hospital Incident	Client Incident
A. __Specimen Problem	A. __Specimen Problem	A. __Specimen Problem
B. __Specimen ID	B. __Specimen ID	B. __Specimen ID
C. __Patient ID	C. __Patient ID	C. __Patient ID
D. __Order Error	D. __Order Error	D. __Order Error
E. __Safety Violation	E. __Safety Violation	E. __Safety Violation
F. __Complaint	F. __Complaint	F. __Complaint
G. __Communication	G. __Communication	G. __Communication
H. __Failure to respond to a STAT	H. __Lack of required information	H. __Lack of required information
I. __Test performed improperly	I. __Technical/procedural error	I. __Technical/Procedural error
J. __Result entry error	J. __Miscellaneous	J. __Miscellaneous
K. __Miscellaneous		
____ Courier	____ Tube system	Service Leader review ____
____ Other		QA Coordinator review ____

Copy of report sent to:

Name ________ Title ________ Dept ________
Name ________ Title ________ Dept ________
Name ________ Title ________ Dept ________

Page 2 of 2

Figure 14–6 Pathology incident report. (Courtesy of Diane Wolff, MLT (ASCP), Phlebotomy Team Leader, Nebraska Methodist Hospital, Omaha, NE.)

Bibliography

Haun, DE, et al: Assessing the competence of specimen-processing personnel. Laboratory Medicine 31:633–637, 2000.

Joint Commission on Accreditation of Healthcare Organizations: Comprehensive Accreditation Manual for Hospitals. JCAHO, Oakbrook Terrace, IL, 2002.

Lewis, MA, and Tamparo, CD: Medical Law, Ethics, and Bioethics for Ambulatory Care, ed. 5. FA Davis, Philadelphia, 2002.

National Academy of Sciences' Institute of Medicine: To Err is Human: Building a Safer Health System. National Academy Press, Washington, D.C., 1999.

National Committee for Clinical Laboratory Standards Approved Guideline 18-A2: Procedures for the Handling and Processing of Blood Specimens. NCCLS, Wayne, PA, 1994.

Study Questions

1. Define QA.

____

____

2. Where must the phlebotomy procedure manual be located?

____

3. State a circumstance in which the procedure manual must be used by the phlebotomist.

____

4. State the role of variables in the development of a QA program.

____

____

____

5. Identify each of the following as a preanalytical, analytical, or postanalytical variable.

   a. __________ Routine complete blood count (CBC) ordered stat

   b. __________ Decimal point misplaced when results are entered into the computer

   c. __________ Hemolyzed specimen

   d. __________ Use of outdated controls for POCT

   e. __________ Increase in contaminated blood cultures

6. Explain how a laboratory reference manual improves the quality of patient testing.

____

____

7. List three preanalytical errors that may be detected by a delta check.

   a. ____

   b. ____

   c. ____

8. How should evacuated tubes be stored in the laboratory?

____

9. True or False. Errors in phlebotomy site collection can affect both patient safety and specimen quality.

____

10. State two ways in which excessive vibration of specimen tubes during transport can affect specimen QA.

    a. ____

    b. ____

11. Within what time frame should plasma or serum be separated from red blood cells?

____

12. State two ways in which specimen quality can be affected when specimens are left uncovered for prolonged periods of time.

    a. ____

    b. ____

13. Briefly describe the QC of centrifuges, refrigerators, and freezers.

____

____

____

14. True or False. It is acceptable to combine plasma collected in lavender and green stopper tubes but not lavender and light blue stopper tubes. Explain your answer.

____

____

15. How is phlebotomy most affected by HIPAA?

____

16. How does QA differ from TQM and CQI?

____

____

17. The primary goal of TQM is

____.

18. Name the four areas assessed by TQM.

    a. ____

    b. ____

c. ______

d. ______

19. Name four customers of the laboratory.

a. ______

b. ______

c. ______

d. ______

20. The worst patient outcome is ______ .

21. State the four dimensions of performance addressed by CQI.

a. ______

b. ______

c. ______

d. ______

22. How do PDMAI and PDCA help an organization meet JCAHO requirements for CQI?

______

23. True or False. Most medical errors are the fault of individuals, not the system.

______

24. Define sentinel event.

______

25. How could a phlebotomist cause a sentinel event?

______

26. List two patient's rights that could result in a lawsuit if the phlebotomist did not observe them.

a. ______

b. ______

27. The principles of right and wrong are called ______ .

28. Describe two incidents that could cause a phlebotomist to be charged with negligence.

a. ______

b. ______

29. What factors must be present to prove negligence?

    a. ______

    b. ______

    c. ______

    d. ______

30. Informed consent is a right of the patient. Explain the role the phlebotomist has in ensuring this right.

    ______

31. List four elements of a risk management program.

    a. ______

    b. ______

    c. ______

    d. ______

32. Name a form used to identify risk patterns in the phlebotomy department.

    ______

Clinical Situations

1. The phlebotomy supervisor completes a study of the specimen ordering patterns initiated as a result of phlebotomy staff dissatisfaction with department organization and complaints about test TAT by the units. State a reason and a corrective action that could be taken for each of the following problems identified by the study.

   a. Increased requests for stat CBCs from the psychiatric unit.

      ______

   b. Patient surveys reveal complaints about phlebotomists frequently returning to perform a second puncture after a short period of time.

      ______

   c. The chemistry department is rejecting an increased number of specimens collected by personnel in the emergency room.

      ______

   d. The medical unit reports delays in the collection of timed tests.

      ______

2. The specimen processing department is cited during an accreditation visit.
   a. What daily equipment documentation could have been missing?

   ____

   b. What documentation on preventive maintenance of equipment could have been missing?

   ____

3. State an error in specimen processing that could cause each of the following problems.
   a. A normal blood alcohol in a noticeably intoxicated person.

   ____

   b. Follow-up on a delta checked flagged result indicates that the specimen was from a different patient.

   ____

   c. Calcium results show a trend that is abnormally high.

   ____

   d. Potassium results are noticeably increased and glucose results are noticeably decreased from specimens collected during morning sweeps.

   ____

4. The laboratory is accused of failure to report a critical result to the intensive care unit. What documentation is requested from the phlebotomist assigned to make the call?

   ____

5. A sentinel event involving a hemolytic transfusion reaction is reported to the JCAHO. The phlebotomy department is identified in the root cause analysis.
   a. What is the most probable cause?

   ____

   b. The phlebotomist insists that the wristband was checked. What else should have been done?

   ____

   c. Suggest an action plan that could be proposed to prevent this event from happening in the future.

   ____

6. A phlebotomist is assigned to the hospital TQM/CQI committee. State a contribution that the phlebotomist can make to each of these areas.
   a. Physical infrastructure

   ____

b. Personnel infrastructure

____

c. Management infrastructure

____

d. Process

____

7. State an example for phlebotomy (other than the one in the book) for each of these performance dimensions.

   a. Doing the wrong thing right

   ____

   b. Doing the wrong thing wrong

   ____

   c. Doing the right thing wrong

   ____

   d. Doing the right thing right

   ____

8. State an action by a phlebotomist that would violate sections 1, 2, 4, and 5 of the Patient's Bill of Rights.

   a. Section 1

   ____

   b. Section 2

   ____

   c. Section 4

   ____

   d. Section 5

   ____

9. A hometown professional football player was admitted to the hospital for blood work. Tests to rule out Hodgkin's disease were ordered. The phlebotomist obtained the blood specimens and delivered them to the laboratory. After work, he or she excitedly told his or her friends of the famous person and the sad reason why he was in the hospital.

   a. Could the phlebotomist face legal charges? Why or why not?

   ____

b. If the football coach calls the laboratory for the test results, can a phlebotomist release the results? Why or why not?

____

c. Under what conditions would HIPAA permit release of these results to the coach?

____

10. Indicate whether a phlebotomist would be accused of libel, slander, assault, battery, invasion of privacy, negligence, or malpractice in the following situations.

a. A phlebotomist tells a patient who refuses to have blood drawn that help will be summoned to forcibly obtain the blood.

____

b. A nurse reports that a patient was found sleeping with a bedrail lowered after the phlebotomist had drawn blood.

____

c. A phlebotomist, angry over recently receiving a speeding ticket, tells a local reporter that the police officer has been to the hospital for an HIV test and it was positive. The hospital has no record of this.

____

d. A phlebotomist pretends to be checking on a celebrity patient who is recovering from surgery.

____

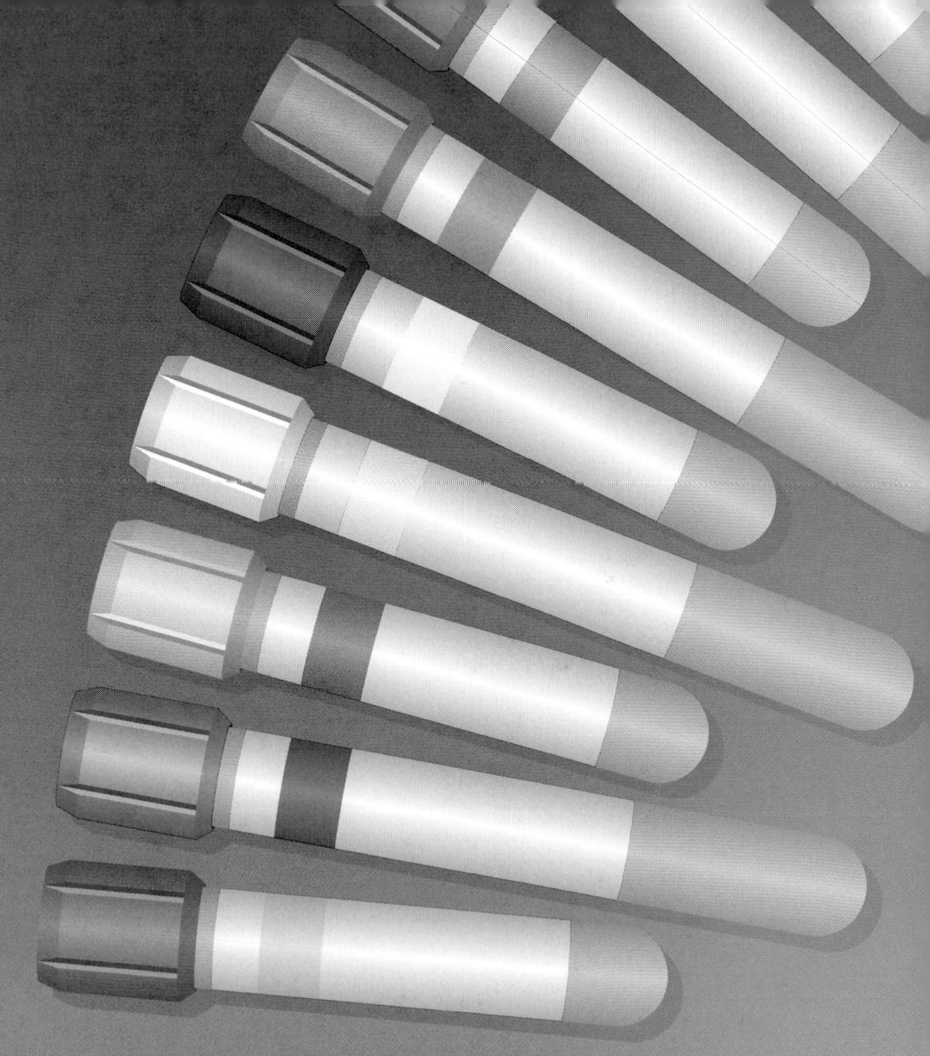

Section Three

Body Systems (Terminology, Anatomy, and Physiology)

Chapter 15

Basic Medical Terminology

Chapter Outline

Prefixes and Suffixes
- Common Prefixes
- Common Suffixes

Word Roots and Combining Forms

Plural Forms

Abbreviations

Learning Objectives

Upon completion of this chapter, the reader will be able to:

1. Define and state the purpose of prefixes, word roots, suffixes, and combining forms.
2. Correctly form medical terms using prefixes, word roots, suffixes, and combining forms.
3. State the meaning of the commonly used prefixes, suffixes, and word roots.
4. Associate common word roots with the corresponding body system.

Medical terminology is derived primarily from the classic Greek and Latin languages. However, it is not necessary to master either of these languages to obtain a solid background in basic medical terminology. Medical terms consist of combinations of three major word parts: prefixes, word roots, and suffixes. The same prefixes and suffixes are frequently used with different word roots. Therefore, knowledge of a small number of commonly used prefixes, word roots, and suffixes can provide the phlebotomist with an extensive medical vocabulary and the medical communication skills necessary for successful job performance.

Prefixes and Suffixes

Prefixes are letters or syllables added to the beginning of a word root to alter its meaning. The prefix usually indicates direction, number, position, or time.

Suffixes are letters or syllables added to the end of a word root to alter its meaning. In medical terminology, suffixes often indicate a condition or a type of procedure.

The most commonly used prefixes and suffixes are presented in this chapter. It is necessary to memorize these common prefixes and suffixes. This process is easier if you relate them to terms that are already familiar to you.

EXAMPLE: In medical terminology, the prefix "post" means "after," just as it does in the term "postgraduate." The suffix "-ectomy" means "surgical removal," and the term "tonsillectomy" is a familiar word to most people.

Common Prefixes

PREFIXES	MEANING
a-, an-, ar-	no, not, without
ab-	away from
acou-	hearing
ad-	toward
af-	to, toward
alba-	white
ambi-	both
ana-	up
aniso-	unequal
ante-	before
anti-, contra-	against
atél-	imperfect, incomplete
auto-	self
bi-	two
bio-	life
blasto-	growth
brachy-	short
brady-	slow
cata-	down
centi-	hundred
chromo-	color
circum-, peri-	around
co-, com-, con-	together, with
contra-	opposite
cyan-	blue
de-	down, from
dia-	through, complete
diplo-	double
dis-	apart, away from
dys-	difficult, painful
ecto-, exo-	outside
edem-	swelling
endo-, intra-	inside, within
epi-	on, over
erythr-	red
eu-	normal, good
ex-	out, away from
exo-	without, outside of
extra-	outside of, in addition to, beyond
fasci-	band
fore-	before, in front
haplo-	single, simple
hemi-	half
hetero-	different
homo-	same
homeo-	unchanged
hydro-	water
hyper-	increased
hypo-	decreased
idio-	distinct, peculiar to an individual
infra-, sub-	below
inter-	between
intra-	within
iso-	equal

lacri-	tears
macro-	large
mal-	bad, ill
medi-	middle
mega-	great
meta-	beyond
micro-	small
milli-	one thousandth
mono-, uni-	one
multi-, poly-	many
narco-	sleep
neo-	new
non-	not
pan-	all
para-	beside, abnormal
per-	through
peri-	around
poly-	many
post-, retro-	after
pre-, ante-	before, in front
primi-	first
pro-	before, in front of
pseudo-	false
quadri-, quadro-	four
retro-	behind, backward
semi-	half
steno-	narrow
sub-	below
supra-, super-	above
sym-	together
syn-	together
tachy-	fast
tox-	poison
trans-	across
tri-	three
ultra-	excessive, extreme

Common Suffixes

SUFFIXES	MEANING
-ac, -al, -ar, -ary, -ic	pertaining to
-ad	toward
-agon	assemble, gather together
-algesia	excessive sensitivity to pain
-algia, -dynia	pain
-an	characteristic of
-ar	relating to
-arche	beginning
-ase	enzyme
-asthenia	lack of strength
-atresia	abnormal closure
-blast	immature cell
-capnia	carbon dioxide
-cele	swelling
-centesis	surgical puncture
-cidal	pertaining to death
-cide	kill
-clast	break
-coccus	spherical
-crine	secrete
-cyte	cell
-cytosis	abnormal condition of cells
-desis	binding, stabilizing, fusion
-dipsia	thirst
-ectasia, -ectasis	distention, expansion
-ectomy	surgical removal
-emesis	vomit
-emia	pertaining to blood
-esthesia	nervous sensation
-form	structure
-gen	producing
-genesis	origin of
-globin, -globulin	protein
-gram	written record
-graph	an instrument for making records
-graphy	method of recording
-gravida	pregnancy
-ia	condition
-iasis	diseased condition
-ile	having qualities of
-ion	process
-ism	condition of
-ist	specialist
-itis	inflammation
-kinesia	movement
-lepsy	seizure
-lith	stone
-logist	one who studies
-logy	study of
-lysis, -rrhexis	rupture
-malacia	softening
-megaly	enlargement
-meter	instrument to measure
-metry	measurement

-ness	state of, quality
-oid	like, similar to
-ole	small, little
-oma	tumor
-opia	eye, vision
-ory	pertaining to
-ose	sugar, having qualities of
-osis, -iasis	abnormal condition
-ostomy	surgical opening
-otomy	cut into, incision into
-ous	pertaining to
-oxia	oxygen level
-paresis	weakness
-pathy	disease
-penia	lack of, deficiency
-pepsia	digestion
-pexy	fixation
-phagia	eating, swallowing
-philia	increase in cell numbers
-phobia	fear
-phonia	voice
-phylaxis	protection
-physis	growth
-plasia	growth
-plasty	surgical repair
-plegia	paralysis
-pnea	breathing
-poiesis	production
-prandial	meal
-ptosis	dropping
-ptysis	spitting
-rrhage	bursting forth
-rrhea	discharge
-scope	instrument for viewing
-scopy	visual examination
-spasm, -stalsis	involuntary contraction
-stasis	controlling, to be still, stop
-sthenia	strength
-stenosis	narrowing, tightening
-stomy	new opening
-taxia	muscle coordination
-tension	pressure
-therapy	treatment
-tome	instrument for cutting
-tomy	incision
-tripsy	crushing
-trophy	development
-tropin	stimulation
-tropic	turning toward
-ula, -ule	small, little
-uria	pertaining to urine
-y	condition, process

Word Roots and Combining Forms

Word roots are the main part of a word and may be combined with prefixes, suffixes, or other roots. The combining form of a word root contains a vowel, usually an "o," which is used to facilitate pronunciation when the word root is combined with another word root or a suffix that does not begin with a vowel.

EXAMPLE: The word root for "heart" is "cardi"

The combining form is "cardi/o"

The suffix "logy" is "study of"

The study of the heart is "cardiology"

A combining vowel is not used when the suffix already begins with a vowel.

EXAMPLE: The word root for "liver" is "hepat"

The suffix for "inflammation" is "itis"

Inflammation of the liver is "hepatitis"

The combining vowel however remains between two word roots even if the second root begins with a vowel.

EXAMPLE: The word root for "electricity" is "electr"

The combining form is "electr/o"

The word root for "brain" is "encephal"

The suffix for "written record" is "gram"

A written record of the electricity of the brain is an "electroencephalogram"

When defining a medical term, begin at the last part of the word (suffix), then define the first part of the word (prefix), and last, define the middle of the word (word root).

Word roots frequently refer to body components. Therefore, common word roots are listed with their corresponding body system in this chapter.

BODY SYSTEM	WORD ROOT OR COMBINING FORM	MEANING
Anatomy	anter/o	front, before
	dist/o	distant
	dors/o	back
	kary/o	nucleus
	later/o	side
	medi/o	middle
	poster/o	back, behind
	proxim/o	near
	viscer/o	internal organs
Integumentary	albin/o	white
	carcin/o	cancer
	cutane/o, dermat/o, derm/o	skin
	erythemat/o	redness
	hidr/o	sweat
	hist/o	tissue
	hydr/o	water
	kerat/o	hard tissue
	melan/o	black
	onych/o	nail
	seb/o	sebum or oily secretion
	squam/o	scalelike
	trich/o	hair
	xanth/o	yellow
Skeletal	arthr/o	joint
	axill/o	armpit
	cephal/o	head
	caud/o	tail
	chrondr/o	cartilage
	cost/o	ribs
	dactyl/o	finger or toe
	fibul/o	fibula
	humer/o	humerus
	mandibul/o	lower jawbone
	maxill/o	upper jawbone
	myel/o	bone marrow
	orth/o	straight
	oste/o	bone
	patell/o	kneecap
	rheumat/o	watery flow
	sacr/o	sacrum
	scapul/o	shoulder blade
	spondyl/o	vertebrae
	synov/i	synovial membrane
Muscular	fibr/o	fibrous connective tissue
	my/o, muscul/o	muscle
	kinesi/o	movement
Nervous	cerebell/o	cerebellum
	cerebr/o	cerebrum
	crani/o	skull
	encephal/o	brain
	gli/o	glue
	mening/o	meninges
	neur/o	nerve
Respiratory	alveol/o	alveolus, air sac
	bronch/o	bronchus
	cyan/o	blue
	nas/o, rhin/o	nose
	olfact/o	sense of smell
	pector/o, thorac/o	chest
	pleur/o	pleura
	pneum/o	air, lung
	pulmon/o	lung
	spir/o	breathe
	steth/o	chest
	trache/o	trachea, windpipe
Digestive	abdomin/o	abdomen
	adip/o, lip/o, steat/o	fat
	amyl/o	starch
	bil/i, chol/o	bile, gall
	bucc/o	cheek
	celi/o, lapar/o	abdomen
	cholecyst/o	gallbladder
	choledoch/o	common bile duct
	cirrh/o	yellow
	col/o	colon
	dent/i, odont/o	tooth
	enter/o	intestine
	esophag/o	esophagus
	gastr/o	stomach
	gingiv/o	gums
	gloss/o, lingu/o	tongue
	gluc/o, glyc/o	glucose
	hepat/o	liver
	icter/o	jaundice
	lith/o	stone
	or/o, stomat/o	mouth
	proct/o	rectum

	sigmoid/o	sigmoid colon
Urinary	cyst/o	urinary bladder
	glomerul/o	glomerulus
	micturit/o	urination
	nephr/o, ren/o	kidney
	noct/i	night
	olig/o	scanty
	pyel/o	renal
	ur/o, urin/o	urine
Endocrine	aden/o	gland
	andr/o	male
	cortic/o	cortex
	crin/o	secrete
	kal/o	potassium
	natr/o	sodium
	somat/o	body
	ster/o	solid structure
	thyr/o	thyroid gland
Reproductive	amni/o	amnion
	balan/o	glans penis
	colp/o	vagina
	episi/o	vulva
	gonad/o	sex glands
	gynec/o	female
	hyster/o	uterus, womb
	lact/o	milk
	mamm/o, mast/o	breast
	men/o	menses, menstruation
	nat/o	birth
	oopho/o, ovul/o	ovary
	orch/o	testes
	ovari/o	ovary
	salping/o	fallopian tubes
	spermat/o	spermatozoa
	test/o	testicle
Circulatory	angi/o	vessel
	arteri/o	artery
	ather/o	fatty substance
	brachi/o	arm
	cardi/o, coron/o	heart
	cyt/o	cell
	erythr/o	red
	leuk/o	white
	scler/o	hardening
	ser/o	serum
	sphygm/o	pulse
	thromb/o	clot
	vas/o	vessel
	ven/o	vein
Lymphatic	immun/o	protection
	lymphaden/o	lymph node
	splen/o	spleen
	tox/o	poison
General	aer/o	air
	agglutin/o	clumping
	ambul/o	to walk
	anis/o	unequal
	audi/o	to hear
	aur/o, ot/o	ear
	bacill/o	rod
	bi/o	life
	coagul/o	clotting
	cry/o	cold
	esthesi/o	feeling
	febr/o	fever
	gen/o	formation
	ger/o	old age
	hem/o, hemat/o	blood
	isch/o	to hold back
	kil/o	thousand
	morph/o	form
	myc/o	fungus
	myring/o	eardrum
	necr/o	death
	nos/o	pertaining to disease
	ocul/o, ophthalm/o	eye
	onc/o	tumor
	opt/o	vision
	path/o	disease
	ped/i	children
	phag/o	eat
	pharmac/o	drug
	phleb/o	vein
	prandi/o	meal
	psych/o	mind
	pur/o, py/o	pus
	radi/o	x-ray, radiant energy

Plural Forms

In writing using medical terms, it is important to know that various medical terms have different plural forms. The phlebotomist should become familiar with the common word endings that have an unusual plural ending.

EXAMPLE: appendix, singular
appendices, plural

SINGULAR WORD ENDING	PLURAL ENDING
-a	-ae
-ax	-aces
-en	-ina
-ex, ix	-ices
-is	-es
-ma	-mata
-nx	-nges
-on	-a
-um	-a
-us	-i
-y	-ies

Abbreviations

Abbreviations are used to shorten words, names, or phrases. Numerous abbreviations are used in the medical field to represent terms, names of organizations, or common medical phrases. Laboratory tests are frequently abbreviated, and phlebotomists must become familiar with these abbreviations.

General medical abbreviations are listed below, and a more extensive list of abbreviations can be found in Appendix III.

ABBREVIATIONS	DEFINITION
ASAP	as soon as possible
bid	twice a day
cc, cm^3	cubic centimeter
cm	centimeter
CPR	cardiopulmonary resuscitation
DOA	dead on arrival
DOB	date of birth
Dx	diagnosis
EKG	electrocardiogram
ER	emergency room
g, gm	gram
Hx	history
IM	intramuscular
IV	intravenous
kg	kilogram
mg	milligram
mL	milliliter
mm	millimeter
NB	newborn
NPO	nothing by mouth
OP	outpatient
post-op	after surgery
pp	postprandial
pre-op	before surgery
PRN	allowable as needed
q	every
qh	every hour
qid	four times a day
QNS	quantity nonsufficient
R/O	rule out
Rx	prescription/treatment
stat	immediately
TPN	total parenteral nutrition (IV feeding)
TPR	temperature, pulse, respiration
Tx	treatment
*u*L	microliter

Bibliography

Gylys, BA, and Wedding, ME: Medical Terminology: A Systems Approach, ed. 3. FA Davis, 1999, Philadelphia.

Masters, RM and Gylys, ME: Introducing Medical Terminology Specialties. FA Davis, 2003, Philadelphia.

Scanlon, V, and Sanders, T: Essentials of Anatomy and Physiology, ed.3. FA Davis, 1999, Philadelphia.

Study Questions

1. To each of the commonly used prefixes add a root to form a word with which you are familiar. It does not have to be medical terminology, but should represent the meaning of the prefix. See the example.

a TYPICAL ____	exo ____	multi ____
ab ____	extra ____	neo ____
ad ____	hetero ____	pan ____
an ____	homo ____	peri ____
ante ____	hydro ____	poly ____
anti ____	hyper ____	post ____
bi ____	hypo ____	pre ____
circum ____	inter ____	pseudo ____
co ____	intra ____	retro ____
con ____	iso ____	sub ____
contra ____	macro ____	super ____
dys ____	mal ____	supra ____
ecto ____	meta ____	trans ____
endo ____	micro ____	uni ____
epi ____	mono ____	

2. Find 10 commonly used suffixes that you can add to a word root or a combining form and create a word that is familiar to you.

   a. ____

   b. ____

   c. ____

   d. ____

e. ______________________________

f. ______________________________

g. ______________________________

h. ______________________________

i. ______________________________

j. ______________________________

3. Define the following medical terms and indicate the body system to which each refers. Underline the root word.

	Definition	Body System
hepatitis	____________	____________
cardiologist	____________	____________
mastectomy	____________	____________
dermal	____________	____________
gastroenterology	____________	____________

4. Complete each medical word.

Incomplete Word Root	Meaning
a. nephr/ ____________	inflammation of a kidney
b. hemat/ ____________	study of blood
c. phleb/o ____________	incision of a vein
d. cardi/o ____________	written record of the heart

5. Find a suffix for each of the following definitions and find the suffix in the word puzzle on page 349 and circle it. Suffixes may be horizontal, vertical, or diagonal, and may be spelled backward.

like ___oid___	surgical puncture ____________
study of ____________	surgical removal ____________
disease ____________	written record ____________

pain ______	method of recording ______
poison ______	surgical repair ______
controlling ______	instrument for cutting ______
enlargement ______	surgical opening ______
tumor ______	instrument for viewing ______
inflammation ______	

C	F	B	I	A	D	X	E	T	M
E	Y	W	Y	L	O	G	Y	S	A
N	T	Q	H	G	P	G	I	T	R
T	S	I	T	I	R	S	X	O	G
E	A	N	A	A	A	Y	A	X	E
S	L	A	P	T	J	M	M	I	C
I	P	H	S	I	H	O	O	C	T
S	Y	M	E	M	O	T	I	U	O
S	C	O	P	E	K	S	I	D	M
Y	L	A	G	E	M	O	H	S	Y

6. Identify the following abbreviations or definitions, and then find the answer in the word puzzle on page 350 and circle it. Answers may be horizontal, vertical, or diagonal and may be spelled backward.

Cm centimeter	as soon as possible ______
Dx ______	intravenous ______
NB ______	four times a day ______
g ______	allowable as needed ______
R/O ______	date of birth ______
immediately ______	quantity nonsufficient ______
prescription ______	nothing by mouth ______
before surgery ______	cardiopulmonary resuscitation ______

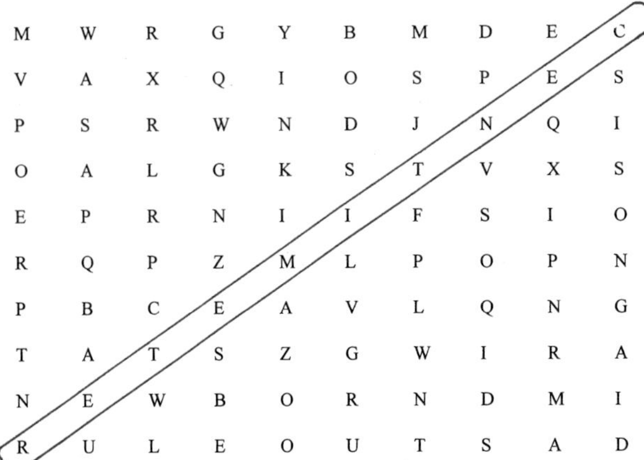

7. Translate the following statements.

   a. A preop patient must be NPO.

   ____

   ____

   b. The stat specimen drawn by the phlebotomist was QNS to R/O a Dx of heart disease.

   ____

   ____

   c. A postop patient receives 25 mg of IV pain medication, PRN.

   ____

   ____

Chapter 16

Basic Anatomy and Physiology

Chapter Outline

Organizational Levels of the Body
- Cells
- Tissues
- Organs
- Body Systems
- Organism

Anatomic Description of the Body
- Directional Terms
- Body Planes
- Body Cavities
- Abdominopelvic Cavity

Body Systems
- Integumentary System
- Musculoskeletal System
- Nervous System
- Respiratory System
- Digestive System
- Urinary System
- Endocrine System
- Reproductive System
- Lymphatic System

Learning Objectives

Upon completion of this unit, the reader will be able to:

1 Explain the levels of organization of the human body.

2 Use directional terms to describe position and location of body structures.

3 List the body cavities and name the main organs contained in each cavity.

4 State the four quadrants and name the nine smaller regions of the abdominopelvic cavity.

5 List all the body systems and identify their functions and major components.

6 List the major disorders associated with each body system.

7 Recognize the major diagnostic tests and commonly used medications associated with each body system.

A basic knowledge of anatomy and physiology is essential for effective work in the healthcare professions. Anatomy is the study of the structure of the body, whereas physiology is the study of how the body functions. Knowing the location and the function of each body part helps the phlebotomist to communicate effectively with coworkers in the medical setting. An understanding of normal physiology will make disorders and diseases easier to understand.

Organizational Levels of the Body

The human body develops into a complex organism through different levels of structure and function, from the simplest to the most complex. Each level includes the previous level to build on. These levels of organization, in ascending order, are cells, tissues, organs, body systems, and the organism.

Cells

The smallest functioning unit of the body is the cell. Over 30 trillion cells provide the basic building blocks for the various structures that make up the human body. The size, shape, and composition of the cell determine cell function. There are several different types of cells, each with a specialized function and the ability to carry out specialized chemical reactions to communicate with other cells throughout the body.

Tissues

Groups of specific cells with similar structure and function form the different types of body tissue and together perform specialized functions. There are four basic types of tissue:

- Epithelial tissue: flat cells in a sheetlike arrangement that cover and line body surfaces
- Connective tissue: blood, bone, and adipose cells that support and connect tissues and organs and provide a support network for the organs
- Muscle tissue: long, slender cells that provide the contractile tissue for movement of the body
- Nerve tissue: cells that are capable of transmitting electrical impulses to regulate body functions

Organs

Organs are body structures formed by the combination of two or more different types of tissue. Each organ is a specialized component of the body (such as the heart, brain, skin, and kidneys) and accomplishes a specific function.

Body Systems

Groups of organs functioning together for a common purpose make up the body systems. The major body systems are the integumentary, skeletal, muscular, nervous, respiratory, digestive, urinary, endocrine, reproductive, circulatory, and lymphatic. Table 16–1 lists the organs and functions of each body system.

Organism

Several body systems make up a complete living entity called an organism. The human body has attained the highest level of organization. The ability of these body systems to work together to sustain life and keep the body functioning normally, in spite of constantly changing internal and external conditions, is an essential function referred to as homeostasis.

Anatomical Description of the Body

Key Terms

Anatomic position	*Sagittal plane*
Frontal plane	*Transverse plane*
Midsagittal plane	

Directional Terms

Healthcare providers effectively communicate with one another and the patient through universally adopted reference systems for the anatomic description of the body. These reference systems include directional terms, body planes, and cavities. The

TABLE 16–1
Summary of Body Systems

System	Function	Organs
Integumentary	Protects against harmful pathogens and chemicals and regulates temperature	Skin, hair, nails, and glands
Skeletal	Supports and protects internal organs, stores minerals, and is the location of blood cell formation	Bones, ligaments, joints, and cartilage
Muscular	Skeletal movement and heat production	Muscles and tendons
Nervous	Recognizes and interprets sensory stimuli and regulates responses to stimuli by coordinating other body systems	Brain, spinal cord, and nerves
Respiratory	Exchanges oxygen and carbon dioxide between the air and circulating blood	Nose, pharynx, larynx, trachea, bronchi, and lungs
Digestive	Breaks down food to usable molecules to be absorbed by the body and eliminates waste products	Mouth, pharynx, esophagus, stomach, small intestine, and large intestine
Urinary	Removes waste products and regulates water and salt balance	Kidneys, ureters, urinary bladder, and urethra
Endocrine	Produces and regulates hormones	Thyroid gland, parathyroid gland, adrenal gland, pancreas, pituitary gland, ovaries, testes, thymus, and pineal gland
Reproductive	Sexual reproduction and development of male and female sexual characteristics	Female: Ovaries, fallopian tubes, uterus, vagina, and breasts Male: Testes, epididymides, vas deferens, seminal vesicles, prostate gland, bulbourethral glands, and penis
Lymphatic	Returns excess tissue fluid to the bloodstream and defense against disease	Lymph vessels, ducts, lymph nodes, spleen, tonsils, and thymus
Circulatory	Transports oxygen, nutrients, and waste products	Heart, arteries, veins, and capillaries

anatomic position for the body is standing erect, the head facing forward and the arms by the sides with the palms facing to the front. When studying anatomic illustrations, note that the right and left sides are opposite your own.

Directional terms indicate the location and position of an area or body part. Table 16–2 contains common directional terms.

Body Planes

An anatomic plane is an imaginary flat surface that divides portions of the body or an organ into front, back, right, left, upper, and lower sections. The ***frontal plane*** divides the body into the **anterior** (front or **ventral**) and **posterior** (back or **dorsal**) portions. The ***sagittal plane*** divides the body vertically into right and left portions. A ***midsagittal plane*** vertically divides the body into equal right and left portions. The ***transverse plane*** is a cross-sectional division separating the body horizontally into upper (**superior**) and lower (**inferior**) portions. Figure 16–1 illustrates the body planes.

Body Cavities

Body cavities are hollow spaces containing the internal organs. Classified into two major groups depending on their location, the anterior and posterior cavities enclose five subcavities (Fig. 16–2). The ventral cavity (anterior) consists of the **thoracic** cavity, abdominal cavity, and pelvic cavity. Pleural membranes line the organs of the thoracic cavity. The parietal pleura lines the chest wall, and the visceral pleura covers the lungs. The **peritoneum** lines the abdominal cavity, and the mesentery covers

TABLE 16-2
Common Directional Terms

Term	Definition	Example
Anterior	in front of or before	The chest is anterior to the spine.
Posterior	toward the back	The spine is posterior to the chest.
Superior	above/in an upward direction	The head is superior to the chest.
Inferior	below/in a downward direction	The chest is inferior to the head.
Proximal	point of attachment near the body center	The knee is proximal to the foot.
Distal	point of attachment further from center	The foot is distal to the knee.
Lateral	to the side	The shoulder is lateral to the chest.
Medial	nearest the midline	The chest is medial to the shoulder.
Ventral	the front side	The chest is on the ventral side of the body.
Dorsal	the back side	The spine is on the dorsal side of the body.
Superficial	toward the surface	The skin is a superficial organ.
Deep	toward the interior	The femoral artery is deep in the body.

the outer surface of the abdominal organs. A muscular wall called the diaphragm separates the thoracic and abdominal cavities. The dorsal cavity (posterior) contains the cranial cavity and spinal cavity. Meninges are the membranes that line these cavities. Table 16–3 lists the main organs contained in these cavities.

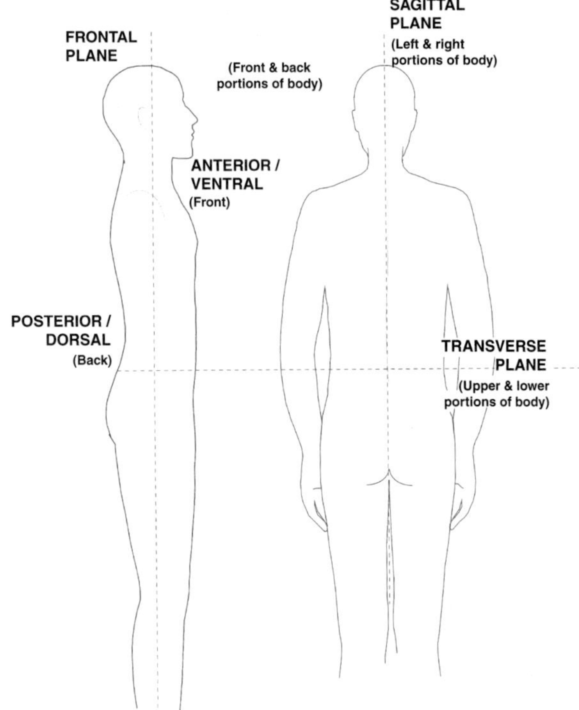

Figure 16–1 The planes of the body.

Abdominopelvic Cavity

The abdominopelvic cavity combines the abdominal and pelvic cavities. An imaginary cross formed by a transverse plane and a midsagittal plane that cross at the **umbilicus** divides the abdominopelvic cavity into four quadrants for clinical evaluation and diagnostic purposes. The four divisions are the right upper quadrant (**RUQ**), right lower quadrant (**RLQ**), left upper quadrant (**LUQ**), and left lower quadrant (**LLQ**). A patient with appendicitis might present with right lower quadrant pain (Fig. 16–3).

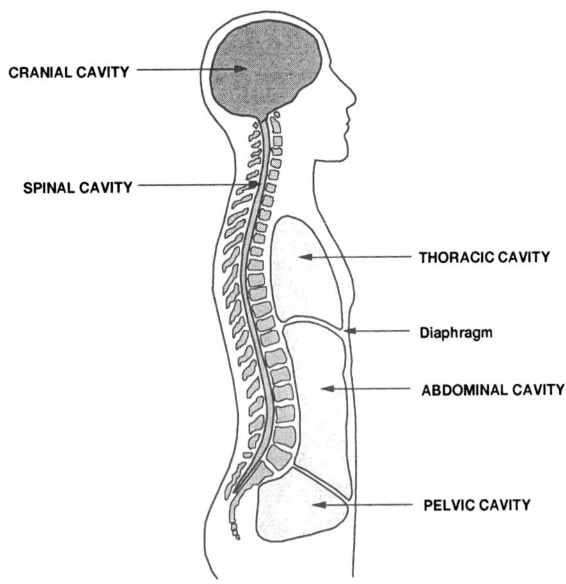

Figure 16–2 The cavities of the body.

TABLE 16-3
Body Cavities and Their Organs

Plane	Cavity	Organs
Anterior	Thoracic	Lungs and heart
	Abdominal	Stomach, small and large intestines, spleen, liver, gallbladder, pancreas, and kidneys
	Pelvic	Bladder, colon, ovaries, and testes
Posterior	Cranial	Brain
	Spinal	Spinal cord

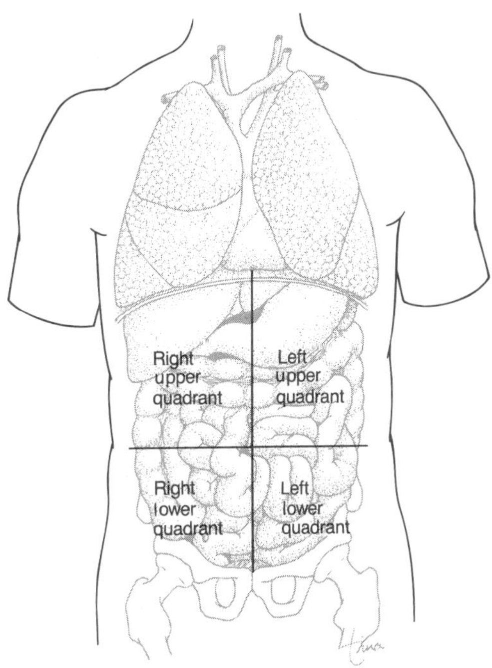

Figure 16–3 Four quadrants of the abdominopelvic cavity. (From Scanlon, VC, and Sanders, T: Essentials of Anatomy and Physiology, ed. 3. FA Davis, Philadelphia, 1999, p. 16, with permission.)

Body Systems

Key Terms

Dermis	***Melanin***
Epidermis	***Sebaceous gland***
Erythema	***Subcutaneous***
Keratin	***Sudoriferous gland***

Integumentary System

The integumentary system consists of the skin, hair, nails, ***sebaceous*** (oil) ***glands***, and ***sudoriferous*** (sweat) ***glands***. The skin is the body's largest organ. On the average adult, it weighs about 7 pounds and, when stretched out, would cover about 18 square feet.

Function

The skin covers the outer surface of the body and provides the functions of protection, regulation, sensation, and secretion.

Skin protects the body against invasion by microorganisms and environmental chemicals, minimizes the loss or entry of water, helps block the harmful effects of sunlight, and helps produce vitamin D.

Skin regulates temperature by insulating the body and raising or lowering body temperature in response to environmental changes. Blood vessels in the skin dilate to bring blood to the surface when the body needs to lose heat and constrict to allow blood to flow to the muscles and organs when the body needs to conserve heat.

Embedded in the skin are sensory receptors to receive the sensations of heat, cold, pain, touch, and pressure that provide information about the external environment.

Millions of glands under the skin produce secretions to lubricate the skin and produce sweat to keep the body cool.

Components

The outer ***epidermis*** and the inner ***dermis*** make up the two main layers of the skin. A layer of ***subcutaneous*** tissue connects the skin to the underlying muscles (Fig. 16–4).

The epidermis is the thinnest layer of skin and contains no blood vessels or nerve endings. It depends on the blood supply in the capillaries of the dermis to provide oxygen and nutrients. Four or five layers of stratified (meaning layered) squamous epithelial cells make up the epidermis. The two most important layers are the innermost layer (**stratum germinativum**) and the outermost layer (**stratum corneum**).

In the inner stratum germinativum, cells undergo cell division (**mitosis**) to continually produce new cells that push the older cells toward the outer skin

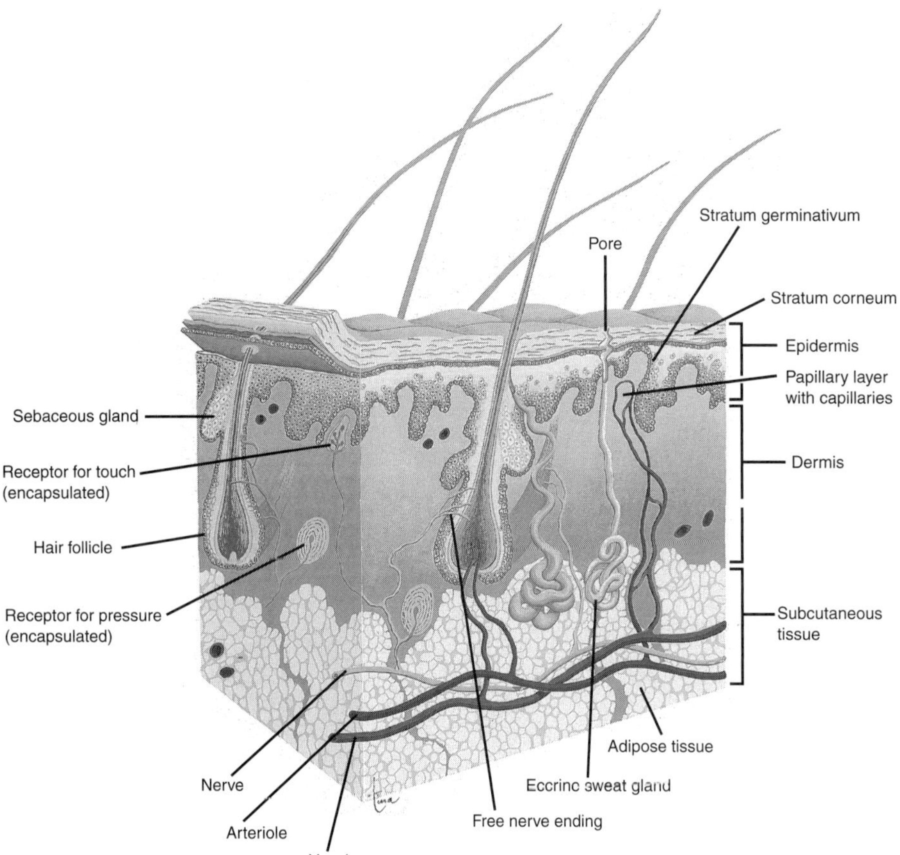

Figure 16–4 Cross-section of the skin. (Adapted from Scanlon, VC, and Sanders, T: Essentials of Anatomy and Physiology, ed. 3. FA Davis, Philadelphia, 1999, p. 85.)

surface. These cells produce the hard protein ***keratin***. As the cells move up to the outermost layer of the epidermis, away from the nutrients in the dermis capillaries, they die. Older skin cells become dry and flake away. A layer of skin replaces itself about once a month.

Melanocytes, the cells that produce the skin pigment ***melanin***, are located in the epidermis. The amount of melanin produced determines the darkness of skin color. Exposure to the ultraviolet (**UV**) rays of the sun stimulates the melanocytes to produce increased amounts of melanin that protect the skin by darkening the color.

The stratum corneum is the outermost layer of the epidermis, consisting of dead cells filled with keratin. Keratin acts as a waterproof coat that prevents the loss or entry of water and resists the entry of pathogens and harmful chemicals.

The dermis lies below the epidermis. The dermis is thicker than the epidermis, and this irregular fibrous connective tissue contains capillaries, lymph vessels, nerve fibers, sudoriferous glands, sebaceous glands, and hair follicles. A layer of dermal papillae acts as peglike projections that help bind the dermis to the epidermis. The uneven ridges and grooves created by this junction form the fingerprints and footprints.

Connective tissue and fat tissue make up the subcutaneous layer located directly beneath the dermis. This tissue connects the skin to the underlying organs, protects and cushions the deep tissues of the body, stores fat for energy, and acts as a heat insulator.

Hair consists of dead cells filled with keratin. Hair fibers grow in sheaths of epidermal tissue called hair follicles. Mitosis takes place in the hair root located at the base of the follicle. The new cells produce keratin, obtain their color from melanin, and grow into the visible portion of the follicle, called the hair shaft. Attached to each hair follicle are tiny smooth muscles called arrector pili or pilomotor. These muscles pull the hair follicles upright to form "goosebumps" when stimulated by cold or fear.

Nails consist of hard keratin plates that cover and protect the fingers and toes. As with the hair fiber, new cells constantly form in the nail root of a nail follicle. The new cells produce keratin and then die to form the nail plate.

Sudoriferous glands are small, coiled glands with ducts extending up through the epidermis to small pores on almost all body surfaces. The forehead, armpits, upper lip, palms, and soles of the feet are the areas of highest concentration. Activated by high external temperature and exercise, the perspiration (sweat) produced by these glands regulates body temperature by evaporation and eliminates waste products through the pores of the skin.

Sebaceous glands are the oil-secreting glands of the skin. Secreted through tiny ducts into hair follicles or directly to the skin surface to prevent drying of the hair and skin is an oily substance called **sebum**. Secretion of sebum varies with age. Adolescents have increased sebum production and older persons often have dry, fragile skin as a result of decreased sebum production.

Disorders

The following are common disorders of the skin.

- Acne: An oversecretion of sebum by sebaceous glands that causes blockage of ducts and formation of pustules. Triggered by hormonal changes of puberty, it is most common in adolescents with oily skin.
- Eczema: An allergic reaction with an itchy rash that may blister and is aggravated by infection, emotional stress, food allergy, and sweating.
- Fever blisters (cold sores): Caused by the herpes simplex virus, usually at the edge of the lip; may become dormant and are triggered by stress or illness.
- Fungal infections: tinea infections such as ringworm, athlete's foot, and jock itch; caused by the dermatophyte fungi that can produce itching, scaling, and ***erythema***.
- Impetigo: A highly contagious bacterial infection caused by *Staphylococcus* or *Streptococcus*, frequently seen in younger children; may present with erythema and progress into blisters that rupture, producing yellow crusts.
- Keloid: Excess collagen scar formation in the area of surgical incisions or skin wounds.
- Psoriasis: A chronic inflammatory skin condition characterized by itchy, scaly, red patches; scales are on top of raised lesions called plaques.
- Skin cancer: Squamous cell carcinoma, basal cell carcinoma, and **malignant** melanoma are the most common (Kaposi's sarcoma is a form of skin cancer associated with acquired immunodeficiency syndrome [AIDS]).
- Warts: Raised, rounded, skin-colored, rough growths usually on the hands and feet, caused by a virus.

Diagnostic Tests

The most frequently ordered diagnostic tests associated with the integumentary system and their clinical correlations are presented in Table 16–4.

Medications

Table 16–5 lists the brand names of the most commonly used medications for the integumentary system and their purpose.

Musculoskeletal System

Bones, joints, and muscles make up the musculoskeletal system. The framework and support for the body is provided by 206 bones, together with the joints, cartilage, and ligaments. More than 600 muscles attached to the bones of the skeleton by tendons move the skeleton and cause the movement of the organs of the body.

TABLE 16–4
Diagnostic Tests Associated with the Integumentary System

Test	Clinical Correlation
Culture and sensitivity (C & S)	Bacterial infection
Fungal culture	Fungal infection
Gram stain	Microbial infection
Potassium hydroxide (**KOH**) prep	Fungal infection
Skin biopsy (**Bx**)	Malignancy

TABLE 16–5
Common Medications for the Integumentary System

Type	Generic and Trade Names	Purpose
Anesthetics	Local: Dyclone, Solarcaine, and Xylocaine	Relieve itching and pain
Antibiotic agents	Bactroban, Mycitracin, Neosporin, and Polysporin	Eliminate infection
Antifungal agents	Desenex, Fungizone, Lotrimin, Mentax, Micatin, and Nystatin	Inhibit growth of fungi and yeast
Anti-inflammatory agents	Steroids: Aristocort, Decadron, hydrocortisone, and Temovate	Relieve redness, swelling, tenderness, and painful inflammation
Antipruritic agents	Atarax, Claritin, Benadryl, Topicort, and Zyrtec	Prevent itching
Antiseptic agents	Betadine, isopropyl alcohol, pHisoHex, and Zephiran	Inhibit growth of pathogens
Antiviral agents	Denavir, Famvir, and Zovirax	Inhibit viral diseases
Emollients	Dermassage, Destin, and Neutroderm	Soothe dry skin
Keratolytics	Carmol, Duofilm, Karalyt, and Saligel	Loosen and destroy outer layers of skin

Skeletal System

Key Terms

Articulation	***Ligament***
Bursa	***Sarcoma***
Cartilage	***Synovial***
Hematopoiesis	***Tendon***

FUNCTION

The five main functions of the skeletal system are support, protection, movement, mineral storage, and blood cell formation (***hematopoiesis***). As the framework of the body, the skeletal system provides support and protects vital organs. Movement is possible because bone is the anchor point for muscles, joints, ***tendons***, and ***ligaments***. Phosphorus and calcium are stored in the bones and are released to the blood as needed. The important function of hematopoiesis takes place in the center (marrow) of bones.

COMPONENTS

The components of the skeletal system are the bones, joints, tendons, ***cartilage***, and ligaments.

BONE COMPOSITION. Bone-forming cells called **osteoblasts** and bone-resorbing cells called **osteoclasts** provide a process by which calcium phosphate deposits are laid down in specific patterns in a gel-like matrix. The osteoblasts produce an enzyme to combine calcium and phosphorus into calcium phosphate, which makes the bones hard and rigid. The osteoclasts remove bone debris and smooth and shape the bones. Cartilage is the flexible part of the

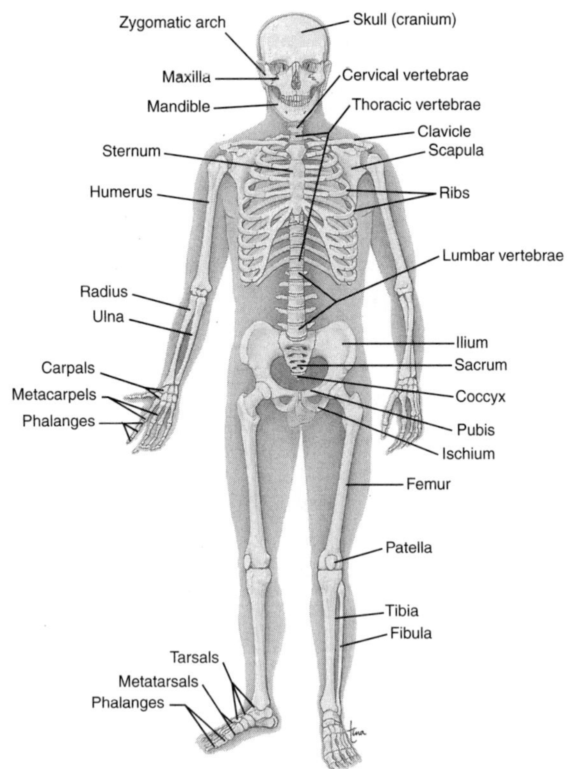

Figure 16–5 The major bones of the body. (From Scanlon, VC, and Sanders, T: Essentials of Anatomy and Physiology, ed. 3. FA Davis, Philadelphia, 1999, p. 106, with permission.)

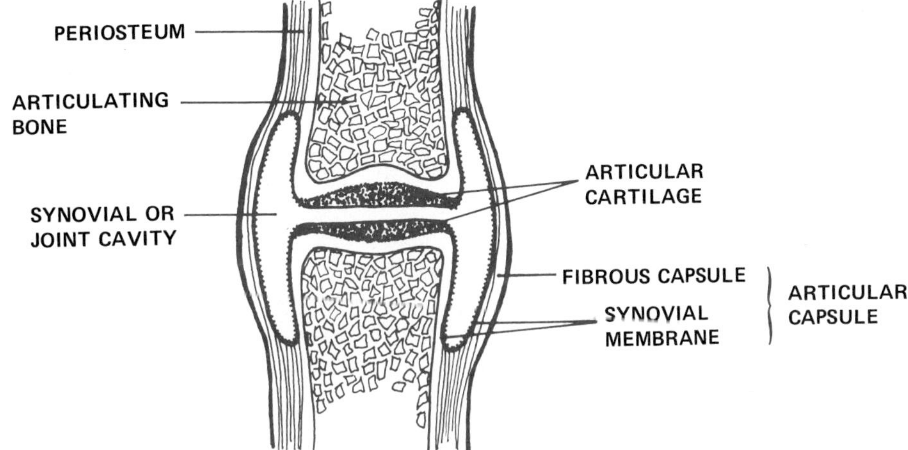

Figure 16–6 Synovial joint. (From Strasinger, SK, and Di Lorenzo, MS: Urinalysis and Body Fluids, ed. 4. FA Davis, Philadelphia, 2001, p. 180, with permission.)

skeletal system and is found where bones come together. Cartilage fibers are imbedded in a gel-like material versus the calcified substance found in bones, and therefore provide greater flexibility.

BONE TYPES. There are four classes of bones, usually based on shape. The *long bones* are found in the extremities. These are the bones of the leg (**femur**, **tibia**, and **fibula**) and the arm bones (**humerus**, **radius**, and **ulna**). *Short bones* are the wrists (**carpals**), hands (**metacarpals**), ankles (**tarsals**), and feet (**metatarsals**). *Flat bones* are for the protection of the inner organs, such as the heart and brain. They have a broad surface for the attachment of muscles. Examples of flat bones are the **cranium**, ribs, **scapula**, and **sternum**. *Irregular bones* have unusual shapes, such as the bones of the vertebrae, **sacrum**, and **coccyx**. Figure 16–5 shows the major bones of the body.

JOINTS. Each bone connects (***articulates***) to another bone by forming an immovable (**synarthrosis**), partially movable (**amphiarthrosis**), or free-moving (**diarthrosis**) joint. The skull bones have immovable joints called cranial sutures, and vertebrae have partially movable joints. However, most joints in the body (knee, hip, elbow, wrist, and foot) are free moving.

All free-moving joints are ***synovial*** joints and consist of a synovial cavity, a joint capsule, and a layer of articular cartilage. Articular cartilage covers the ends of each bone, providing a smooth surface, and acts as a cushion against jolts. The synovial cavity is the space between the bones at the joint and is separated by a joint capsule. The joint capsule fits over the ends of the two bones and secures the joint together tightly by ligaments (strong connective tissue). The synovial membrane lining the joint capsule secretes synovial fluid, a thick and slippery fluid that prevents friction and allows easy movement of bones. Small sacs of synovial fluid called ***bursae*** located between the joint and tendons allow tendons to slide easily across joints. Figure 16–6 illustrates a synovial joint.

DISORDERS

The following are common disorders of the skeletal system.

- Ankylosing spondylitis: Pain and stiffness in the joints of the lower back
- Arthralgia: Pain without swelling or redness in the joints; can be caused by tension, virus infections, unusual exertion, or accidents.
- Arthritis: Inflammation of the joint, causing swelling, redness, warmth, and pain on movement. The four most common types are osteoarthritis, rheumatoid arthritis, gout, and ankylosing spondylitis.
- Bursitis: Inflammation of the bursae (sacs of synovial fluid) located between the joints and the tendons, commonly causing swelling and pain in the shoulder, elbow, and heel.
- Fractures (**Fx**): Breaking of bone caused by stress, cancer, or metabolic disease. The different types of fractures are:
  - Comminuted fracture: The bone has been splintered into many pieces by two or more intersecting breaks.

- Compound (open) fracture: The bone is broken with fragments protruding through the skin.
- Greenstick fracture: The bone is partially bent and partially broken; often seen in children.
- Impacted fracture: The bone fragment is driven into another bone.
- Simple (closed) fracture: The bone is broken with no puncture through the skin.

- Gout: Painful metabolic condition caused by uric acid crystals forming in the joints, frequently the big toe, the ankle, or the knee; occurs mostly in men.
- Lyme disease: Result of an infection caused by a spirochete bacterium carried by deer ticks. An oval rash, fever, headache, stiff neck, and backache can develop 3 to 20 days after the bite of an infected tick. The synovial membrane becomes infected, producing joint, neurologic, or cardiac problems.
- Osteoarthritis: Occurs in later life and causes swelling and pain, primarily in weight-bearing joints.
- Osteoma: A benign or malignant bone tumor. Malignant tumors, called ***sarcomas***, are named for the specific tissue affected:
  - Fibrosarcoma: Fibrous connective tissue
  - Lymphosarcoma: Lymphoid tissue
  - Chondrosarcoma: Cartilage
  - Osteosarcoma: Bone
  - Ewing's sarcoma: Shaft of the long bones
- Osteomalacia: Softening of the bones resulting from inability to absorb calcium, caused by a vitamin D deficiency; often called rickets. It is seen in infants and children, and may result in bone deformity.
- Osteomyelitis: Inflammation of the bones and bone marrow caused by a bacterial infection; often caused by local trauma to the bone such as improper microtechniques in phlebotomy.
- Osteoporosis: Bone disease involving decreased bone density, producing porous bones that can become brittle and easily broken; causes include a lack of protein, calcium, or vitamin D; high doses of corticosteroids; or lack of estrogen in postmenopausal women.
- Paget's disease: A metabolic disorder in which new abnormal bone replaces spongy bone, resulting in deformity of flat bones and bowing of the legs; usually affects adults older than 35 years.
- Rheumatoid arthritis (RA): Chronic inflammation of the joints caused by an autoimmune reaction involving the joint connective tissue. The inflammation causes painful swelling and can produce crippling deformities as it spreads from the inflamed synovial membrane to the cartilage of a joint. RA usually starts in middle life and is diagnosed with a blood test to determine the presence of the autoantibody [rheumatoid factor (**RF**)].
- Scoliosis: Lateral curvature of the spine with deviation either to the right or left that gives the spine the shape of an "S." It can be **congenital** or develop in early teen years as a result of poor posture.
- Spina bifida: Congenital disorder characterized by an abnormal closure of the spinal canal resulting in the malformation of the spine.
- Systemic lupus erythematosus (**SLE**): Autoimmune disease affecting the connective tissue: cartilage, bones, ligaments and tendons; usually seen in women of childbearing age. A hallmark of the disease is the classic butterfly rash that appears across the cheeks and the bridge of the nose.

DIAGNOSTIC TESTS

The most frequently ordered diagnostic tests associated with the skeletal system and their clinical correlations are presented in Table 16–6.

MEDICATIONS

Table 16–7 lists the brand names of the most commonly used medications for the skeletal system and their purpose.

Muscular System

Key Terms

Cardiac muscle	*Skeletal muscle*
Insertion	*Smooth muscle*
Origin	*Striated*

The muscular system works in conjunction with the skeletal and nervous systems to provide body movement. Composed of long slender cells called fibers, muscles make up 42% of body weight. Each muscle

TABLE 16–6
Diagnostic Tests Associated with the Skeletal System

Test	Clinical Correlation
Alkaline phosphatase (ALP)	Bone disorders
Antinuclear antibody (ANA)	Systemic lupus erythematosus
Arthroscopy	Joint trauma
Calcium (Ca)	Bone disorders
Computerized axial tomography (CT scan)	Body structure examination
Culture and sensitivity (C & S)	Microbial infection
Fluorescent antinuclear antibody (FANA)	Systemic lupus erythematosus
Gram stain	Microbial infection
Magnetic resonance imaging (MRI)	Body structure examination
Phosphorus (P)	Skeletal disorders
Rheumatoid arthritis (RA)	Rheumatoid arthritis
Synovial fluid analysis	Arthritis
Uric acid	Gout
X-ray	Bone structure

consists of fibers held together by connective tissue enclosed in a fibrous sheath.

FUNCTION

Muscles are attached to the bones of the skeleton by tendons. The ability of the muscle to contract provides the body with movement, posture, and heat production. A special type of contraction called **tonicity** maintains posture. A partial contraction of skeletal muscles shortens only a few muscles and does not allow movement. Muscles held in position resist the pull of gravity. Heat produced through chemical changes involved during muscle contraction maintains a constant body temperature. Muscles not only provide skeletal movement but also pass food through the digestive system, propel blood through blood vessels, and contract the bladder to expel urine.

COMPONENTS

The three types of muscle found in the body are skeletal, smooth, and cardiac. They are classified by their function and appearance. The three types of muscle are shown in Figure 16–7.

Skeletal muscle is a ***striated*** voluntary muscle that attaches to bones and is responsible for movement of the body. It is called a voluntary muscle because a person has control over its activity. It is a striated muscle because of its cross-striped appearance when examined microscopically.

Smooth muscle is an unstriated involuntary (**visceral**) muscle that lacks the cross-striped appearance microscopically. It is controlled by the autonomic nervous system. Found in the walls of veins and arteries and in the internal organs of the digestive, respiratory, and urinary systems, smooth muscle functions without conscious control.

TABLE 16–7
Common Medications for the Skeletal System

Type	Generic and Trade Names	Purpose
Analgesics	Non-narcotic: Aleve, aspirin, Motrin, Nuprin, and Tylenol Narcotic: Demerol, morphine sulfate, Percocet, and Vicodin	Relieve swelling, fever, and pain
Anti-inflammatory agents	Nonsteroidal: Anapox, aspirin, Bextra, Celebrex, Motrin, and Naprosyn Steroids: Celestone, Decadron, and Kenalog	Relieve bone and joint pain
Antirheumatic agents	Enbrel, gold therapy, Imuran, Plaquenil, and Rheumatrex	Treat rheumatoid arthritis

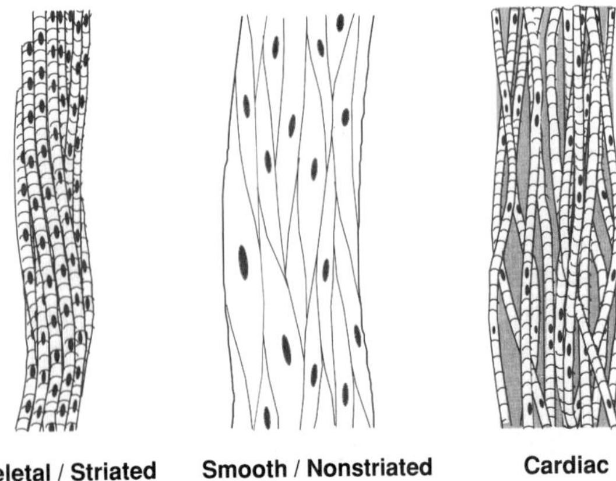

Figure 16–7 The three types of muscle.

Cardiac muscle is the muscle of the heart wall. Like skeletal muscle, it is a striated muscle. However, it is also an involuntary muscle. Controlled by the autonomic nervous system, cardiac muscle rhythmically contracts without conscious control.

MUSCLE MOVEMENT Tendons, cords of fibrous connective tissue, attach skeletal muscle to bones. A muscle attaches to a stationary bone, the ***origin***, and to a movable bone, the ***insertion***. As the muscle contracts and shortens, the insertion bone moves toward the stationary bone. A muscle pulls when it contracts, but it cannot push. An opposing muscle contracts to pull the bone in the other direction. A muscle that produces movement is the prime mover, and the opposing muscle is an antagonist. Table 16–8 lists the major muscle movements. The concept of muscular movement is illustrated in Figure 16–8.

TABLE 16–8
Major Muscle Movements*

Motion	Action
Abduction	Moving away from the middle of the body
Adduction	Moving toward the middle of the body
Extension	Straightening of a limb
Flexion	Bending of a limb
Pronation	Turning the palm down
Supination	Turning the palm up
Dorsiflexion	Elevating the foot
Plantar flexion	Lowering the foot
Rotation	Moving a bone around its longitudinal axis

* Grouped in pairs of antagonistic function (except for rotation)

DISORDERS

The following are common disorders of the muscular system.

- Atrophy: Wasting away of muscle caused by inactivity.
- Carpal tunnel syndrome (**CTS**): Characterized by pain and tingling in the fingers and hand, may radiate to the shoulder. Caused by pressure on the median nerve as it passes through the ligaments, bones, and tendons.
- Fibromyalgia syndrome (**FMS**): A condition with chronic muscle pain, fatigue, sleep problems, irritable bowel syndrome, morning stiffness, anxiety, and memory problems.
- Muscular dystrophy (**MD**): An inherited disorder in which the muscles are replaced by fat and fibrous tissue and progressively weaken.
- Myalgia: Muscle pain that can be caused by tension, viral infections, exertion, accidents, or (in rare cases) cancer or thyroid disease.
- Myasthenia gravis: A neuromuscular disorder of the skeletal muscle that affects the transmission of nerve impulses to the muscles of the eyes, face, and limbs.
- Poliomyelitis: Viral infection of the nerves controlling skeletal movement, resulting in muscle weakness and paralysis.

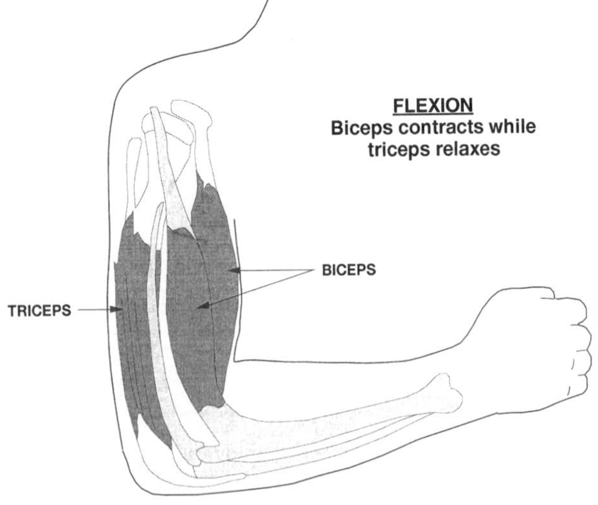

Figure 16–8 An example of muscular movement.

TABLE 16-9
Diagnostic Tests Associated with the Muscular System

Test	Clinical Correlation
Computerized axial tomography (CT scan)	Soft-tissue examination
Creatinine kinase [CK(CPK)]	Muscle damage
Creatinine kinase isoenzymes (**CK-MM, MB**)	Muscle damage
Electromyogram (**EMG**)	Muscle function
Lactic acid	Muscle fatigue
Magnesium (**Mg**)	Musculoskeletal disorders
Magnetic resonance imaging (MRI)	Soft-tissue examination
Myoglobin	Muscle damage
Potassium (K)	Muscle function

- Tendinitis: Inflammation of the tendons caused by excess exertion; common locations are the rotator cuff around the shoulder, biceps, and the Achilles tendon (large tendon that connects the calf muscles to the back of the heel).

DIAGNOSTIC TESTS

The most frequently ordered diagnostic tests associated with the muscular system and their clinical correlations are presented in Table 16–9.

MEDICATIONS

Table 16–10 lists the brand names of the most commonly used medications for the muscular system and their purpose.

Nervous System

The nervous system is the communication system for the body. It controls and regulates all body systems to maintain homeostasis. Nerve impulses cause muscles to contract to move bones and enable one to hear, see, taste, think, and react.

Key Terms

Afferent neuron	*Meninges*
Autonomic nervous system	*Myelin sheath*
Axon	*Neuroglia*
Central nervous system	*Neuron*
Dendrite	*Peripheral nervous system*
Efferent neuron	*Synapse*

Function

The primary functions of the nervous system are to recognize sensory stimuli, to interpret these sensations, and to initiate the appropriate response that provides the communication, integration, and control of all body functions. Electrical nerve impulses traveling by way of a nerve fiber and the release of a chemical substance called a neurotransmitter accomplish these functions. The specialized cell of the nervous system is the ***neuron***, whose type varies depending on the function it performs.

Components

The nervous system is divided into the ***central nervous system*** (**CNS**) and the ***peripheral nervous system*** (**PNS**). The CNS lies in the center of the body and consists of the brain and the spinal cord. The PNS consists of nerves located outside the skull and spinal column that extend out into the body and connect the brain and spinal cord to all parts of the body.

Two types of cells are present in the nervous system. The main functioning cell that conducts nerve impulses is the neuron. The second type of cell is the ***neuroglia***, which acts as nerve glue or connective support for neurons and does not

TABLE 16-10
Common Medications for the Muscular System

Type	Generic and Trade Names	Purpose
Analgesics	Non-narcotic: Aleve, aspirin, Motrin, Nuprin, and Tylenol	Relieve swelling, fever, and pain
Muscle relaxants	Flexeril, Paraflex, Parafon Forte DSC, Robaxin, Skelaxin, Soma, and Zanaflex	Relax muscle spasms
Neuromuscular blocking agent	Flaxedil, Norcuron, and Tracriun	Relax muscles

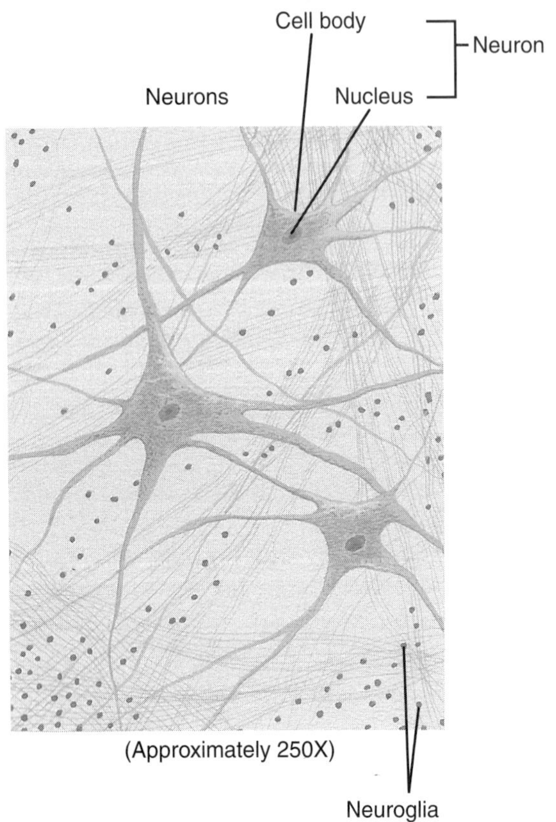

Figure 16–9 The nerve cells. (From Scanlon, VC, and Sanders, T: Essentials of Anatomy and Physiology, ed. 3. FA Davis, Philadelphia, 1999, p. 76, with permission.)

conduct nerve impulses. Figure 16–9 illustrates the nerve cells.

Different types of neurons are classified by the way they transmit impulses. Sensory neurons, also called ***afferent neurons***, transmit impulses from the sensory organs to the brain and spinal cord. Motor or ***efferent neurons*** transmit impulses away from the brain and spinal cord to the muscles and glands to produce a response of either contraction or secretion. Central neurons or **interneurons** transmit impulses from sensory neurons to motor neurons.

A neuron consists of three main parts: ***dendrites***, a cell body, and an ***axon***. Several dendrites branch out to receive and carry impulses to the cell body. The axon, which is a single long projection, extends out and carries impulses away from the cell body. Axons are covered by a protective ***myelin sheath*** that acts as a special insulator and can accelerate electrical impulses. Because myelin is a white fatty substance, the axons have a white appearance and are therefore called the white matter. Gray matter consists of all the fibers, dendrites, and nerve cell bodies that are not covered with the myelin sheath and have a gray appearance.

The point at which the axon of one neuron and the dendrite of another neuron come together is called a ***synapse***. Nerve impulses are transmitted at the synapse. The nerve impulse from an axon stops at the synapse, chemical signals are sent across the gap, and the impulse then continues along the dendrites, cell body, and the axon of the next neuron.

The CNS, consisting of the brain and spinal cord, is the communication center of the nervous system. It receives impulses from all parts of the body, processes the information, and initiates a response. The brain and spinal cord are continuous through an opening in the base of the skull.

The brain is one of the largest organs in the body and is the center for regulating body functions. The major structures of the brain are the **cerebrum**, the **cerebellum**, the **diencephalon**, and the **brain stem**. The cerebrum is the largest part of the brain, and consists of two hemispheres divided by a longitudinal fissure (groove). Each hemisphere is divided into lobes that have the same name as the cranial bone they are near (frontal, parietal, temporal, and occipital). The cerebrum governs all sensory and motor activity. The cerebellum is located in the posterior part of the brain and coordinates voluntary movement, equilibrium, and balance. The diencephalon consists of the **thalamus** and **hypothalamus**. The thalamus relays all sensory impulses, except olfactory, and affects emotional behavior. The hypothalamus regulates autonomic nerve impulses and endocrine activity. The brainstem consists of the midbrain, **medulla oblongata**, and **pons**. It is the conduction pathway between the brain and the spinal cord.

The spinal cord has an ascending nerve tract to carry sensory impulses to the brain. A descending nerve tract carries motor impulses away from the brain to the muscles and organs.

The skull bones provide protection for the brain and the vertebrae provide protection for the spinal cord. Three layers of connective tissue membranes called ***meninges*** cover the brain and spinal cord to provide additional shock-absorbing protection. The thick outermost layer is the **dura mater**, which lines the skull and vertebral canal. The middle layer is the **arachnoid membrane**. The innermost layer is the **pia mater**, which is a thin membrane covering the surface of the brain and spinal cord. The subarachnoid space located between the arachnoid and pia mater contains fluid called **cerebrospinal fluid** (CSF). CSF circulates through the inner ventricles of the brain, the central canal of the spinal cord, and the subarachnoid space to cushion the brain and spinal cord from shocks that could cause injury. It also supplies nutrients to the cells.

The nerve network branching throughout the body from the brain and spinal cord is the PNS. The 12 pairs of cranial nerves connect to the brain by passing through openings to the skull. Cranial nerves distribute to the head and neck regions of the body, except for the tenth cranial nerve, called the vagus, which controls the structures of the neck, chest, and abdomen. The 31 pairs of spinal nerves pass through the openings in the vertebral column. Spinal nerves distribute in a bandlike fashion to the trunk and to the upper and lower extremities.

The PNS includes the ***autonomic nervous system*** (**ANS**). It consists of the motor neurons to control the involuntary bodily functions such as heartbeat, stomach contractions, respiration, and gland secretions. The ANS has two divisions, the sympathetic and parasympathetic. They function opposite one another and are controlled by the hypothalamus to keep the body in a state of homeostasis. The sympathetic division controls stress situations such as anger or fear by increasing the heart rate and dilating vessels. The parasympathetic controls relaxed situations by decreasing the heart rate and the other body activities to normal levels.

Disorders

The following are common disorders of the nervous system.

- Alzheimer's disease: Characterized by diminished mental capabilities, including memory loss, anxiety, and confusion.
- Amyotrophic lateral sclerosis (**ALS**): A disorder of the motor neurons in the brain and spinal cord that causes skeletal and muscular weakness; also called Lou Gehrig's disease.
- Bell's palsy: Inflammation of a facial nerve that causes paralysis and numbness of the face.
- Cerebral palsy: A condition associated with birth defects, marked by partial paralysis and poor muscle coordination.
- Cerebrovascular accident (**CVA**): Stroke, which can be caused by a cerebral hemorrhage or arteriosclerosis (hardening of the arteries). A decrease in the flow of blood to the brain causes destruction of the brain tissue from lack of oxygen.
- Encephalitis: Inflammation of the brain caused by a virus; symptoms are lethargy, stiff neck, or convulsions. A **lumbar puncture** (**LP**), used to analyze the CSF, can confirm the diagnosis.
- Epilepsy: Recurring seizure disorder resulting from abnormal electrical activity or malfunctioning of the chemical substances of the brain.
- Meningitis: Inflammation of the membranes of the brain or spinal cord caused by a variety of microorganisms; severe headaches, fever, and a stiff neck are common symptoms.
- Multiple neurofibromatosis: Fibrous tumors throughout the body causing crippling deformities.
- Multiple sclerosis (**MS**): A chronic degenerative disease of the CNS that destroys the myelin sheath of the brain and spinal cord; the myelin sheath is replaced by hard plaquelike lesions that interfere with the transmission of nerve impulses, resulting in diminished motor control. Muscle weakness, poor coordination, and paralysis may occur.
- Myelitis: Inflammation of the spinal cord.
- Neuralgia: Pain of the nerves.
- Neuritis: Inflammation of nerves associated with a degenerative process.
- Parkinson's disease: Chronic disease of the nervous system characterized by muscle tremors, muscle weakness, and loss of equilibrium; frequently a disease of the older population, with stiffness of joints, unblinking eyes, and slowness of movement.
- Reye's syndrome: An acute disease that causes edema of the brain and fatty infiltration of the liver and other organs; viral in origin; seen in children after aspirin administration.
- Shingles (herpes zoster): An acute viral disease caused by varicella zoster, the virus that causes chicken pox, which can remain dormant in the body and reappear in the form of shingles. Painful herpeslike blister eruptions occur along

TABLE 16–11
Diagnostic Tests Associated with the Nervous System

Test	Clinical Correlation
Cerebrospinal fluid (CSF) analysis	
Cell count/Differential	Neurological disorders or meningitis
Culture and Gram stain	Meningitis
Glucose and protein	Neurological disorders or meningitis
Computerized axial tomography (CT scan)	Soft-tissue examination
Creatinine kinase isoenzymes (**CK-BB**)	Brain damage
Culture and sensitivity (C & S)	Microbial infection
Drug screening	Therapeutic drug monitoring or drug abuse
Electroencephalogram (**EEG**)	Brain function
Gram stain	Microbial infection
Lead	Neurological function
Lithium (Li)	Antidepressant drug monitoring
Lumbar puncture (LP)	Cerebrospinal fluid analysis
Magnetic resonance imaging (MRI)	Soft-tissue examination
Myelogram	Spinal cord examination
X-ray	Organ examination

the peripheral nerves, usually at or above the waist.

Diagnostic Tests

The most frequently ordered diagnostic tests associated with the nervous system and their clinical correlations are presented in Table 16–11.

Medications

Table 16–12 lists the brand names of the most commonly used medications for the nervous system and their purpose.

Respiratory System

Key Terms

Deoxyhemoglobin
External respiration
Hemoglobin
Internal respiration
Oxyhemoglobin
Pleura

TABLE 16–12
Common Medications for the Nervous System

Type	Generic and Trade Names	Purpose
Analgesics	Non-narcotic: Levoprome, Nubain, and Stadol Narcotic: codeine, Darvon, Demerol, Dilaudid, and morphine sulfate	Relieve pain
Anesthetics	Local: Novocainal, Nupercain, Solarcaine, Tronolane, and Xylocaine General: Fluothane, nitrous oxide, Penthrane, and Pentothal	Produce loss of sensation
Anticonvulsants	Depakene, Diamox, Dilantin, Mesantoin, Neurontin, Topamax, and Tridione	Reduce the severity of convulsive seizures
Antipyretics	Aspirin, ibuprofen, Naprosyn, and Tylenol	Reduce fever and relieve pain
Sedatives and hypnotics	Nonbarbiturates: Ambien, Dalmane, Halcion, Noctec, Placidyl, and Restoril Barbiturates: Amytal, Buticaps, Luminal, Nembutal, and Seconal	Calm nerves and induce sleep

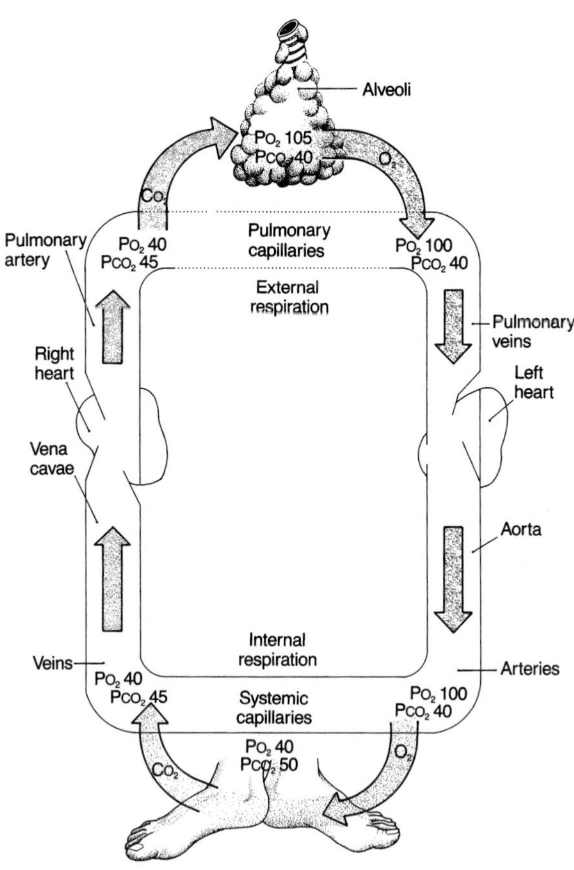

Figure 16–10 External and internal respiration. (From Scanlon, VC, and Sanders, T: Essentials of Physiology, ed. 3. FA Davis, Philadelphia, 1999, p. 338, with permision.)

The respiratory system, in conjunction with the circulatory system, furnishes oxygen (O_2) for individual tissue cells and removes carbon dioxide (Co_2). This system is crucial to the survival of cells, which is accomplished by breathing air in and out of the lungs, where respiration, the exchange of oxygen and carbon dioxide, occurs.

Function

The function of the respiratory system is to exchange the gases oxygen and carbon dioxide between the circulating blood and the air and tissues. Oxygen is a colorless, odorless, combustible gas found in the air; carbon dioxide is a colorless, odorless, incombustible gas that is a waste product of cell metabolism.

The exchange of gases involves two types of respiration processes: ***external respiration*** and ***internal respiration***. External respiration is the exchange of gases in the blood by the lungs; internal respiration is the exchange of gases in the body between the blood and tissue cells. In external respiration, ventilated lungs receive oxygen from the air that enters the bloodstream through capillaries in the lungs, and at the same time, carbon dioxide leaves the bloodstream and is expelled into the air by the lungs. In internal respiration, the oxygen leaves the blood and enters the tissue cells, and carbon dioxide from the tissue cells enters the bloodstream (Fig. 16–10).

Components

The respiratory system consists of the upper respiratory tract, which includes the organs outside the chest cavity; and the lower respiratory tract, which includes the organs within the chest cavity. The nose, **pharynx**, **larynx**, and upper **trachea** make up the upper respiratory tract. The lower trachea, bronchi, and lungs constitute the lower respiratory tract (Fig. 16–11).

Air enters and leaves the respiratory system through the nose, which acts as the primary filter. The nose moistens and warms the inhaled air, helps to produce sound, and contains the **olfactory receptors** (sensory organs for smell).

Air from the nose passes into the pharynx (throat), which is a tubelike structure that acts as a passageway for food and air. The pharynx is divided into three portions: the nasopharynx, the oropharynx, and the laryngopharynx. The laryngopharynx opens anteriorly to the larynx (voicebox) and posteriorly into the esophagus. Food passes to the esophagus, which leads to the stomach, and air passes to the larynx, which leads to the lungs.

Located in the larynx are vocal cords, which determine the quality of voice sounds. A leaf-shaped piece of cartilage on top of the larynx, the **epiglottis**, blocks the opening to the larynx during swallowing to prevent food or liquid from entering the trachea.

From the larynx, the air passes to the trachea (windpipe), which provides the opening through which outside air can reach the lungs. The trachea divides into two main branches called primary bronchi, which lead to the right and left lungs. These bronchi continue to subdivide into smaller and smaller treelike secondary branches until they reach the smallest branches, called **bronchioles,** which extend to all parts of the lung. Attached to the bron-

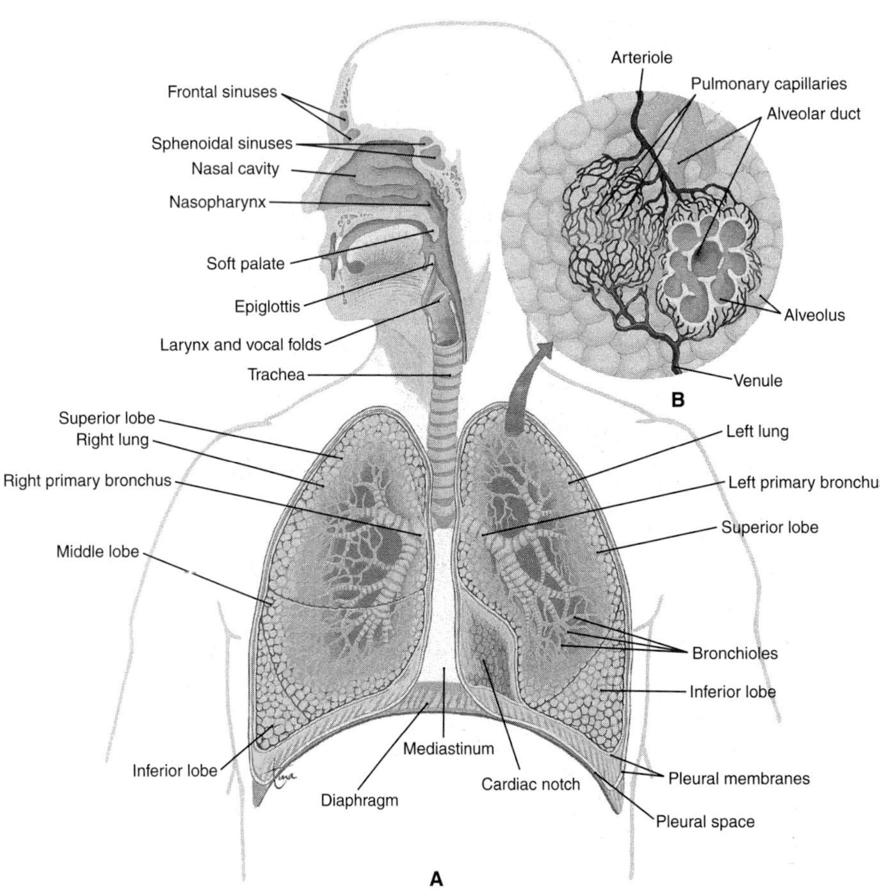

Figure 16–11 The respiratory system. (*A*) Anterior view of the upper and lower respiratory tracts. (*B*) Microscopic view of alveoli and pulmonary capillaries. (From Scanlon, VC, and Sanders, T: Essentials of Anatomy and Physiology, ed. 3. FA Davis, Philadelphia, 1999, p. 330, with permission.)

chioles are alveolar ducts that terminate in clusters of air sacs called **alveoli**.

The lungs lie on either side of the heart, enclosed in a serous membrane called the ***pleura***. The right lung is divided into three lobes and the left lung into two lobes. The main function of the lung is to bring air into contact with the blood to exchange oxygen and carbon dioxide. To facilitate this exchange, each lung contains around 300 million alveoli. Effective gas exchange occurs between the alveoli and surrounding capillaries because the walls of the alveoli and capillaries are composed of a one-cell layer of epithelium. Surfactant, a fluid that coats the thin walls, reduces surface tension to stabilize the walls and allows inflation of the alveoli. Blood in the lung capillaries is low in oxygen and high in carbon dioxide. Oxygen from the alveoli diffuses into the blood in the capillaries, whereas carbon dioxide diffuses from the capillaries into alveoli to be exhaled.

Blood transports oxygen and carbon dioxide through the ***hemoglobin*** in red blood cells. Hemoglobin with oxygen attached is called ***oxyhemoglobin*** and is carried to the tissues for use by the body cells. Carbon dioxide attaches to hemoglobin to form ***deoxyhemoglobin***, which is carried to the lungs, where the carbon dioxide is expelled.

Gaseous pressure determines how oxygen or carbon dioxide associates with (attaches to) or dissociates from (releases) hemoglobin. The concentration of each gas in a particular site is expressed as a value called partial pressure. In the lungs, the partial pressure of oxygen is high and the partial pressure of carbon dioxide is low. Therefore, in the lungs, oxygen attaches to hemoglobin and carbon dioxide dissociates from hemoglobin. In the tissues, the partial pressure of oxygen is low and the partial pressure of carbon dioxide is high, so that oxygen dissociates from hemoglobin and carbon dioxide attaches to hemoglobin. Arterial blood gases tests measure the partial pressure of oxygen and carbon dioxide in the blood.

Disorders

The following are common disorders of the respiratory system.

- Asthma: Swelling or constriction of the bronchial tubes causing wheezing, a feeling of chest constriction, and difficulty in breathing; most common in children and adolescents, triggered by infection, emotional upset, cold air, air pollution, or allergens
- Bronchitis: Chronic inflammation of the bronchial tubes causing a deep cough that can produce sputum.
- Chronic obstructive pulmonary disease (COPD): Inflammation or obstruction of the bronchi and/or alveoli over a long period; wheezing and progressive irreversible damage cause chronic bronchitis and emphysema.
- Cystic fibrosis: A hereditary disorder causing production of viscous mucus that blocks the bronchioles; can result in chronic respiratory infections and pulmonary failure.
- Emphysema: Chronic inflammation resulting in destruction of the bronchioles caused by cigarette smoke or air pollutants; symptoms are shortness of breath (**SOB**) and enlargement of the chest cavity.
- Infant respiratory distress syndrome (**IRDS**): A condition affecting prematurely born infants, caused by a lack of surfactant in the alveolar air sacs in the lungs. Surfactant coats the alveolar walls to lower the surface tension so that air moves easily in and out of the lungs. Without surfactant, the alveoli collapse and breathing is difficult.
- Lung cancer: Masses form and block air passages; the most frequent sites are the bronchi, and the cancer can spread rapidly to other parts of the body; symptoms are coughing and sputum production.
- Pleurisy: Inflammation of the pleural membrane covering the chest cavity and the outer surface of the lungs; symptoms are chest pain and worsening pain with a deep breath or cough.
- Pneumonia: Acute infection of the alveoli of the lungs in which the alveoli fill with fluid so that the air spaces are blocked and it is difficult to exchange oxygen and carbon dioxide; characterized by fever, chills, cough, and headache.
- Pulmonary edema: Accumulation of fluid in the lungs; frequently a complication of congestive heart failure.
- Rhinitis: Inflammation of the nasal mucous membranes resulting in a runny nose, caused by viruses, allergies, or prolonged use of nose drops.
- Strep throat: Inflammation of the pharynx caused by streptococcal group A bacteria; symptoms are sore throat, fever, swollen lymph glands, scarlet fever rash, and abdominal pain.
- Tuberculosis (**TB**): Infectious disease decreasing respiratory function, caused by *Mycobacterium tuberculosis.*
- Upper respiratory infection (**URI**): Infection of the nose, pharynx, or larynx, including the common cold; symptoms include sore throat, runny nose, congested ears, hoarseness, swollen glands, and fever.

Diagnostic Tests

The most frequently ordered diagnostic tests associated with the respiratory system and their clinical correlations are presented in Table 16–13.

Medications

Table 16–14 lists the brand names of the most commonly used medications for the respiratory system and their purpose.

Digestive System

Key Terms

Alimentary tract	***Digestion***
Amino acids	***Feces***
Bile	***Insulin***
Bilirubin	***Nausea***
Diarrhea	***Peristalsis***

Food provides the energy required for the growth, repair, and maintenance of body cells. A meal of meat and mashed potatoes with butter provides complex proteins, carbohydrates, and fat. However, the body cells cannot absorb food in this complex form. The digestive system converts the protein from meat to ***amino acids***, the carbohydrate from the potatoes to a simple sugar (glucose), and the fat from the butter to fatty acids and triglycerides. These simple

TABLE 16–13
Diagnostic Tests Associated with the Respiratory System

Test	Clinical Correlation
Arterial blood gases (ABGs)	Acid-base balance
Bronchoalveolar lavage	Microbial infection
Bronchoscopy	Lung examination or biopsy
Cold agglutinins	Atypical pneumonia
Complete blood count (CBC)	Pneumonia
Computerized axial tomography (CT scan)	Soft-tissue examination
Electrolytes (Lytes)	Acid-base balance
Gram stain	Microbial infection
Lung biopsy (Bx)	Malignancy
Magnetic resonance imaging (MRI)	Soft-tissue examination
Pleural fluid analysis	Infection or malignancy
Pulmonary function tests (**PFTs**)	Respiratory disorders
Purified protein derivative (**PPD**)	Tuberculosis (TB) screening
Sweat chloride test	Cystic fibrosis
Thoracentesis	Pleural effusions
Throat and sputum cultures	Bacterial infection
X-ray	Organ examination

molecules are absorbed and used by the body. The digestive system eliminates waste products formed during this process as *feces*.

Function

The digestive system performs three major functions: ***digestion***, absorption of nutrients, and elimination of waste products. Digestion occurs by both mechanical and chemical processes. The mechanical breakdown begins in the mouth, where the teeth and tongue physically alter the food into smaller pieces. Saliva moistens and lubricates the food to facilitate swallowing. The food continues to break down mechanically by churning in the stomach, where it mixes with digestive fluids. Digestive enzymes and acids further break down the larger molecules into smaller molecules in chemical digestion. Enzymes in the saliva, gastric fluid, pancreatic fluid, and intestinal fluid speed up these chemical reactions, whereas specific enzymes exist to break down carbohydrates,

TABLE 16–14
Common Medications for the Respiratory System

Type	Generic and Trade Names	Purpose
Antihistamines	Allegra, Benadryl, Claritin, Hismanal, Periactin, and Zyrtec	Relieve nasal passage swelling and inflammation
Antituberculosis agents	Myambutol, Nydrazid, and Rifamate	Treat tuberculosis
Antitussives	Non-narcotic: Benylin, Delsym, Robitussin, and Tessalon Narcotic: codeine, Endal-HD, and Tussar	Suppress coughing
Bronchodilators	aminophylline, ephedrine sulfate, and Proventil	Improve bronchial airflow
Decongestants	Afrin, Coricidin, Sinutab, and Sudafed	Reduce nasal congestion
Expectorants	Deconsal, Entex, Isoclor, and Robitussin	Remove lower respiratory tract secretions
Inhalation corticosteroids	Azmacort, Beclovent, and Decadron	Treat allergies and bronchial asthma
Mucolytics	Duratuss, Humibid, and Mucomyst	Liquefy mucus

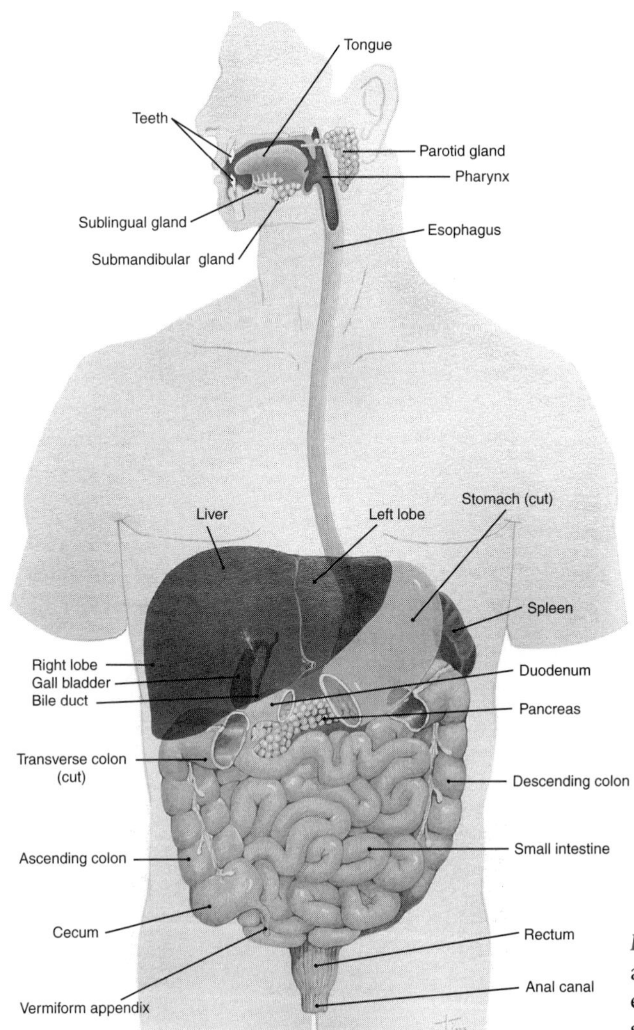

Figure 16–12 The digestive system. (From Scanlon, VC, and Sanders, T: Essentials of Anatomy and Physiology, ed. 3. FA Davis, Philadelphia, 1999, p. 353, with permission.)

proteins, and fats. Carbohydrates such as starch are broken down to simple sugars by the enzyme **amylase**, proteins are digested to amino acids by the peptidase enzymes, and fats are converted to fatty acids and glycerol by the enzyme **lipase**. Other chemicals facilitate the process and help food pass through the digestive tract.

Absorption of the digested products of food occurs through the walls of the small intestine into the blood and lymph, which transport the nutrients to the other parts of the body to produce energy and nourish body cells. Sugars and amino acids are absorbed into the bloodstream; fatty acids and triglycerides enter the lymphatic vessels.

Elimination of waste products is the third function of the digestive system. Unusable products of digestion are concentrated as feces in the large intestine, from which they pass out of the body through the anus.

Components

The components of the digestive system (Fig. 16–12) form a 30-foot continuous tube in adults that begins with the mouth and ends at the anus. This tube is commonly known as the gastrointestinal tract or ***alimentary tract***. The organs of the gastrointestinal tract include the mouth, pharynx, esophagus, stomach, small intestine, large intestine, **rectum**, and anus. The pharynx and esophagus act as a passageway through which food is propelled to the stomach by wavelike muscular contractions called ***peristalsis***. The stomach is a large saclike organ that stores food and continues to digest it with hydrochloric acid and other gastric juices. The small intestine has three parts: the **duodenum**, the **jejunum**, and the **ileum**. Digestion takes place in the mouth, stomach, and small intestine; nutrient absorption occurs mainly in the small intestine. The large intestine is divided into the **cecum**, colon, rectum, and anal canal. The **appendix** is attached to the cecum and does not have a known function in the digestive process. The colon consists of four parts: the ascending, transverse, descending, and sigmoid colon. Elimination of waste products begins in the colon and ends at the rectum and anus.

Accessory organs that assist in the breakdown of food include the teeth, salivary glands, tongue, liver, gallbladder, and pancreas. The teeth and tongue break food into small pieces. The salivary glands (the parotid, submandibular, and sublingual) provide saliva to dissolve and moisten food and produce salivary amylase. The liver secretes ***bile*** to aid in fat digestion and absorption. The gallbladder concentrates and stores excess bile. The pancreas secretes the digestive enzymes lipase, amylase, and trypsin, and produces ***insulin***. The liver, the largest internal organ in the body, has several important functions. It converts glucose to glycogen and back to glucose as needed; assists in protein breakdown; manufactures fibrinogen, prothrombin, heparin, and the blood clotting proteins; stores vitamins; forms ***bilirubin***; and detoxifies harmful substances such as alcohol.

Disorders

The following are common disorders of the digestive system.

- Appendicitis: Inflammation of the appendix requiring surgical removal; symptoms are acute pain in the right lower quadrant of the abdomen, ***nausea*** or vomiting, and fever.
- Cholecystitis: Inflammation of the gallbladder caused by gallstones blocking the bile duct; if gallstones cannot pass through the gallbladder, severe pain radiating to the right shoulder and obstructive jaundice may occur. Removal of the gallbladder may be necessary.
- Cirrhosis: Chronic inflammation of the liver caused by alcoholism, hepatitis, or malnutrition, resulting in degeneration of liver cells. Jaundice and liver failure may occur.
- Colitis: Acute or chronic inflammation of the colon; causes abdominal cramping, ***diarrhea***, or possible ulceration, producing blood and mucus-streaked stools.
- Crohn's disease: Autoimmune disorder producing chronic inflammation of the intestinal tract accompanied by diarrhea and malabsorption.
- Diverticulosis: Inflammation of the pouches in the walls of the colon with pain presenting in the left lower quadrant of the abdomen, tenderness, and fever.
- Gastritis: Inflammation of the stomach lining.
- Gastroenteritis: Inflammation of the stomach and intestinal tracts, producing nausea, vomiting, diarrhea, and abdominal cramps.
- Hemorrhoids: Enlargement of the veins in the anorectum; may be internal or external and produce bleeding, inflammation, and pain.
- Hernia: Protrusion of an organ or structure through the wall of the body cavity in which it is contained.
- Hepatitis: Acute inflammation of the liver caused by exposure to toxins or the hepatitis viruses A, B, or C. Symptoms include loss of appetite, nausea, fatigue, and jaundice.
- Pancreatitis: Inflammation of the pancreas resulting from abdominal injury, toxins, gallstones, drugs, or alcoholism; results in pancreas tissue destruction caused by an accumulation of pancreatic digestive fluids.
- Peritonitis: Inflammation of the lining of the abdominal cavity (the peritoneum); frequently caused by a ruptured appendix or a perforated ulcer.
- Ulcer: Open lesion in the gastric mucosa, caused by increased acid secretion or bacterial infection, that may cause pain, hemorrhage, or perforation of the walls of the stomach or duodenum.

Diagnostic Tests

The most frequently ordered diagnostic tests associated with the digestive system and their clinical correlations are presented in Table 16–15.

Medications

Table 16–16 lists the brand names of the most commonly used medications for the digestive system and their purpose.

TABLE 16–15
Diagnostic Tests Associated with the Digestive System

Test	Clinical Correlation
Alanine aminotransferase [ALT(SGPT)]	Liver disorders
Albumin	Malnutrition or liver disorders
Alcohol	Intoxication
Alkaline phosphatase (ALP)	Liver disorders
Ammonia	Severe liver disorders
Amylase	Pancreatitis
Aspartate aminotransferase [AST(SGOT)]	Liver disorders
Barium enema (**BaE**)	Colon abnormalities
Bilirubin	Liver disorders
Carcinoembryonic antigen (**CEA**)	Carcinoma detection and monitoring
Cholecystogram	Gallbladder function
Colonoscopy	Colon examination or biopsy
Complete blood count (CBC)	Appendicitis or other infection
Computerized axial tomography (CT scan)	Soft-tissue examination
Gamma-glutamyl transferase (GGT)	Early liver disorders
Gastrin	Gastric malignancy
Gastrointestinal (**GI**) series	Gastrointestinal tract obstruction or abnormalities
Hepatitis A, B, and C immunoassays	Hepatitis A, B, and C screening
Lactic dehydrogenase [LD(LDH)]	Liver disorders
Lipase	Pancreatitis
Liver biopsy (Bx)	Malignancy
Magnetic resonance imaging (MRI)	Soft-tissue examination
Occult blood	Gastrointestinal bleeding or intestinal malignancy
Ova and parasites (O & P)	Parasitic infection
Peritoneal fluid analysis	Bacterial infection
Stool culture	Pathogenic bacteria
Total protein (TP)	Liver disorders
Ultrasonogram	Organ examination

Urinary System

Key Terms

Nephron
Renal
Renal dialysis
Uremia

The urinary system removes waste products of metabolism, excess dietary chemicals, and excess water from the body in the form of urine. Urine is continually produced by the kidney, flows through the **ureters** to the bladder, and leaves the body through the **urethra**. This process maintains normal homeostasis of body fluids.

TABLE 16–16
Common Medications for the Digestive System

Type	Generic and Trade Names	Purpose
Antacids	Amphojel, Mylanta, sodium bicarbonate, and Tums	Neutralize excess stomach acid and relieve indigestion
Antidiarrheal agents	Imodium, Kaopectate, Lomotil, and Pepto-Bismol	Relieve diarrhea
Antiemetics	Antivert, Compazine, Dramamine, Phenergan, and Tigan	Suppress vomiting
Laxatives	Dulcolax, Ex-Lax, Metamucil, Milk of Magnesia, and Senokot	Relieve constipation

Function

Urine is formed in the ***nephrons*** of the kidney by a process of filtration and reabsorption. Blood enters the kidney through the ***renal*** artery, which branches into arterioles leading to the nephrons, and then into a collection of capillaries called the **glomerulus**. The filtration process takes place in the glomerulus, where small substances such as water, sodium and chloride ions, urea, creatinine, and uric acid are filtered out of the blood and collect in the **Bowman's capsule**. Large proteins and cells remain in the blood.

Reabsorption of water, glucose, sodium, and other essential nutrients required by the body begins as the glomerular filtrate passes through the **proximal convoluted tubule** and continues in the descending and ascending **loop of Henle**. The final adjustment of urinary composition occurs in the **distal convoluted tubule** and **collecting duct** (Fig. 16–13). Substances not filtered by the glomerulus are secreted by the tubules into the urinary filtrate. Urine consists of 95% water and 5% solid substances. Normal urine is clear yellow to amber in color, with a specific gravity of 1.010 to 1.025, and a slightly acid pH.

The actual amount of urine produced depends on the body's state of hydration and normally averages about 1000 mL (1 liter) per 24 hours. An average adult bladder can retain about 800 mL of urine. Normally, an adult feels the urge to void when the bladder contains around 300 mL of urine.

The ability of the kidneys to reabsorb previously filtered substances from the blood back into the bloodstream regulates the acid-base and fluid balance of the body.

The kidneys also produce hormones, such as **renin** to control blood pressure, and **erythropoietin** to regulate the production of red blood cells.

Components

The urinary system consists of two kidneys, two ureters, the urinary bladder, and the urethra.

The kidneys are bean-shaped organs containing an outer cortex region and an inner medulla region. The functioning unit of the kidney is the nephron, which consists of the Bowman's capsule, the glomerulus, the proximal convoluted tubule, the loop of Henle, the distal convoluted tubule, and

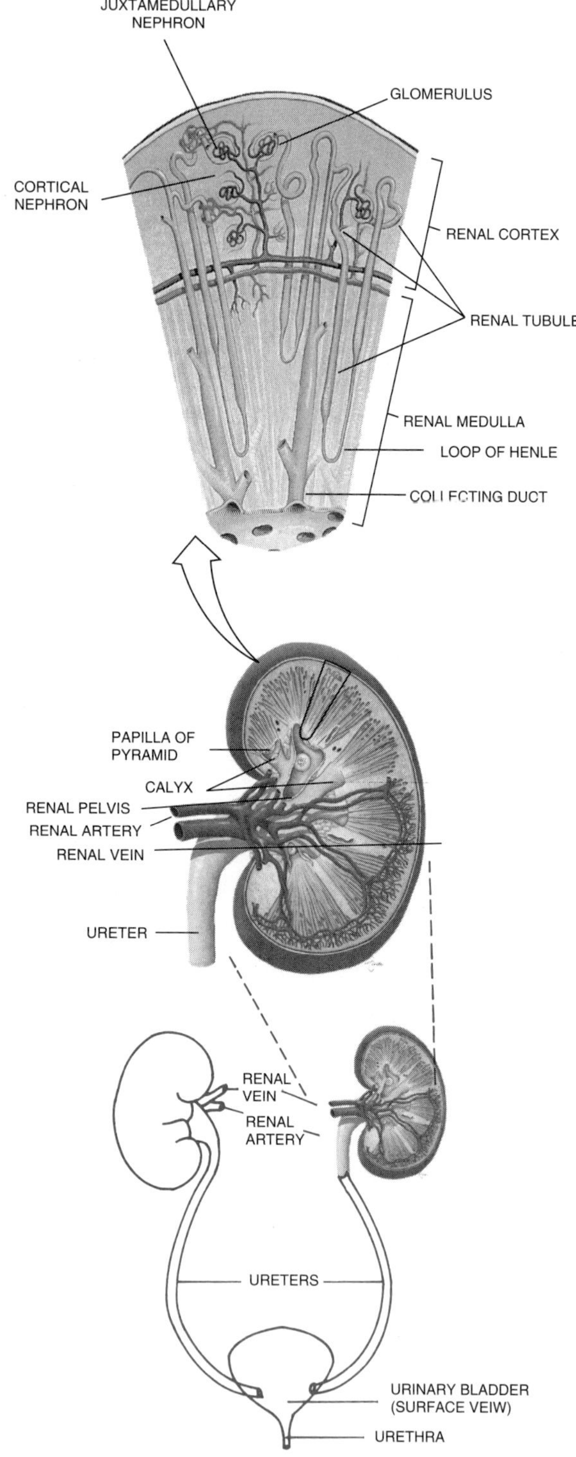

Figure 16–13 The relationship of the nephron to the kidney and excretory system. (Adapted from Scanlon, VC, and Sanders, T: Essentials of Anatomy and Physiology, ed. 3. FA Davis, Philadelphia, 1999, p. 405.)

collecting duct. Each kidney contains approximately one million nephrons.

The two ureters are muscular tubes that conduct urine from the kidney to the bladder. The urinary bladder is an expandable sac located in the anterior portion of the pelvic cavity. The bladder stores the urine formed by the nephron. When the bladder becomes full, muscles in the bladder walls squeeze urine into the urethra for elimination. The urethra is a tube extending from the bladder to an external opening, called the urinary meatus. The male urethra transports urine and semen. The female urethra carries only urine.

Disorders

The following are common disorders of the urinary system.

- Cystitis: Inflammation of the urinary bladder, usually caused by a bacterial infection. The most common symptoms are pain or burning on urination, frequent urgent urination, and blood in the urine.
- Glomerulonephritis: Inflammation of the glomerulus of the kidney caused by an immune disorder or infection; symptoms are dark brown urine containing blood and protein, headache, elevated blood pressure, renal failure, and ***uremia***. Acute glomerulonephritis can be caused by a delayed immune response to a streptococcal infection.
- Pyelonephritis: Inflammation of the renal pelvis and connective tissue of the kidney, usually caused by a bacterial infection; symptoms at onset are chills, fever, nausea, and vomiting. Urinalysis reveals the presence of bacteria, white bloods cells, white blood cell casts, and red blood cells.
- Renal calculi: Stones composed of calcium, phosphate, uric acid, oxalate, or other chemicals that crystallize within the kidney.
- Renal failure: Complete cessation of renal function resulting in the need for ***renal dialysis*** and kidney transplantation.
- Uremia: Excess urea, creatinine, uric acid, and other metabolic waste products in the blood.
- Urinary tract infection **(UTI)**: Bacterial infection involving any of the organs of the urinary system; includes urethritis, cystitis, and pyelonephritis.

Diagnostic Tests

The most frequently ordered diagnostic tests associated with the urinary system and their clinical correlations are presented in Table 16–17.

TABLE 16–17
Diagnostic Tests Associated with the Urinary System

Test	Clinical Correlation
Albumin	Kidney disorders
Antistreptolysin O (ASO) titer	Acute glomerulonephritis
Blood urea nitrogen (BUN)	Kidney function
Computerized axial tomography (CT scan)	Soft-tissue examination
Creatinine	Kidney function
Creatinine clearance	Glomerular filtration
Cystoscopy	Bladder examination or biopsy
Electrolytes (Lytes)	Fluid balance
Intravenous pyelogram **(IVP)**	Kidney disease
Kidney biopsy (Bx)	Malignancy
Magnetic resonance imaging (MRI)	Soft-tissue examination
Osmolality	Fluid and electrolyte balance
Routine urinalysis (UA)	Renal or metabolic disorders
Total protein (TP)	Kidney disorders
Ultrasonogram	Organ examination
Uric acid	Kidney function
Urine culture	Bacterial infection

TABLE 16-18
Common Medications for the Urinary System

Type	Generic and Trade Names	Purpose
Antibacterial agents	Bactrim, Cipro, Floxin, Gantanol, Gantrisin, Levaquin, Septra, and Thiosulfil	Treat urinary tract infection
Diuretics	Aldactone, Bumex, Demadex, Diuril, Dyrenium, HydroDIURIL, and Lasix	Promote urination

Medications

Table 16-18 lists the brand names of the most commonly used medications for the urinary system and their purpose.

Endocrine System

Key Terms

Endocrine
Gland
Homeostasis
Hormone
Hyperglycemia
Polydipsia
Polyphagia

The ***endocrine*** system produces and regulates ***hormones***. Hormones regulate activities such as metabolism, growth and development, reproduction, and responses to stress. Hormones maintain ***homeostasis*** through the regulation of body fluids, acid-base balance, and energy production.

Function

The endocrine system interacts with the nervous system to communicate, regulate, and control body functions. Unlike the nervous system, which commands and controls with nerve impulses, the ***glands*** of the endocrine system direct long-term changes in body activities by secreting chemical substances called hormones. Endocrine glands are ductless glands that secrete hormones directly into the bloodstream to circulate throughout the body until they reach a target organ. Hormones bind to a specific receptor site located on the cell membrane of a target organ and cause specific chemical reactions to occur. A feedback system regulated by supply and demand stimulates or decreases the release of hormones.

Components

The endocrine glands include the thyroid gland, four parathyroid glands, two adrenal glands, pancreas, pituitary gland, two female ovaries, two male testes, thymus, and pineal gland (Fig. 16-14). Each gland produces hormones that perform a specific function as listed in Table 16-19.

The secretions of the gastrointestinal mucosa, the placenta, and the kidney also provide endocrine function. The stomach lining secretes **gastrin** to stimulate gastric acid secretion; the placenta secretes chorionic gonadotropin hormone, **estrogen**, and **progesterone** during pregnancy. The kidney secretes erythropoietin to stimulate red blood cell production and renin to increase blood pressure.

Disorders

The following are common disorders of the endocrine system.

PITUITARY

- Acromegaly: Marked enlargement of the bones in the hands, feet, and face caused by hypersecretion of **growth hormone (GH)** in adulthood.
- Diabetes insipidus (**DI**): Hyposecretion of **antidiuretic hormone (ADH)**, causing a failure of the kidneys to reabsorb water and resulting in excessive urination and thirst.
- Dwarfism: Abnormally small body size caused by hyposecretion of GH in childhood. Bones are underdeveloped but well proportioned to the body; sexual immaturity.
- Gigantism: Marked increase in body size caused by hypersecretion of GH in childhood.

THYROID

- Cretinism: Congenital deficiency in the secretion of the thyroid hormones **triiodothyronine** (T_3) and **thyroxine** (T_4) (hypothyroidism) resulting in mental retardation, impaired growth, and abnormal bone formation.
- Goiter: An enlargement of the thyroid gland

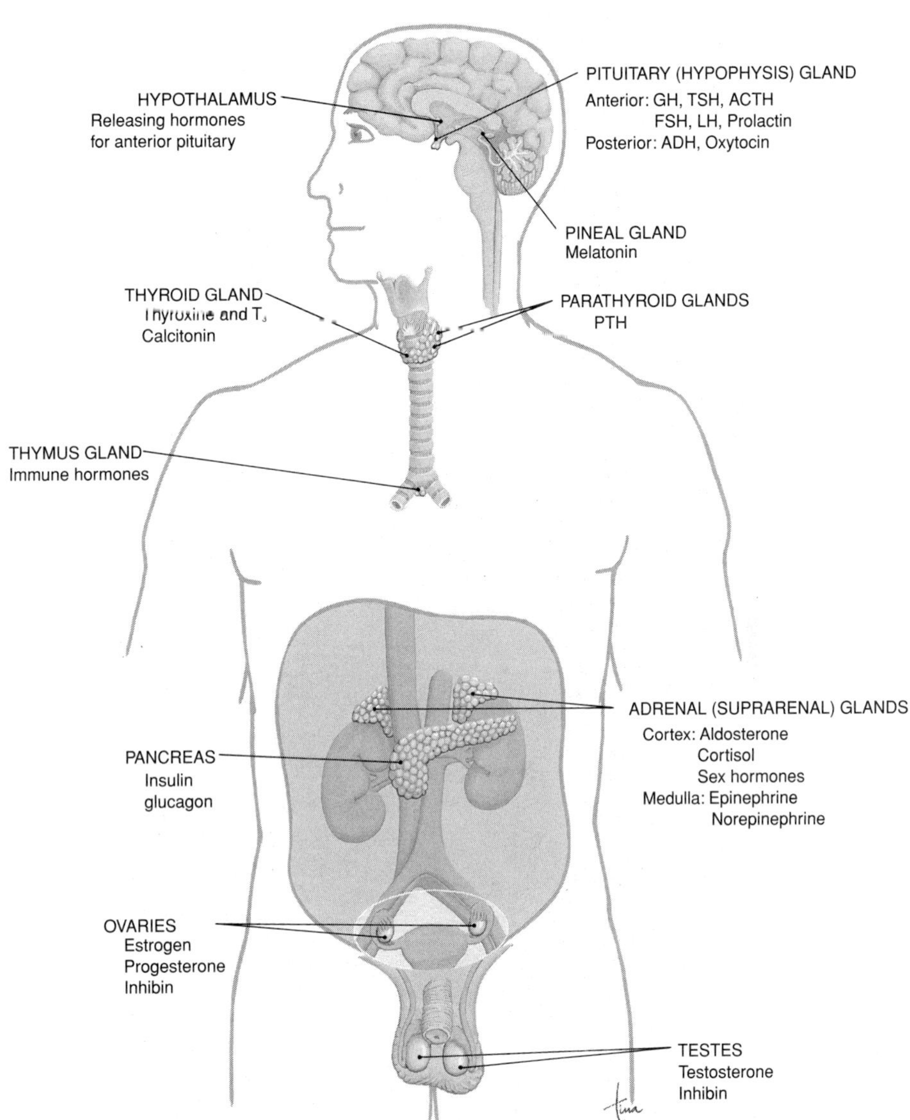

Figure 16–14 The endocrine system. (From Scanlon, VC, and Sanders, T: Essentials of Anatomy and Physiology, ed. 3. FA Davis, Philadelphia, 1999, p. 211, with permission.)

caused by hyperthyroidism; sometimes caused by dietary deficiency of iodine.

- Graves' disease: Increased cellular metabolism caused by excessive production of the thyroid hormones T_3 and T_4 (hyperthyroidism); characteristics include **exophthalmos** (protrusion of the eyeballs caused by swelling behind the eyes), weight loss, increased appetite, nervousness, excessive perspiration, rapid heart rate, and fatigue.
- Myxedema: A condition of subcutaneous tissue swelling caused by hypothyroidism that develops in adulthood; symptoms of the lowered metabolic rate are lethargy, weight gain, loss of hair, mental apathy, muscle weakness, slow heart rate, and puffiness of the face.

PARATHYROID

- Hyperparathyroidism: Excessive **parathyroid hormone (PTH)** secretion, often caused by a benign tumor, leading to kidney stones, bone weakness, osteoporosis, and hypercalcemia (increased blood calcium levels).
- Hypoparathyroidism: Deficient PTH secretion caused by injury or surgical removal of the

TABLE 16–19
Summary of Endocrine Hormones

Gland	Hormone	Function
Anterior pituitary	Growth hormone (GH) (Somatropin)	Stimulates bone and body growth
	Thyroid-stimulating hormone **(TSH)**	Stimulates the thyroid gland hormones thyroxine (T_4) and triiodothyronine (T_3)
	Adrenocorticotropic hormone (ACTH)	Stimulates adrenal cortex to secrete cortisol
	Follicle-stimulating hormone (FSH)	Stimulates growth of ovarian follicles in females and sperm production in males
	Luteinizing hormone (LH)	Stimulates ovulation in females and produces testosterone in males
	Prolactin **(PRL)**	Stimulates milk production by mammary glands and promotes growth of breast tissue
	Melanocyte-stimulating hormone **(MSH)**	Regulates melanin deposits that influence skin pigmentation
Posterior pituitary	Antidiuretic hormone (ADH)	Stimulates water reabsorption by the kidney to maintain body hydration
	Oxytocin	Stimulates uterine contraction and milk secretion by the mammary gland
Thyroid	Triiodothyronine (T_3) and thyroxine (T_4)	Regulate cell metabolism and increase energy production
	Calcitonin	Decreases the reabsorption of calcium and phosphate from bones into the blood
Parathyroid	Parathyroid hormone (PTH)	Increases the reabsorption of calcium and phosphate from the bones into the blood
Adrenal cortex	Aldosterone	Regulates sodium and potassium levels in the blood
	Cortisol	Regulates metabolism of proteins, carbohydrates, and fats and suppresses inflammation
	Androgens and estrogens	Maintain secondary sex characteristics
Adrenal medulla	Epinephrine (adrenaline)	Increases cardiac activity
	Norepinephrine (noradrenalin)	Constricts blood vessels and increases blood pressure
Pancreas	Insulin	Lowers blood sugar by transporting glucose from blood to the cells
	Glucagon	Increases blood sugar levels by converting glycogen to glucose
Ovaries	Estrogen and progesterone	Maintain female reproductive system and develop secondary female sex characteristics
Testes	Testosterone	Promotes maturation of spermatozoa and development of male secondary sex characteristics
Thymus	Thymosin	Promotes maturation of T lymphocytes and development of the immune system
Pineal	Melatonin	Regulates the body's internal clock

gland, decreasing blood calcium levels (hypocalcemia) and resulting in muscle spasms called tetany.

ADRENAL

- Addison's disease: Caused by hyposecretion of the adrenal cortex hormone cortisol, resulting in decreased blood sugar levels, muscle weakness, weight loss, nausea, low blood pressure, and dehydration.
- Cushing's disease: Hypersecretion of the adrenal cortex hormone cortisol as a result of

increased adrenal cortex stimulation by ACTH from the pituitary gland, caused by a tumor of the pituitary gland or adrenal cortex gland, or excessive administration of corticosteroids for medical reasons. Patients develop a round "moonface" and a buffalo hump on the thoracic region of the back because of the redistribution of fat. Skin and bones become thin and fragile.

PANCREAS

- Diabetes mellitus **(DM)**: Insulin deficiency that prevents sugar from leaving the blood and entering the body cells, resulting in **hyperglycemia** and **glucosuria**; symptoms include frequent urination **(polyuria)**, excessive thirst **(polydipsia)**, extreme hunger **(polyphagia)**, weight loss, fatigue, and blurred vision.
- Hyperinsulinism: Increased secretion of insulin by the pancreas, decreasing the blood sugar level.
- Hypoglycemia: Abnormally decreased blood sugar level that is associated with nervousness, headaches, and confusion.

Diagnostic Tests

The most frequently ordered diagnostic tests associated with the endocrine system and their clinical correlations are presented in Table 16–20.

Medications

Table 16–21 lists the brand names of the most commonly used medications for the endocrine system and their purpose.

Reproductive System

Key Terms

Gamete	*Ova*
Gonads	*Ovulation*
Menopause	*Semen*
Menstruation	*Spermatozoa*

The purpose of the reproductive system is the perpetuation of future generations of the human species. The organs and hormones specific to the male and female reproductive systems ensure sexual reproduction and the development of male and female secondary sex characteristics.

Function

The vital functions of the male and female reproduction systems are to produce ***gametes***, to enable fertilization, and to provide a nourishing environment for the developing embryo/fetus. The male and female reproductive glands, called the ***gonads***, produce and store the gametes, or sex cells. In men, the testes produce the gametes called ***spermatozoa,***

TABLE 16–20
Diagnostic Tests Associated with the Endocrine System

Test	Clinical Correlation
Adrenocorticotropic hormone (ACTH)	Adrenal and pituitary gland function
Calcium (Ca)	Parathyroid function
Catecholamines	Adrenal function
Computerized axial tomography (CT scan)	Soft-tissue examination
Cortisol	Adrenal cortex function
Glucose	Hypoglycemia or diabetes mellitus
Glucose tolerance test (GTT)	Hypoglycemia or diabetes mellitus
Growth hormone (GH)	Pituitary gland function
Insulin	Glucose metabolism and pancreatic function
Magnetic resonance imaging (MRI)	Soft-tissue examination
Parathyroid hormone (PTH)	Parathyroid function
Phosphorus (P)	Endocrine disorders
Testosterone	Testicular function
Thyroid function (T_3, T_4, TSH) studies	Thyroid function
Thyroid scan	Thyroid tumors

TABLE 16–21
Common Medications for the Endocrine System

Type	Generic and Trade Names	Purpose
Antithyroid hormone	Tapazole	Increases metabolic rate
Insulin	Humulin, Novolin, and Velosulin	Lowers blood sugar level
Oral hypoglycemics	Actos, Avandia, DiaBeta, Glucophage, Glucotrol, Glyset, Micronase, and Tolinase	Stimulate insulin secretion
Thyroid hormones	Cytomel, Euthroid, Levothroid, Synthroid, and Thyrolar	Increase metabolic rate

and in women, the ***ovaries*** produce the gametes called ***ova*** or eggs. Reproduction occurs through **fertilization** between the ovum and the spermatozoa, usually in the fallopian tubes. This produces an embryo that develops for 9 months in the uterus of women during pregnancy. If fertilization does not occur, the uterine lining sheds, which is indicated by bleeding called ***menstruation***.

The ovaries begin to release ova (***ovulation***) at puberty and continue to release them until ***menopause***. Hormones from the pituitary gland stimulate the ovaries to secrete estrogen and progesterone. These hormones facilitate menstruation, pregnancy, and the development of the secondary sex characteristics. During pregnancy, the placenta produces the hormone human chorionic gonadotropin (HCG). Detection of HCG in serum or urine provides the diagnostic test to confirm pregnancy.

Beginning at puberty and continuing throughout life, the male testes produce billions of spermatozoa and secrete the hormone testosterone for the development of secondary male sex characteristics.

Components

The female reproductive system consists of two ovaries for the production of ova (eggs); two **fallopian tubes** that transport an egg or fertilized embryo to the **uterus**; the uterus for embryo development; the vagina, which receives sperm during intercourse, discharges menstrual blood, and acts as the birth canal during delivery of a fetus; external genitalia (vulva) for sexual stimulation and lubrication; and mammary glands (breasts) to produce milk for the newborn (Fig. 16–15).

The male reproductive organs are shown in Figure 16–16 and include: two **testes** (enclosed in the **scrotum**), which manufacture sperm and produce **testosterone**; two **epididymides** for sperm maturation and storage; two **vasa deferentia**, which convey sperm to the ejaculatory duct; two **seminal vesicles**, which produce fluid to nourish the sperm; the **prostate gland**, which secretes fluid to maintain sperm motility; two **bulbourethral glands**, which secrete fluid before ejaculation; and the urethra within the penis, which carries the sperm out of the body. ***Semen*** is the transporting medium for the sperm discharged during ejaculation. Sperm and the secretions of the seminal vesicles, prostate gland, and the bulbourethral glands constitute semen.

Disorders

The following are common disorders of the male and female reproductive systems.

- Carcinoma: Malignant tumors of the cervix **(Cx)**, ovary, prostate, or testes.
- Endometriosis: Increased endometrial (uterine lining) tissue that migrates outside the uterus;

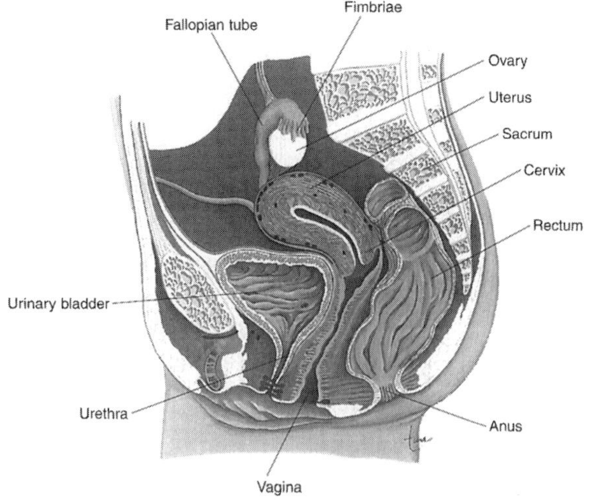

Figure 16–15 The female reproductive system. (Adapted from Scanlon, VC, and Sanders, T: Essentials of Anatomy and Physiology, ed. 3. FA Davis, Philadelphia, 1999. p. 446.)

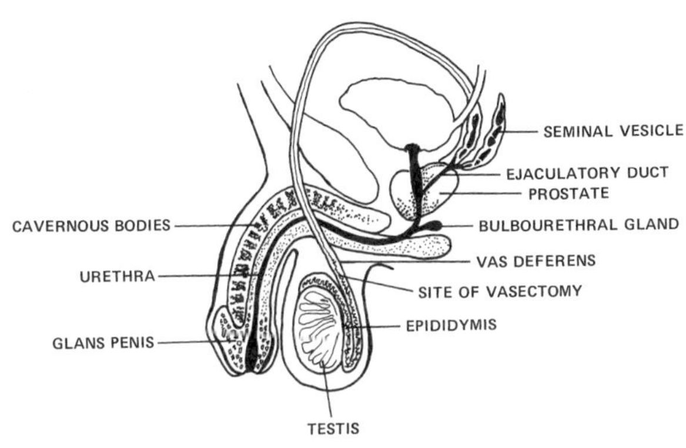

Figure 16–16 The male reproductive system. (Adapted from Strasinger, SK, and Di Lorenzo, MS: Urinalysis and Body Fluids, ed. 4. FA Davis, Philadelphia, 2001, p. 170.)

associated with **dysmenorrhea**, pelvic pain, and inability to become pregnant.

- Fibroids: **Benign** uterine tumors that may cause excessive uterine bleeding.
- Pelvic inflammatory disease (**PID**): Inflammation of the ovaries, cervix, uterus, or fallopian tubes, caused by infection that may result in infertility or septicemia.
- Premenstrual syndrome (**PMS**): Characterized by symptoms including depression, irritability, mood swings, weight gain, breast tenderness, water retention, and nervousness occurring 7 to 14 days before menstruation.
- Sexually transmitted diseases (**STDs**): Diseases transmitted by sexual contact such as chlamydiosis, gonorrhea, herpes genitalis, syphilis, trichomoniasis, and AIDS.
- Toxic shock syndrome (TSS): Systemic shock symptoms caused by a *Staphylococcus aureus* infection in menstruating women using superabsorbent tampons; characterized by high fever, confusion, syncope, headache, skin rash, and markedly decreased blood pressure.

Diagnostic Tests

The most frequently ordered diagnostic tests associated with the reproductive system and their clinical correlations are presented in Table 16–22.

TABLE 16–22
Diagnostic Tests Associated with the Reproductive System

Test	Clinical Correlation
Amniocentesis	Fetal maturity or genetic defects
Chorionic villus sampling (**CVS**)	Genetic defects
Computerized axial tomography (CT scan)	Soft-tissue examination
Estradiol, estriol, and estrogen	Ovarian or placental function
Fluorescent treponemal antibody-absorbed (FTA-ABS)	Syphilis
Genital culture	Bacterial infection
Gram stain	Microbial infection
Human chorionic gonadotropin (HCG)	Pregnancy
Laparoscopy	Abdominal exploration or ovarian or fallopian tube disorders
Magnetic resonance imaging (MRI)	Soft-tissue examination
Mammogram	Breast cancer detection
Pap smear (Pap)	Cervical or vaginal carcinoma
Prostate-specific antigen (PSA)	Prostatic cancer
Prostatic acid phosphatase (**PAP**)	Prostatic cancer
Rapid plasma reagin (RPR)	Syphilis
Rubella titer	Immunity to German measles
Semen analysis	Fertility or effectiveness of a vasectomy
Toxoplasma antibody screening	*Toxoplasma* infection
Ultrasonogram	Organ examination
Vaginal wet prep	Microbial infection
Venereal Disease Research Laboratory (VDRL)	Syphilis

TABLE 16–23
Common Medications for the Reproductive System

Type	Generic and Trade Names	Purpose
Contraceptives	Oral: Alesse, Brevicon, Cyclesse, Desogen, Demulen, Estrostep, Levlen, Loestrin, Lo/Ovral, Micronor, Norplant System, Ortho-Novum, Ovulen, Orthotricyclen, and Triphasil Injectable: Depo-Provera and Lunelle	Prevent ovulation
Female hormones	Activella, Aygestin, Estrace, Estraderm, Evista, Gesterol, Norinyl, Norulate, Ogen, Orthoprefest, Premarin, Provera	Treat amenorrhea, dysfunctional bleeding, and menopausal hormone replacement therapy
Uterine relaxants	Ethanol and Yutopar	Delay labor
Uterine stimulants	Oxytocin and Pitocin	Control postpartum bleeding and induce labor

Medications

Table 16–23 lists the brand names of the most commonly used medications for the reproductive system and their purpose.

Lymphatic System

Key Terms

B lymphocytes	*Lymph*
Cell-mediated immunity	*Lymph nodes*
Humoral immunity	*T lymphocytes*

The lymphatic system is the body's "other" vessel system and connects to the circulatory system. Lymphatic vessels, called capillaries and veins, extend throughout the body to propel ***lymph*** fluid back to the circulatory system. Lymph forms from **interstitial fluid**, the tissue fluid that leaks from blood capillaries and surrounds the body cells. It is a clear, colorless fluid consisting of 95% water, proteins, salts, sugar, lymphocytes, monocytes, and waste products of metabolism. It does not contain platelets or red blood cells. Lymph flows through the lymphatic vessels, entering the bloodstream through ducts that connect to veins in the upper chest.

Function

The lymphatic system has three major functions. It drains excess fluid from the tissue spaces and transports the nutrients and waste products back to the bloodstream. It provides a defense mechanism against disease by storing lymphocytes and monocytes that protect the body from foreign substances through phagocytosis and the immune response. It acts as the passageway for the absorption of fats from the small intestine into the bloodstream.

Components

The parts of the lymphatic system are the lymph vessels, right lymphatic duct, thoracic duct, ***lymph nodes***, tonsils, thymus, and spleen. Lymph capillaries collect the fluid from the interstitial spaces. Lymph capillaries join with larger lymph vessels, the venules and veins, where the lymph enters two terminal vessels, the **right lymphatic duct** and **thoracic duct**. The right lymphatic duct receives lymph from the upper right quadrant of the body and empties into the right subclavian vein. The thoracic duct receives lymph from the left upper quadrant of the body and lower body and returns it to the blood in the left subclavian vein. Valves in the lymph vessels allow the lymph to flow in only one direction toward the chest cavity by skeletal muscle contraction. Figure 16–17 displays the relationship between the lymphatic and circulatory systems.

Lymph nodes located along the lymphatic pathway filter the lymph as it flows through the lymphatic vessels. Lymph nodes store lymphocytes and monocytes to phagocytize bacteria and foreign substances, stimulate the immune response, and recognize and destroy cancer cells. The major lymph nodes are the cervical (neck), axillary (armpits), inguinal (groin), and mediastinal (chest) nodes.

The tonsils, thymus gland, and spleen also contain lymphoid tissue to store lymphocytes and monocytes. The tonsils (located in the pharynx)

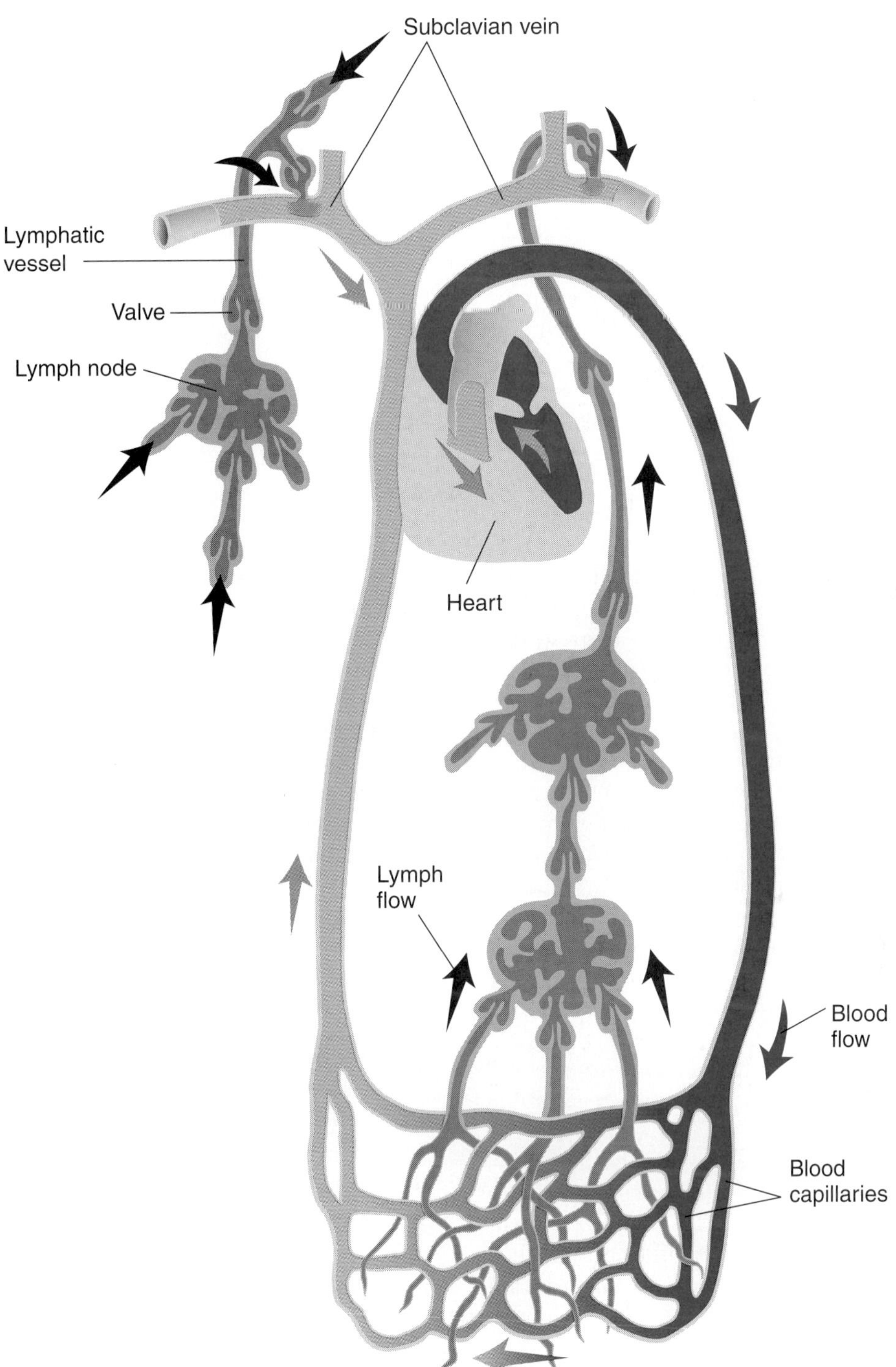

Figure 16–17 The relationship of lymphatic vessels to the cardiovascular system. (From Scanlon, VC, and Sanders, T: Essentials of Anatomy and Physiology, ed. 3. FA Davis, Philadelphia, 1999, p. 305, with permission.)

filter bacteria at the entrance of the respiratory and digestive tracts. The thymus gland, located between the lungs, controls the immune system. It produces T cells to provide cellular immunity. The spleen, located in the upper left quadrant of the abdomen, filters cell debris, bacteria, parasites, and old red blood cells.

Immune System

The lymphatic system controls the body's immune system by the recognition of foreign antigens filtered through the lymph nodes and spleen, and the maintenance of a high concentration of ***B*** and ***T lymphocytes***. An antigen is a large molecule located on cells that stimulates the formation of antibodies. Cells are recognized as "self" or foreign by the antigens present on the cell membrane. Foreign antigens are present on bacteria, toxins, viruses, fungi, and cancer cells, and cause the B or T lymphocytes to activate either a humoral or cellular immune response.

An antibody (immunoglobulin) is a protein that is produced by exposure to antigens. ***Humoral immunity*** or antibody-mediated immunity involves the production of antibodies to specific antigens by B lymphocytes in the spleen and lymph nodes. Helper T cells recognize foreign antigens and then activate B cells to transform into plasma cells that produce specific antibodies to the antigens to destroy them. Humoral immunity is the major immune response against bacterial infections.

T lymphocytes produce chemical substances (**lymphokines**) rather than antibodies for the destruction of foreign antigens in cellular or ***cell-mediated immunity***. T cells differentiate into helper T cells to recognize a foreign antigen and suppressor T cells to control the immune response by stopping the immune response once the foreign antigen has been destroyed. Natural killer (NK) cells chemically destroy foreign cells, cells infected with viruses, and cancer cells by disrupting the cell membrane. Cell-mediated immunity is the major protection against intracellular microorganisms, such as viruses, and tumor cells. It also can cause rejection of transplanted tissue.

In AIDS, it is the helper T cells that are infected by the human immunodeficiency virus (HIV). Without the helper T cells, the immune system is severely compromised. Foreign antigens are not recognized, B cells are not activated, and natural killer T cells are not stimulated to proliferate.

Disorders

The following are common disorders of the lymphatic system.

- AIDS: A suppressed immune system caused by the pathogen HIV, transmitted through sexual contact, blood products and needles, or from mother to infant perinatally. Conditions frequently associated with AIDS are *Pneumocystis carinii* pneumonia, Kaposi's sarcoma, and a variety of fungal and viral diseases.
- Hodgkin's disease: A malignant tumor of the lymphatic tissue that produces painless enlarged lymph nodes, splenomegaly, fever, weakness, anemia, weight loss, and night sweats.
- Infectious mononucleosis (IM): Infectious disease caused by the Epstein-Barr virus characterized by enlarged lymph nodes, increased lymphocytes, weakness, fatigue, fever, and sore throat; occurs mostly in young adults.
- Lymphoma: A solid tumor, frequently malignant, of the lymphatic tissue such as Burkitt's lymphoma and non-Hodgkin's lymphoma.
- Lymphosarcoma: A diffuse malignant tumor of the lymphatic tissue.
- Multiple myeloma: Malignant proliferation of plasma cells in the bone marrow that produces painful nodules, impaired hematologic and immune system functions, and destruction of bone.

Diagnostic Tests

The most frequently ordered diagnostic tests associated with the lymphatic system and their clinical correlations are presented in Table 16–24.

Medications

Table 16–25 lists the brand names of the most commonly used medications for the lymphatic system and their purpose.

Bibliography

Scanlon, VC, and Sanders, T: Essentials of Anatomy and Physiology, ed. 3. FA Davis, Philadelphia, 1999.

Strasinger, SK, and Di Lorenzo, MS: Urinalysis and Body Fluids, ed. 4. FA Davis, Philadelphia, 2001.

Strasinger, SK, and Di Lorenzo, MS: Skills for the Patient Care Technician. FA Davis, Philadelphia, 1999.

TABLE 16–24
Diagnostic Tests Associated with the Lymphatic System

Test	Clinical Correlation
Anti-HIV	Human immunodeficiency virus
Antinuclear antibody (ANA)	Systemic lupus erythematosus
Complete blood count (CBC)	Infectious mononucleosis
Computerized axial tomography (CT scan)	Soft-tissue examination
Fluorescent antinuclear antibody (FANA)	Systemic lupus erythematosus
Immunoglobin (Ig) levels	Immune system function
Lymph node biopsy (Bx)	Malignancy
Magnetic resonance imaging (MRI)	Soft-tissue examination
Monospot	Infectious mononucleosis
Protein electrophoresis	Multiple myeloma
T-cell count	Immune function/AIDS monitoring
Western blot	Human immunodeficiency virus

TABLE 16–25
Common Medications for the Lymphatic System

Type	Generic and Trade Names	Effect
Anti-AIDS drugs	Abacavir, Epivir, Indinavir, Invirase, lamivudine, stavudine, and zidovudine (ZDV, AZT)	Inhibit viral replication
Antihistamines	Atarax, Benadryl, Periactin, and Zyrtec	Relieve allergic symptoms
Anti-inflammatories	Decadron, Feldene, Indocin, and Lodine	Relieve swelling
Antineoplastics	Cytoxan, methotrexate, Nolvadex (tamoxifen), and Taxol	Destroy malignant cells, prevent metastasis
Biologicals	Gamulin, Hep-B-gammagee, and vaccines	Provide immunity
Immunosuppressives	Imuran, Progal, and Sandimmune (cyclosporine)	Prevent transplant rejection
Multiple sclerosis agents	Avonex and Betaseron	Inhibit autoimmune myelin destruction

Study Questions

1. Name and define the four types of tissue in the body.
   a. ______
   b. ______
   c. ______
   d. ______

2. Name the body system associated with each of the following functions:
   a. Directs body activities through hormones ______
   b. Protects the body against the invasion of harmful pathogens and chemicals ______
   c. Provides skeletal movement ______
   d. Exchanges oxygen and carbon dioxide between the air and blood ______
   e. Removes urea from the blood ______

3. Name the plane that divides the body into equal right and left halves.

   ______

4. Define the following directional terms:
   a. Anterior

      ______

   b. Posterior

      ______

   c. Proximal

      ______

   d. Distal

      ______

   e. Dorsal

      ______

5. Name the cavity lined by each of the following membranes:
   a. Parietal pleura ______
   b. Peritoneum ______
   c. Meninges ______

6. What is the largest organ in the body?

____

7. Describe the two layers of skin.

   a. _______________

   ____

   ____

   b. _______________

   ____

   ____

8. Name the pigment that determines skin color and the cell that produces it.

   a. Pigment _______________

   b. Cell _______________

9. Name the two types of skin glands and the function of each.

Type	Function
a. ________	________
b. ________	________

10. The vitamin produced by the skin is

_______________.

11. List four classifications of bones and give an example of each.

Classification	Example
a. ________	________
b. ________	________
c. ________	________
d. ________	________

12. The fluid within the joint cavity that prevents friction is

_______________.

13. The action of moving a body part toward the midline is _______________.

14. Name the three types of muscle tissue.

    a. ______________________________

    b. ______________________________

    c. ______________________________

15. The connective tissues that attach skeletal muscle to bones are

    ______________________________.

16. Name the two divisions of the nervous system.

    a. ______________________________

    b. ______________________________

17. List and describe the three major parts of the neuron.

Part	Description
a. ______________	______________
b. ______________	______________
c. ______________	______________

18. Name the two types of neurons and describe their function.

Type	Function
a. ______________	______________
b. ______________	______________

19. The fluid that circulates through the brain and spinal cord is

    ______________________________.

20. Differentiate between external and internal respiration.

    ____

    ____

    ____

    ____

21. The air sacs of the lung are the ______________________________.

22. The cartilage that blocks the larynx during swallowing is the

    ______________________________.

23. Name three digestive enzymes.

 a. ______________________________

 b. ______________________________

 c. ______________________________

24. State four functions of the liver.

 a. ______________________________

 b. ______________________________

 c. ______________________________

 d. ______________________________

25. Name the organ in the GI tract where absorption mainly occurs.

 ____

26. The functioning unit of the kidney is the ______________________________ .

27. The organs that transport urine from the kidneys to the bladder are the ______________ .

28. Define and state the function of an endocrine gland.

 ____

 ____

29. The chemical substances secreted by endocrine glands are ______________________ .

30. The hormone that maintains normal blood sugar is ______________________ .

31. The endocrine gland known as the master gland is the ______________________ .

32. The male sex hormone produced by the testes is ______________________ .

33. The gonad for the female reproductive system is the ______________________ .

34. List the three functions of the reproductive system.

 a. ______________________________

 b. ______________________________

 c. ______________________________

35. List the three functions of the lymphatic system.

 a. ______________________________

 b. ______________________________

 c. ______________________________

36. The predominant lymphocyte produced in humoral immunity is the

____.

37. List two types of T lymphocytes.

    a. ____

    b. ____

38. The immune response that is stimulated in an organ transplant is

____.

Appendix 1

Laboratory Tests and the Required Type of Anticoagulants and Volume of Blood

This is a list of anticoagulant and specimen requirements for the most common test requests at Nebraska Methodist Hospital, Omaha, NE. Each laboratory has specific test protocols.

Test	Collection Tube	Minimum Amount	Comments
Ammonia	Lavender	3 mL	Send on ice
Amylase	Light green PST/Gold SST	3 mL	
Antibiotic assay (Gent, Tob, Vanco)	Red clot/Clear nongel Microtainer	5 mL/(0.5 mL)	No SST tubes
Antibody ID/Screen	Lavender	7 mL	Blood bank ID
Beta HCG/Quant.	Light green PST/Gold SST	3 mL	
Bilirubin	Gold SST/Amber Microtainer	1.5 mL/(0.5 mL)	Protect from light
B_{12}	Gold SST/Red clot	3 mL	
CBC	Lavender	3 mL	
Cortisol	Gold SST/Red clot	2 mL	Serum only
Crossmatch	Lavender	7 mL	Blood bank ID remains on for 72 hours
D-Dimer	Light blue	4.5 mL	Tube must be full (stable for 4 hours)
Ethanol/alcohol	Red clot/Gray	3 mL	Do not open tube until testing
Fibrinogen	Light blue	4.5 mL	Tube must be full
Folate	Gold SST/Red clot	3 mL	
Glucose	Light green PST/Gold SST	3 mL	
Hgb A1C	Lavender/Lavender Microtainer	1 mL/(0.3 mL)	
Hgb/Hct	Lavender	3 mL	
Hepatitis panel	Gold SST/Red clot	6 mL	
Ionized calcium	Gold SST/Red clot/ Arterial gas syringe	7 mL	Tube must be full; may use arterial gas syringe
Lactate	Green/Arterial gas syringe	5 mL	Send on ice; analyze in 15 minutes
Lead	Tan EDTA	2 mL	
Lipase	Light green PST/Gold SST	3 mL	

Test	Collection Tube	Minimum Amount	Comments
Lithium	Gold SST/Red clot	5 mL	Draw 12 hours post dose
MI panel (myo, CK-MB, troponin)	White PPT	3 mL	Stable 4 hours
Monospot	Gold SST/Red clot	3 mL	
pH	Green	3 mL	Send on ice
Platelet	Lavender	3 mL	
Prothrombin time (PT)	Light blue	4.5 mL	Full tube; stable 4 hours refrigerated
PTT/APTT	Light blue	4.5 mL	Full tube; stable 4 hours refrigerated
Protein electrophoresis	Gold SST/Red clot	3 mL	
Reticulocyte count	Lavender	3 mL	
Therapeutic drugs (digoxin, Theo, Pheno, Pheny, Carb, Val Ac)	Red clot/Clear nongel Microtainer	3 mL/Full Microtainer	No SST tubes
TSH/Free T_4	Light green PST/Gold SST	3 mL	
Quant. Proteins (C3, C4, IgG, IgA, IgM, haptoglobin)	Gold SST/Red clot	3 mL	
Sedimentation rate (ESR)	Lavender	5 mL	Stable 4 hours at room temperature
Chemistry panels (renal, hepatic, comprehensive, metabolic)	Light green PST/Gold SST	3 mL	
Lipid panel (HDL, Chol, Trig)	Gold SST	5 mL	

APTT = activated partial thromboplastin time; Carb = carbamazepine; CBC = complete blood count; Chol = cholesterol; CK-MB = isoenzyme of creatine kinase with muscle and brain subunits; ESR = erythrocyte sedimentation rate; Gent = gentamicin; HCG = human chorionic gonadotropin; Hct = hematocrit; HDL = high-density lipoprotein; Hgb = hemoglobin; ID = identification; Ig = immunoglobin; MI = myocardial infarction; myo = myoglobin; pH = hydrogen ion concentration; Pheno = phenobarbital; Pheny = phenytoin; PST = plasma separator tube; PTT = partial thromboplastin time; Quant. = quantitative; SST = serum separator tube; T_4 = thyroxine; Theo = theophylline; Tob = tobramycin; Trig = triglycerides; TSH = thyroid-stimulating hormone; Val Ac = valproic acid; Vanco = vancomycin.

Courtesy of Diane Wolff, MLT(ASCP), Phlebotomy Team Leader, Nebraska Methodist Hospital, Omaha, NE

Appendix 2

Intravenous Infusion: Blood Specimen Collection from Vascular Access Device

Use the following table to determine the necessary flush volumes.

Intravenous Access: Blood Draws/Flush Protocols

								Arterial Lines		
		Peripheral	**Central Venous Catheters**	**Hickman**	**Groshong**	**Implanted Ports**	**PICC**	**Radial Arterial Lines**	**Femoral Line**	**Midline Catheter**
	Flush each lumen	An indwelling peripheral catheter is not routinely used for blood specimen collection	5 mL NS if IV solution will interfere with lab studies 10 mL NS	10 mL NS if IV solution will interfere with lab studies	10 mL NS if TPN or blood and if blood coagulation studies ordered; flush with 20 mL NS	10 mL NS if IV solution will interfere with lab studies	If TPN, flush with 20 mL NS	Turn stopcock off to pressure bag. DO NOT use line for blood cultures.	Turn stopcock off to pressure bag	A midline catheter is routinely used for blood draws 10 mL NS
With IV infusing	Clamp each lumen/tubing before blood draw		1 minute	1 minute	**DO NOT** clamp. Stop all IVs infusing for 1 minute	1 minute	1 minute			1 minute
	Discard		10 cc	10 mL	10 mL	10 mL	10 mL	10 mL with syringe	10 mL with syringe	10 mL
	Withdraw blood sample		Based on test	Based on test	Based on test	Based on test	Based on test	According to lab specimen	According to lab specimen	Based on test

(*Continued on following page*)

Intravenous Access: Blood Draws/Flush Protocols

		Peripheral	Central Venous Catheters	Hickman	Groshong	Implanted Ports	PICC	*Arterial Lines*		Midline Catheter
								Radial Arterial Lines	Femoral Line	
	Flush each lumen after draw		5–10 mL NS, resume infusion in all lumens	10 mL NS, resume infusion	10 mL NS, resume infusion	10 mL NS, resume infusion	10 mL NS, resume infusion	Turn stopcock toward patient; flush stop-cock using sterile syringe; replace with new sterile cap; then flush line via trans-ducer manu-ally until line is clear and verify wave form	Turn stopcock toward patient; flush stop-cock using sterile syringe; replace with new sterile cap; then flush line via trans-ducer manu-ally until line is clear and verify wave form	10 cc NS resume infu-sion
Without IV infusing	Flush each lumen		10 mL NS	10 mL NS	10 mL NS	10 mL NS	10 mL NS			8–10 mL NS
	Discard		8–10 mL NS							8–10 mL NS
	Withdraw blood sample		Based on test	Based on test	Based on test	Based on test	Based on test			Based on test

(*Continued on following page*)

Intravenous Access: Blood Draws/Flush Protocols

							Arterial Lines		
	Peripheral	Central Venous Catheters	Hickman	Groshong	Implanted Ports	PICC	Radial Arterial Lines	Femoral Line	Midline Catheter
Flush each lumen after draw		5–10 mL NS followed by 1.5 mL heparinized saline (100 units/mL)	10 mL NS followed by 1.5 mL heparinized saline (100 units/mL)	10 mL NS	If close-ended, flush with 10 mL NS. If open-ended, flush with 10 mL NS and follow with 5 mL heparinized saline (100 units/mL)	If close-ended, flush with 10 mL NS. If open-ended, follow with 5 mL heparinized saline (100 units/mL)			10 mL NS

IV = intravenous; NS = normal saline; PICC = peripherally inserted central catheter.

Note: If patient is undergoing transplant, question patient about using normal saline for flushing instead of heparin because heparin interferes with immunological response.

If patient is undergoing heparin therapy in the IV line, **DO NOT** use this line for collection of coagulation factor studies.

Courtesy of Diane Wolff, MLT(ASCP), Phlebotomy Team Leader, Nebraska Methodist Hospital, Omaha, NE.

Appendix 3

Abbreviations

AABB	American Association of Blood Banks
Ab	Antibody
ABGs	Arterial blood gases
ABO	Blood group
ACD	Acid citrate dextrose
ACT	Activated clotting time
ACTH	Adrenocorticotropic hormone
ADH	Antidiuretic hormone
AFB	Acid-fast bacteria
Ag	Antigen
AIDS	Acquired immunodeficiency syndrome
ALP	Alkaline phosphatase
ALS	Amyotrophic lateral sclerosis
ALT (SGPT)	Alanine aminotransferase
AMT	American Medical Technologists
ANA	Antinuclear antibody
ANS	Autonomic nervous system
APTT (PTT)	Activated partial thromboplastin time
ARD	Antimicrobial removal device
ASAP	As soon as possible
ASCLS	American Society for Clinical Laboratory Science
ASCP	American Society of Clinical Pathology
ASO	Antistreptolysin O
ASPT	American Society of Phlebotomy Technicians
AST (SGOT)	Aspartate aminotransferase
AV	Atrioventricular
BaE	Barium enema
BB	Blood bank
bid	Twice a day
BNP	Brain natriuretic peptide
BP	Blood pressure
BSI	Body substance isolation
BT	Bleeding time
BUN	Blood urea nitrogen
Bx	Biopsy
C & S	Culture and sensitivity
Ca	Calcium
CAP	College of American Pathologists
CAT/CT scan	Computerized tomography
CBC	Complete blood count
CBGs	Capillary blood gases
cc, cm^3	Cubic centimeter
CCU	Cardiac care unit
CDC	Centers for Disease Control and Prevention
CEA	Carcinoembryonic antigen
CEU	Continuing education unit
CHF	Congestive heart failure
CK (CPK)	Creatine kinase
CK-BB, MB, and MM	Creatine kinase isoenzymes
Cl	Chloride
CLIA '88	Clinical Laboratory Improvement Amendments of 1988
CLPlb	Certified Laboratory Phlebotomist
CLS	Clinical Laboratory Scientist
CLT	Clinical Laboratory Technician
cm	Centimeter
CMS	Centers for Medicare and Medicaid Services
CMV	Cytomegalovirus
CNA	Certified Nursing Assistant
CNS	Central nervous system

CO_2	Carbon dioxide
COLA	Commission on Laboratory Assessment
COPD	Chronic obstructive pulmonary disease
CPR	Cardiopulmonary resuscitation
CPT	Certified Phlebotomist Technician
CPT	Current Procedural Terminology
CQI	Continuous quality improvement
CRP	C-reactive protein
CSF	Cerebrospinal fluid
CT	Cytologist
CTS	Carpal tunnel syndrome
CVA	Cerebrovascular accident
CVAD	Central venous access device
CVS	Chorionic villus sampling
Cx	Cervix
DAT	Direct antihuman globulin test
DI	Diabetes insipidus
DIC	Disseminated intravascular coagulation
Diff	Differential
DM	Diabetes mellitus
DNR	Do not resuscitate
DOA	Dead on arrival
DOB	Date of birth
DRG	Diagnosis-related group
Dx	Diagnosis
ECG/EKG	Electrocardiogram
EDTA	Ethylenediaminetetra-acetic acid
EEG	Electroencephalogram
EIA	Enzyme immunoassay
EMG	Electromyogram
EMLA	Eutectic mixture of local anesthetics
ER	Emergency room
ESR	Erythrocyte sedimentation rate
FANA	Fluorescent antinuclear antibody
FDA	Food and Drug Administration
FDP	Fibrin degradation product
FMS	Fibromyalgia syndrome
FSH	Follicle-stimulating hormone
FTA-ABS	Fluorescent treponemal antibody—absorbed
FUO	Fever of unknown origin
Fx	Fracture
g	Gravitational force
g, gm	Gram
GGT	Gamma glutamyl transferase
GH	Growth hormone
GI	Gastrointestinal
GTT	Glucose tolerance test
HBIG	Hepatitis B immune globulin
HB_sAg	Hepatitis B surface antigen
HBV	Hepatitis B virus
HCG	Human chorionic gonadotropin
Hct	Hematocrit
HCV	Hepatitis C virus
HDL	High-density lipoprotein
HDN	Hemolytic disease of the newborn
Hgb	Hemoglobin
HIPAA	Health Insurance Portability and Accountability Act of 1996
HIV	Human immunodeficiency virus
HLA	Human leukocyte antigen
HMO	Health maintenance organization
HT	Histology technician
HTL	Histology technologist
Hx	History
ICD-9	International Classification of Disease, 9th Edition
ICU	Intensive care unit
Ig	Immunoglobulin
IM	Intramuscular
IM	Infectious mononucleosis
INR	International Normalized Ratio
IRDS	Infant respiratory distress syndrome
IV	Intravenous
IVP	Intravenous pyelogram
JCAHO	Joint Commission on Accreditation of Healthcare Organizations
K	Potassium
K_2EDTA	Dipotassium ethylenediamine-tetra-acetic acid
K_3EDTA	Tripotassium ethylenediamine-tetra-acetic acid
kg	Kilogram
KOH	Potassium hydroxide
L & D	Labor and delivery
LD (LDH)	Lactic dehydrogenase
LDL	Low-density lipoprotein
LH	Luteinizing hormone
Li	Lithium
LIMS (LIS)	Laboratory information management system (laboratory information system)
LLQ	Left lower quadrant

LP	Lumbar puncture
LPN	Licensed Practical Nurse
LUQ	Left upper quadrant
Lytes	Electrolytes
MCH	Mean corpuscular hemoglobin
MCHC	Mean corpuscular hemoglobin concentration
MCV	Mean corpuscular volume
MD	Muscular dystrophy
mg	Milligram
Mg	Magnesium
MI	Myocardial infarction
mL	Milliliter
MLT	Medical Laboratory Technician
mm	Millimeter
mm Hg	Millimeters of mercury
MRI	Magnetic resonance imaging
MS	Multiple sclerosis
MSDS	Material Safety Data Sheet
MSH	Melanocyte-stimulating hormone
MT	Medical Technologist
Na	Sodium
NB	Newborn
NCA	National Credentialing Agency for Medical Laboratory Personnel
NCCLS	National Committee for Clinical Laboratory Standards
NFPA	National Fire Protection Association
NPA	National Phlebotomy Association
NPO	Nothing by mouth
O & P	Ova and parasites
O_2	Oxygen
OP	Outpatient
OR	Operating room
OSHA	Occupational Safety and Health Administration
OT	Occupational therapy
P	Phosphorus
Pap	Papanicolaou stain for cervical cancer
PAP	Prostatic acid phosphatase
PBT	Phlebotomy Technician
Pco_2	Partial pressure of carbon dioxide
PEP	Postexposure prophylaxis
PF3	Platelet factor 3
PFT	Pulmonary function test
pH	Negative log of the hydrogen ion concentration (less than 7 is acid and above 7 is alkaline)
PICC	Peripherally inserted central catheter
PID	Pelvic inflammatory disease
PKU	Phenylketonuria
Plt	Platelet
PMS	Premenstrual syndrome
PNS	Peripheral nervous system
Po_2	Partial pressure of oxygen
POCT	Point-of-care testing
POL	Physician office laboratory
post-op	After surgery
pp	Postprandial
PPD	Purified protein derivative
PPE	Personal protective equipment
PPM	Provider-performed microscopy
PPT	Plasma preparation tube
pre-op	Before surgery
PRL	Prolactin
PRN	Allowable as needed
PSA	Prostate-specific antigen
PST	Plasma separator tube
PT	Physical therapy
PT	Prothrombin time
PTH	Parathyroid hormone
q	Every
QA	Quality assurance
QC	Quality control
qh	Every hour
qid	Four times a day
QNS	Quantity nonsufficient
RA	Rheumatoid arthritis
RBC	Red blood cell
RCF	Relative centrifugal force
RDS	Respiratory distress syndrome
RDW	Red cell distribution width
Retic	Reticulocyte
RF	Rheumatoid factor
Rh	The D (Rhesus) antigen on red blood cells
RIA	Radioimmunoassay
RLQ	Right lower quadrant
RN	Registered Nurse
R/O	Rule out
rpm	Revolutions per minute
RPR	Rapid plasma reagin
RPT	Registered Phlebotomy Technician
RUQ	Right upper quadrant
Rx	Prescription/treatment
SA	Sinoatrial

SG	Specific gravity
SLE	Systemic lupus erythematosus
SOB	Shortness of breath
SPS	Sodium polyanetholesulfonate
SST	Serum separator tube
stat	Immediately
STD	Sexually transmitted disease
T & C	Type and crossmatch
T_3	Triiodothyronine
T_4	Thyroxine
TAT	Turn-around time
TB	Tuberculosis
TC	Throat culture
TC/HDL	Total cholesterol/high density lipoprotein
TcB	Transcutaneous bilirubin
TDM	Therapeutic drug monitoring
TP	Total protein
tPA	Tissue plasminogen activator
TPN	Total parenteral nutrition (IV feeding)
TPR	Temperature, pulse, respiration
TQM	Total quality management
TSH	Thyroid-stimulating hormone
TSS	Toxic shock syndrome
TT	Thrombin time
Tx	Treatment
UA	Routine urinalysis
*u*L	Microliter
URI	Upper respiratory infection
UTI	Urinary tract infection
UV	Ultraviolet
VDRL	Venereal Disease Research Laboratory
VLDL	Very low density lipoprotein
WBC	White blood cell
ZDV	Zidovudine

Glossary

Accreditation Process by which a program or institution documents meeting established guidelines

Accuracy Closeness of the measured result to the true value

Adrenocorticotropic hormone Hormone produced by the anterior pituitary gland to stimulate secretion of adrenal cortex hormones

Aerosol Fine suspension of particles in air

Afferent neuron Nerve cell carrying impulses to the brain and spinal cord (sensory neuron)

Airborne precautions Isolation practices associated with airborne diseases

Aldosterone Hormone produced by the adrenal cortex to regulate electrolyte and water balance

Alimentary tract Digestive tract

Aliquot Portion of a sample

Alternative medicine Medical procedures not generally considered to be proven by conventional scientific methods

Alveoli Air sacs in the lungs where the exchange of O_2 and Co_2 occurs

Amino acids Building blocks for protein

Amniotic fluid Fluid surrounding the fetus in the uterus

Amphiarthrosis Slightly movable joint

Amylase Pancreatic enzyme to digest starch

Analytical variables Processes that occur during testing of a sample

Anatomic position Body position used in anatomic descriptions (the body is erect and facing forward with the arms at the side and the palms facing forward)

Androgen Male hormone produced by the adrenal cortex to maintain secondary sex characteristics

Anemia Deficiency of red blood cells

Antecubital Area of the arm opposite the elbow (location of the large veins used in phlebotomy)

Antecubital fossa Indentation of the midarm opposite the elbow (location of the large veins used in phlebotomy)

Anterior (ventral) Pertaining to the front of the body

Antibody Protein produced by exposure to antigen

Anticoagulant Substance that prevents blood from clotting

Antidiuretic hormone Hormone produced by the posterior pituitary gland to stimulate retention of water by the kidney

Antigen Substance that stimulates the formation of antibodies

Antiglycolytic agent Substance that prevents the breakdown of glucose

Antiseptic Substance that destroys or inhibits the growth of microorganisms

Aortic semilunar valve Structure that prevents backflow of blood from the aorta to the left ventricle

Apheresis Removal of specific cellular components or plasma from a person's blood

Appendix Accessory organ of the digestive system that extends from the cecum

Arachnoid membrane Middle layer of the meninges

Arteriole Small arterial branch leading into a capillary

Arteriospasm Spontaneous constriction of an artery

Artery Blood vessel carrying oxygenated blood from the heart to the tissues

Articulation Joint

Aseptic Free of contamination by microorganisms

Assault Attempt or threat to touch or injure another person

Atrioventricular valve Structure that prevents backflow of blood from the right ventricle to the right atrium

Atrium One of two upper chambers of the heart

Autoimmunity Condition in which a person produces antibodies that react with the person's own antigens

Autologous donation Donation of a unit of blood designated to be available to the donor during surgery

Autologous transfusion Transfusion of a person's own previously donated blood

Autonomic nervous system System regulating the body's involuntary functions by carrying impulses from the brain and spinal cord to the muscles, glands, and internal organs

Axon Fiber of nerve cells that carries impulses away from the cell body of the neuron

B lymphocytes Lymphocytes that transform into plasma cells to produce antibodies

Bacteria One-cell microorganisms

Bacteriology The study of bacteria

Bacteriostatic Capable of inhibiting the growth of bacteria

Bar code Computer identification system

Basal state Metabolic condition after 12 hours of fasting and lack of exercise

Basilic vein Vein located on the underside of the arm

Battery Unauthorized physical contact

Benign Noncancerous

Bevel Area of the needle point that has been cut on a slant

Bicuspid valve Structure that prevents backflow of blood from the left ventricle to the left atrium

Bile Digestive juice to break up fat

Bilirubin Yellow-pigmented hemoglobin degradation product

Biohazardous Pertaining to a hazard caused by infectious organisms

Biopsy Removal of a representative tissue for microscopic examination

Blood group Classification based on the presence or absence of A or B antigens on the red blood cells

Body substance isolation Guideline stating that all moist body substances are capable of transmitting disease

Bowman's capsule Structure that encloses the glomerulus and collects filtered substances from the blood

Brainstem Portion of the brain that consists of the medulla, pons, and midbrain

Bronchioles Smallest air passageways within the lungs

Bulbourethral glands Glands on either side of the prostate gland that produce a mucous secretion before ejaculation

Bundle of His Muscle fibers connecting the atria with the ventricles of the heart

Bursa Sac of synovial fluid located between a tendon and a bone to decrease friction

Butterfly Winged infusion set used for small veins

Calcaneus Heel bone

Calcitonin Hormone produced by the thyroid gland to reduce calcium levels in the blood

Calibration Standardization of an instrument used to perform diagnostic tests

Cannula Tube that can be inserted into a cavity

Capillary Small blood vessel connecting arteries and veins that allows the exchange of gases and nutrients between the cells and the blood

Carcinogenic Capable of causing cancer

Cardiac muscle Striated muscle of the heart

Cardiologist Specialist in the study of the heart

Cardiovascular Pertaining to the heart and blood vessels

Carpals/metacarpals Bones of the wrist and hands

Cartilage Flexible connective tissue surrounded by gel (located where bones come together)

Cast Protein structure formed in the tubules of the kidney

Catheter Tube inserted into the body for injecting or withdrawing fluids

Cecum First part of the large intestine

Cell-mediated immunity Immune response by T lymphocytes to directly destroy foreign antigens

Central nervous system Brain and spinal cord

Central Venous Access Device Catheter inserted into the superior vena cava

Centrifuge Instrument that spins test tubes at high speeds to separate the cellular and liquid portions of blood

Cephalic vein Vein located on the thumb side of the arm

Cerebellum Back part of the brain, responsible for voluntary muscle movements and balance

Cerebrospinal fluid Fluid surrounding the brain and spinal cord

Cerebrum Largest part of the brain, responsible for mental processes

Certification Documentation assuring that an individual has met certain professional standards

Chain of custody Documentation of the collection and handling of forensic specimens

Civil lawsuit Court action between individuals, corporations, government bodies, or other organizations (compensation is monetary)

Clot Blood that has coagulated

Clot activator Clot-promoting substance such as glass particles, silica, and celite

Coccyx Last four of five tiny vertebrae at the base of the spine (tailbone)

Collecting duct Part of the renal tubule that extends from the distal convoluted tubule to the renal pelvis

Collateral circulation Additional vessels supplying circulation to a particular area

Compatibility/crossmatch Procedure that matches patient and donor blood before a transfusion

Confidentiality Maintaining the privacy of information

Congenital Existing at birth but not hereditary

Contact precautions Isolation practices to prevent the spread of disease caused by patient contact

Continuous quality improvement Institutional program focusing on customer expectations

Control Substance of known concentration used to monitor the accuracy of test results

Cortisol Hormone produced by the adrenal cortex to regulate the use of sugars, fats, and proteins by cells

Coumadin Anticoagulant monitored by the prothrombin time

Cranium Bones of the skull enclosing the brain

Criminal lawsuit Court action brought by the state for committing a crime against public welfare (punishment is imprisonment and/or a fine)

Critical value Laboratory test result critical to patient survival

Cross-training Instruction to acquire additional patient care skills

Cryoprecipitate Component of fresh plasma that contains clotting factors

Culture and sensitivity Microbiology test to identify microorganisms and determine antibiotic susceptibility

D-dimer Product of fibrinolysis

Decentralization Performance of procedures in various locations

Delta check Comparison of a patient's current results with previous results

Dendrite Fiber of nerve cells that carries impulses to the cell body of the neuron

Deoxyhemoglobin Oxygen-poor hemoglobin

Dermal Pertaining to the skin

Dermis Inner layer of the skin

Diagnosis-related group Government classification of a medical disorder for purposes of cost reimbursement

Diarrhea Watery stools

Diarthrosis Freely movable joint

Diastole Relaxation phase of the heartbeat

Diencephalon Second portion of the brain, contains the thalamus and hypothalamus

Digestion Breakdown of complex foods to simpler forms so that they can be used by cells

Disinfectant Substance that destroys microorganisms (usually used on surfaces rather than on skin)

Distal convoluted tubule Part of the renal tubule between the loop of Henle and the collecting duct

Diurnal variation Normal changes in blood constituent levels at different times of the day

Documentation Recording of pertinent information such as test results, quality control, and observations

Droplet precautions Isolation practices to prevent the spread of microorganisms carried in fluid droplets

Duodenum First part of the small intestine

Dura mater Outermost layer of the meninges

Dysmenorrhea Painful menstruation

Ecchymoses Hemorrhagic discoloration

Edema Accumulation of fluid in the tissues

Efferent neuron Nerve cell carrying impulses away from the brain and spinal cord (motor neuron)

Electrocardiography Recording of variations in the electrical activity of the heart muscle

Electroencephalography Recording of electrical changes in various areas of the brain

Electrolytes Ions in the blood (primarily sodium, potassium, chloride, and carbon dioxide)

Electrophoresis Method of separation by electrical charge

Endocardium Inner lining of the heart

Endocrine Pertaining to ductless glands that secrete hormones directly into the bloodstream to affect other organs

Enzyme Protein capable of producing a chemical reaction with a specific substance (substrate)
Epicardium Outer layer of the heart
Epidermis Outer layer of the skin
Epididymides Coiled organs of the testes where sperm mature
Epiglottis Leaf-shaped cartilage that covers the larynx during swallowing
Epinephrine (adrenalin) Hormone produced by the adrenal medulla to increase heart rate and blood pressure
Erythema Redness from inflammation of the skin
Erythrocyte Red blood cell
Erythropoietin Hormone produced by the kidney to increase red blood cell production
Estrogen Female hormone produced by the adrenal cortex and the ovaries to maintain secondary sex characteristics
Ethics Principles of personal and professional conduct
Evacuated tubes Blood collection tubes containing a premeasured amount of vacuum
Exchange transfusion Removal of blood and replacement with an equal volume of donor blood
Exophthalmos Abnormal protrusion of the eyeball
External respiration Exchange of O_2 and CO_2 at the lungs

Fallopian tubes Tubes connecting the ovaries and uterus
Fasting Abstinence from food and liquids (except water) for a specified period
Feathered edge Area of the blood smear where the microscopic examination is performed
Feces Waste product of digestion
Femur Long bone of the upper leg
Fertilization Union of the sperm and ovum
Fibrin Protein substance produced in the coagulation process to form the foundation of a clot
Fibrinolysis Breakdown of a fibrin clot
Fibula Smaller long bone of the lower leg
First morning specimen The first voided urine specimen collected immediately upon arising; recommended screening specimen
Fistula Permanent surgical connection between an artery and a vein (used for dialysis)
Follicle-stimulating hormone Hormone produced by the anterior pituitary gland to stimulate estrogen secretion and egg production by the ovaries and sperm production by the testes
Forensic Pertaining to legal proceedings
Fresh frozen plasma Plasma collected from a unit of blood and immediately frozen
Frontal plane Vertical plane dividing the body into the anterior (front) and the posterior (back) portions

Gamete Male or female sex cell
Gastrin Hormone produced by the gastric mucosa to stimulate gastric acid secretion
Gauge Unit of measure assigned to the diameter of a needle bore
Geriatric Pertaining to old age
Gland Organ that secretes a substance
Glomerulus Collection of capillaries enclosed by the Bowman's capsule where filtration occurs
Glucagon Hormone produced by the pancreas to stimulate conversion of glycogen to glucose
Glucosuria Glucose in the urine
Glycolysis Breakdown of glucose
Glycosuria Glucose in the urine (glucosuria)
Gonads Ovaries and testes
Gram stain Stain used to classify bacteria
Growth hormone Hormone produced by the anterior pituitary gland to stimulate growth of the bones and tissues

Hematoma Discoloration produced by leakage of blood into the tissue
Hematopoiesis Formation of blood cells in the bone marrow
Hematuria/hemoglobinuria Blood or hemoglobin in the urine
Hemochromatosis Excessive accumulation of iron in the body
Hemoconcentration Increase in the ratio of formed elements to plasma
Hemoglobin Red blood cell protein that transports O_2 and CO_2 in the bloodstream
Hemolysis Destruction of red blood cells
Hemolytic disease of the newborn Rh incompatibility between mother and fetus that can cause hemolysis of fetal red blood cells
Hemostasis Stoppage of blood flow from a damaged blood vessel
Hemostat Surgical clamp
Heparin Anticoagulant monitored by the activated partial thromboplastin time
Heparin lock Device inserted into a vein for administering medications and collecting blood

Homeostasis State of equilibrium in the body

Hormone Substance produced by a ductless gland and transported to parts of the body via the blood to control and regulate body functions

Human chorionic gonadotropin Hormone produced by the placenta during pregnancy to stimulate the ovaries to produce estrogen and progesterone

Humerus Long bone of the upper arm

Humoral immunity Immune response that produces antibodies

Hyperbilirubinemia Increased serum bilirubin

Hyperglycemia Elevated glucose levels in the blood

Hypodermic Under the skin

Hypotension Low blood pressure

Hypothalamus Part of the brain that regulates body temperature and the secretions of the pituitary gland

Hypothyroidism Reduced thyroid function

Iatrogenic Pertaining to a condition caused by treatment, medications, or diagnostic procedures

Icteric Appearing yellow

Identification band Bracelet worn by patients that contains specific identification information

Ileum Last part of the small intestine

Immunochemistry Chemical analysis performed using antigens and antibodies

Immunoglobulin Another name for antibody

Immunohematology The study of blood cell antigens and their antibodies

Immunology The study of the immune system

Incident report Detailed report of a condition that affected patient care or worker safety, documenting the incident and actions taken

Indwelling line Tube inserted into an artery or vein (primarily for administering fluids)

Infection Multiplication of microorganisms in body tissues

Inferior Pertaining to a position below another structure

Informed consent Patient's right to know the method and risks before agreeing to treatment

Insertion Movable attachment point of a muscle to a bone

Insulin Hormone produced by the pancreas to promote the use of glucose by the body

Internal respiration Exchange of O_2 and Co_2 between the blood and the cells of the body

International Normalized Ratio Standardized prothrombin time reporting system to equate results among reagent manufacturers

Interneuron Nerve cell entirely within the central nervous system

Interstitial fluid Fluid located in the spaces between cells

Invasion of privacy Unauthorized release of information

Iontophoresis Electrical stimulation of soluble salt ions used in the collection of sweat electrolyte specimens

Isoenzyme Specific form of an enzyme

Jaundiced Appearing yellow

Jejunum Second part of the small intestine

Keratin Tough protein found in the outer skin, hair, and nails

Ketonuria Ketones in the urine

Labile Biologically or chemically unstable

Laboratory reference manual Document providing laboratory information to other areas of the hospital

Larynx Organ between the pharynx and the trachea containing the vocal cords

Leukemia Malignant overproduction of white blood cells

Leukocyte White blood cell

Ligament Fibrous connective tissue that binds bones together at the joint

Lipase Pancreatic enzyme that digests fats

Lipemic Pertaining to turbidity from lipids

Litigation Law suit

Local anesthetic Substance that paralyzes nerve endings in the area of the injection

Loop of Henle Part of the renal tubule between the proximal convoluted tubule and the distal convoluted tubule

Lot Group of products manufactured at the same time under the same conditions

Luer tip Part of a syringe that attaches to the needle

Lumen Cavity of an organ or tube, such as a blood vessel or a needle

Lumbar puncture Procedure used to remove cerebrospinal fluid from the lower spine

Luteinizing hormone Hormone produced by the anterior pituitary gland to stimulate ovulation

Lymph Fluid in the lymphatic vessels

Lymph node Lymph tissue that filters lymph as it passes to the circulatory system
Lymphedema Retention of excess lymph fluid
Lymphokines Chemicals released by activated T cells that attract macrophages
Lymphostasis Stoppage of lymph flow

Macrophage Cell derived from monocytes capable of phagocytosis of pathogens, damaged cells, and old red blood cells
Magnetic "flea" Small metal filing
Malignant Cancerous
Malpractice Medical care that does not meet a reasonable standard and results in harm
Mastectomy Excision of the breast
Median cubital vein Vein located in the center of the antecubital area
Medulla oblongata Part of the brain that regulates heart rate, respiration, and blood pressure
Melanin Black pigment in the outer skin
Melanocyte-stimulating hormone Hormone produced by the anterior pituitary gland to stimulate pigmentation of the skin
Melatonin Hormone produced by the pineal gland that influences circadian rhythms
Meninges Protective membranes around the brain and spinal cord
Menopause Permanent end of the monthly menstrual cycle
Menstruation Monthly shedding of the uterine lining
Metabolic Pertaining to the chemical changes taking place in the body
Microbiology The study of microorganisms
Microorganism One-cell organism such as a bacterium or virus
Microsample A sample less than 1 mL in size
Midsagittal plane Vertical plane dividing the body into equal right and left portions
Mitosis Cell division
Mitral valve Valve between the left atrium and left ventricle of the heart
Mnemonics Memory-aiding abbreviations
Mycology The study of fungi
Myelin sheath Tissue around the axon of the peripheral nerves
Myocardium Muscle layer of the heart

Nausea Unpleasant sensation producing the urge to vomit
Necrosis Death of cells
Negligence Failure to perform duties according to accepted standards
Neonatal Pertaining to the first 4 weeks after birth
Nephron Functional unit of the kidney that forms urine
Neuroglia Connective tissue cells of the nervous system that do not carry impulses
Neuron Nerve cell
Norepinephrine (noradrenalin) Hormone produced by the adrenal medulla to constrict blood vessels and increase blood pressure
Nosocomial infection Infection acquired in the hospital

Occluded Obstructed
Olfactory receptors Sensory receptors in the nasal cavity that provide the sense of smell
Origin Stationary attachment point of a muscle to a bone
Osteoblast Bone-producing cell
Osteoclast Bone-resorbing cell
Osteomyelitis Inflammation of the bone
Ovaries Female gonads that produce ova
Ovulation Release of the egg cell from the ovary
Ovum (pl. ova) Female reproductive cell
Oxyhemoglobin Hemoglobin with O_2 attached
Oxytocin Hormone produced by the posterior pituitary gland to stimulate contraction of the uterus at delivery and the release of milk into the breast ducts

Package insert Testing procedure information provided by the manufacturer of the testing materials
Packed cells Blood from which the plasma has been removed
Palmar Pertaining to the palm of the hand
Palpation Examination by touch
Parasitology The study of parasites
Parathyroid hormone Hormone produced by the parathyroid gland to regulate calcium levels in the blood
Partial pressure Amount of pressure exerted by an individual gas within a mixture of gases
Pathogen Microorganism capable of producing disease
Pathology Branch of medicine specializing in the study of disease
Patient's Bill of Rights Document written by the

American Hospital Association stating the patient's rights during treatment

Patient-focused care Patient care that does not require transporting the patient to various locations

Peak level specimen Specimen collected when a serum drug level is highest

Pericardium Membrane surrounding the heart

Peripheral nervous system All nerves outside the brain and spinal cord

Peristalsis Wavelike muscular contractions to propel material through the digestive tract

Peritoneum Membrane lining the abdominal cavity

Personal protective equipment Apparel worn to prevent contact with and transmission of pathogenic microorganisms

Petechiae Small red spots appearing on the skin

Phagocytosis Ingestion of bacteria or other foreign particles by a cell

Pharynx Tubelike structure located behind the nose that is a passageway for air and food (throat)

Phenylalanine Naturally occurring amino acid

Phenylketonuria Presence of abnormal phenylalanine metabolites in the urine

Phlebotomy Puncture or incision into a vein to obtain blood

Pia mater Innermost layer of the meninges

Pilocarpine Sweat-inducing chemical

Plantar Pertaining to the sole of the foot

Plasma Liquid portion of blood

Plasma cell Cell derived from an activated B cell that produces antibodies to a specific antigen

Platelet Small, irregularly shaped disk formed from particles of a very large cell in the bone marrow called the megakaryocyte

Platelet plug Initial blockage of a vascular puncture by platelets

Pleura Double-folded membrane surrounding each lung

Pneumatic tube system Air-driven transport system

Point-of-care testing Laboratory tests performed in the patient care area

Polycythemia Markedly increased numbers of red blood cells

Polydipsia Excessive thirst

Polyphagia Excessive desire to eat

Polyuria Marked increase in the urine flow

Pons Part of the brain stem that influences respiration

Postanalytical variables Processes that affect the reporting and interpretation of test results

Postexposure prophylaxis Preventive measures taken when a person is exposed to infectious disease

Posterior (dorsal) Pertaining to the back of the body

Postprandial After eating

Preanalytical variables Processes that occur before collection of a sample

Precision Reproducibility of a test result

Procedure manual Detailed documentation of procedures and methods used in performing tests

Professionalism Conduct and qualities that typify a professional

Proficiency testing Performance of tests on specimens provided by an external monitoring agency

Progesterone Female hormone produced by the adrenal cortex and the ovaries to promote conditions suitable for pregnancy

Prolactin Hormone produced by the anterior pituitary gland to stimulate breast development and milk secretion

Prostate gland Gland that surrounds the first inch of the male urethra and secretes an alkaline fluid to maintain sperm motility

Proteinuria Protein (albumin) in the urine

Prothrombin Protein converted to thrombin in the coagulation process

Proximal convoluted tubule Part of the renal tubule between the Bowman's capsule and the loop of Henle

Pulmonary circulation Flow of blood from the heart to the lungs and back to the heart

Pulmonary semilunar valve Structure that prevents backflow of blood from the pulmonary arteries to the right ventricle

Pulse Measurement of the rhythm of ventricle contraction

Quality assurance Methods used to guarantee quality patient care

Quality control Methods used to monitor the accuracy of procedures

Radioactivity Emission of radiant energy

Radioisotope Substance that emits radiant energy

Radius Shorter bone of the lower arm located on the lateral or thumb side

Reagent Substance used to produce a chemical reaction

Reagent strip/dipstick Chemical-impregnated plastic strip used for analysis of urine
Rectum End part of the colon
Renal Pertaining to the kidney
Renal dialysis Procedure to remove waste products from the blood when the kidneys are not functioning
Renin Hormone produced by the kidney to increase blood pressure
Requisition Form detailing orders for patient testing
Respiration rate Number of breaths per minute
Right lymphatic duct Duct that collects the lymph fluid from the upper right quadrant to return it to the blood
Root cause analysis Evaluation of the causative factors of variation in performance

Sacrum Five fused sacral vertebrae at the base of the spine
Sagittal plane Vertical plane dividing the body into left and right portions
Sarcoma Malignant tumor containing embryonic connective tissue
Scapula Flat bone forming the back of the shoulder (shoulder blade)
Sclerosed Hardened
Scrotum Sac that contains the male testes
Sebaceous gland Oil-producing gland
Sebum Oily secretion of the sebaceous gland
Semen Fluid containing spermatozoa
Seminal vesicles Glands that secrete alkaline fluid that becomes part of semen
Sentinel event An unanticipated death or permanent loss of function not related to a patient's illness or underlying condition
Septicemia Pathogenic microorganisms in the blood
Septum Partition between the right and left sides of the heart
Serology The study of serum
Serum Clear yellow fluid that remains after clotted blood has been centrifuged and separated
Shift Abrupt change in the mean of quality control results
Shock Sudden decrease in blood flow interfering with heart and tissue function
Sinoatrial node Mass of pacer cells considered the dominant pacemaker of the heart
Skeletal muscle Striated voluntary muscle that moves bones
Smooth muscle Unstriated involuntary muscle of the internal organs and blood vessels
Spermatozoa Sperm cells / male gametes
Sphygmomanometer Instrument that measures blood pressure
Standard precautions Guidelines describing personnel protective practices
Steady state A 30-minute period of controlled stable oxygen consumption and no physical exercise
Sterile Free of microorganisms
Sternum Breastbone (alternate site for the collection of bone marrow specimens)
Stethoscope Instrument used for listening to sounds produced within the body
Stratum corneum Outermost layer of the epidermis, consisting of dead cells filled with keratin
Stratum germinativum Innermost layer of the epidermis in which cell division occurs
Streptokinase Clot lysis activator
Striated Marked with grooves or stripes
Subcutaneous layer Innermost layer of skin, composed of connective tissue and fat
Sudoriferous gland Sweat-producing gland
Superficial On the surface
Superior Pertaining to a position above another structure
Supine Lying on the back
Sweat electrolytes test Diagnostic test for the detection of cystic fibrosis
Synapse Point at which an impulse is transmitted from one neuron to another
Synarthrosis Immovable joint
Syncope Fainting
Synovial Pertaining to lubricating fluid secreted by membranes in joint capsules
Systemic circulation Flow of blood between the heart and the tissues
Systole Contraction phase of the heartbeat

T lymphocytes Lymphocytes that act directly on an antigen to destroy it
Tachometer Instrument for measuring speed
Tarsals/metatarsals Bones of the ankles and feet
Tendon Connective tissue that binds muscles to bones
Testes Male gonads that produce sperm
Testosterone Hormone produced by the testes that is responsible for the development of male sexual characteristics

Thalamus Part of the brain that regulates subconscious sensations

Therapeutic phlebotomy Collection of a unit of blood performed as a patient treatment

Thixotropic gel Substance that undergoes a temporary change in viscosity during centrifugation

Thoracic Pertaining to the chest

Thoracic duct Duct that collects the lymph from the lower body and upper left quadrant to return it to the blood

Thrombin Enzyme that converts fibrinogen to fibrin

Thrombocyte Cell involved with clotting (platelet)

Thrombolytic therapy Administration of medication to enhance clot lysis

Thrombosis Formation of blood clots within the vascular system

Thrombus Clot formed on the inner wall of a vein

Thymosin Hormone produced by the thymus gland for the maturation of T cells

Thyroid-stimulating hormone Hormone produced by the anterior pituitary gland to stimulate secretion of thyroid hormones

Thyroxine Hormone produced by the thyroid gland to stimulate metabolism of cells

Tibia Larger long bone of the lower leg

Tonicity Active resistance to stretching in muscles (maintains posture)

Tort Wrongful act committed by one person against another person or property

Total quality management Institutional policy to provide customer satisfaction

Toxicology Study of poisons

Trachea Organ that provides the opening between the larynx and the bronchi

Transmission-based precautions Isolation procedures based on airborne, droplet, and contact disease transmission

Transverse plane Horizontal plane dividing the body into upper and lower portions

Trend Gradual change above or below the mean of quality control results

Tricuspid valve Valve between the right atrium and right ventricle

Triiodothyronine Hormone produced by the thyroid gland to stimulate metabolism of cells

Trough level specimen Specimen collected when a serum drug level is lowest

Tunica adventitia Outer layer of blood vessels, composed of connective tissue

Tunica intima Inner layer of blood vessels, composed of endothelial cells

Tunica media Middle layer of blood vessels, composed of smooth muscle tissue

Turn-around-time Amount of time between the request for a test and the reporting of results

Ulna Larger long bone of the forearm opposite the thumb

Umbilicus The navel

Unit of blood 405 to 495 mL of blood collected from a donor for a transfusion

Universal precautions Guideline stating that all patients are capable of transmitting bloodborne disease

Uremia Increased urea in the blood

Ureters Tubes that carry urine from the kidney to the bladder

Urethra Organ that carries urine from the bladder to the outside of the body

Urinalysis Physical, chemical, and microscopic analysis of urine

Urokinase Clot lysis activator

Uterus Female organ that forms a placenta to nourish a developing embryo

Valve Structure in veins and the heart that closes an opening so blood will flow in only one direction

Variable Measurable condition used to evaluate the quality of patient care or laboratory specimens

Vas deferens Tube that carries sperm from the epididymides to the ejaculatory duct

Vascular Pertaining to blood vessels

Vasovagal reaction Stimulation of the blood vessels by the vagus nerve

Vector Carrier that transfers an infective agent from one host to another

Vein Blood vessel carrying deoxygenated blood from the tissues to the heart

Ventilation device Apparatus to control the amount of oxygen inhaled

Ventricle One of two lower chambers of the heart

Venule Small vein leading from a capillary to a vein

Virology The study of viruses

Visceral Pertaining to organs within a body cavity

Volar Pertaining to the palm side of the forearm

Waived test Laboratory test requiring no special training

Winged infusion set A stainless steel needle and tubing apparatus attached to plastic wings

Index

An "f" following a page number indicates a figure; a "b" following a page number indicates a box; and a "t" following a page number indicates a table.